Dedicated to:

My mother and father and also to my husband and children.

Copyright © 2017 by Mulunesh Belay

Photography by Merrill Peterson
Writing by Carol Yoon and Merrill Peterson
Book design and production by Emiko Peterson-Yoon
Oromo flag image (p. 11) courtesy of Wikimedia Commons.

All rights reserved. This book or any portion thereof may not be reproduced or used in any manner whatsoever without the express written permission of the publisher except for the use of brief quotations in a book review.

Printed in the United States of America

Yoon Works Inc

ISBN 978-0-9974026-0-5

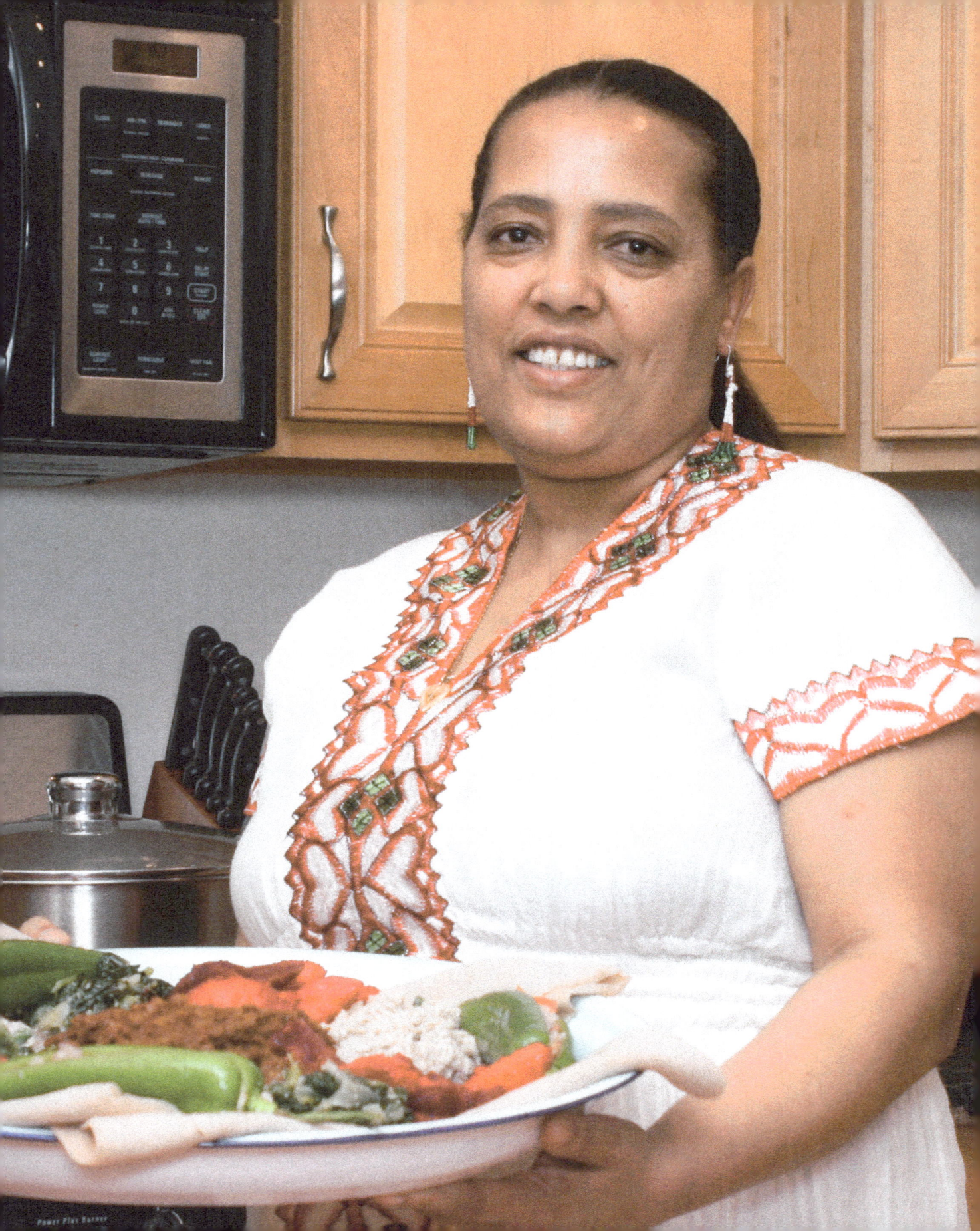

ETHIOPIAN FEAST

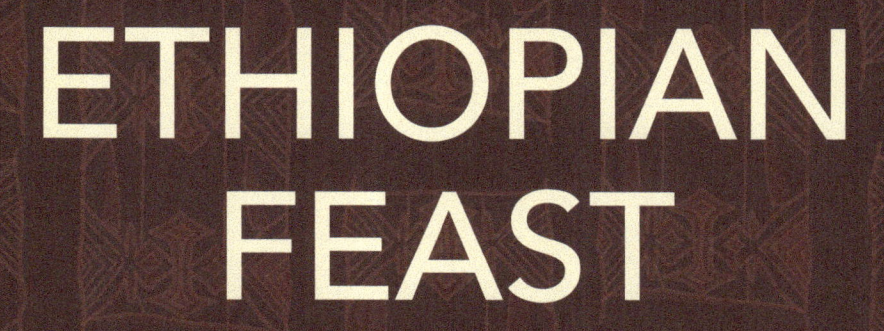

The Crown Jewel of African Cuisine

by Mulunesh Belay

with Merrill Peterson
and Carol Yoon

TABLE OF CONTENTS

Introduction

Welcome 5

My Culinary Journey 7

Useful Equipment 12

Ethiopian Meals 13

Ingredients 15

Recipes

- The Basics: Spices and Seasonings 19
- The Staff of Life: Injera and other Breads and Grains 31
- The Most Admired of Foods: Meat and Seafood Main Dishes 57
- Farm Fresh: Cheese and Eggs 109
- Hearty Vegetables: Lentil Stews 121
- Straight from the Garden: Leaf and Root Vegetables 147
- Just a Nibble: Snacks and Treats 177
- Thirst Quenchers: Ethiopian Drinks .191

Acknowledgements 202

Index 203

About the Authors 208

Key: (V) = Vegetarian   (VG) = Vegan   (GF) = Gluten Free   (DF) = Dairy Free

WELCOME

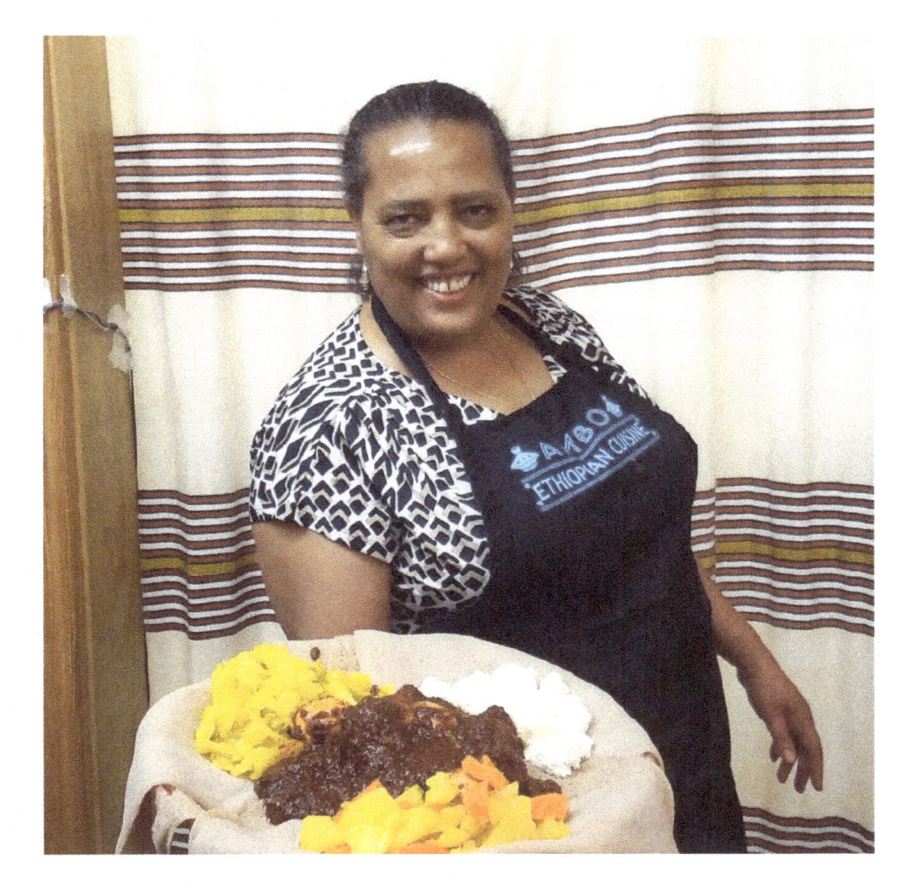

Welcome, friends, to the world of Ethiopian cooking!

Ethiopian food is a special cuisine from a special place. I am so proud of my country. Our land is beautiful and rugged, full of mountains and great plateaus and rivers that give us water and life. Our country is also home to many different tribes and ancient cultures. I am from the Oromo tribe or Oromo people, the largest ethnic group in my country. Like other tribes, we have our own unique language and distinct culture. Despite my country's cultural variety, we Ethiopians are all bound by one great culinary tradition.

Ethiopian food is very special among African foods perhaps, because of the unusual geography of our country. With mountains shoring up our borders, our cuisine has been able to develop in some isolation from our other African neighbors. Some people say it is also the most truly African of cuisines, because our country's long political independence has left our cooking largely untouched by European and Asian culinary influences. But more important, our food is wonderful! The flavors are lush and complex, full of unique and subtle spicing. Beautiful, delicious, aromatic - Ethiopian food is a feast for the senses. Every meal begins with our famous Injera, a delicate sourdough flatbread, on top of which are mounded spiced vegetables, fragrant greens, sauced meats and tart homemade cheeses. It truly is the crown jewel of African cuisine.

An Ethiopian meal is more than delicious tastes. It is a celebration of connection, of family and friends. When we eat, we do not sit quiet and polite along long tables, with a clink clink of forks on plates in silence. An Ethiopian meal is family and friends sitting crowded around a big colorful woven basket called a mesob. On top of the basket sits a great round plate with Injera and every kind of food. Everyone eats from the same great communal plate, laughing, talking, bumping shoulders.

In recent years, I have seen a big change in how others view Ethiopian food. It used to be that few people outside of our country knew about our food. Now, Ethiopian food is talked about everywhere. People see how good our food is for all kinds of people. It is delicious but it is also traditionally gluten-free. And because meat has often been only a special food for

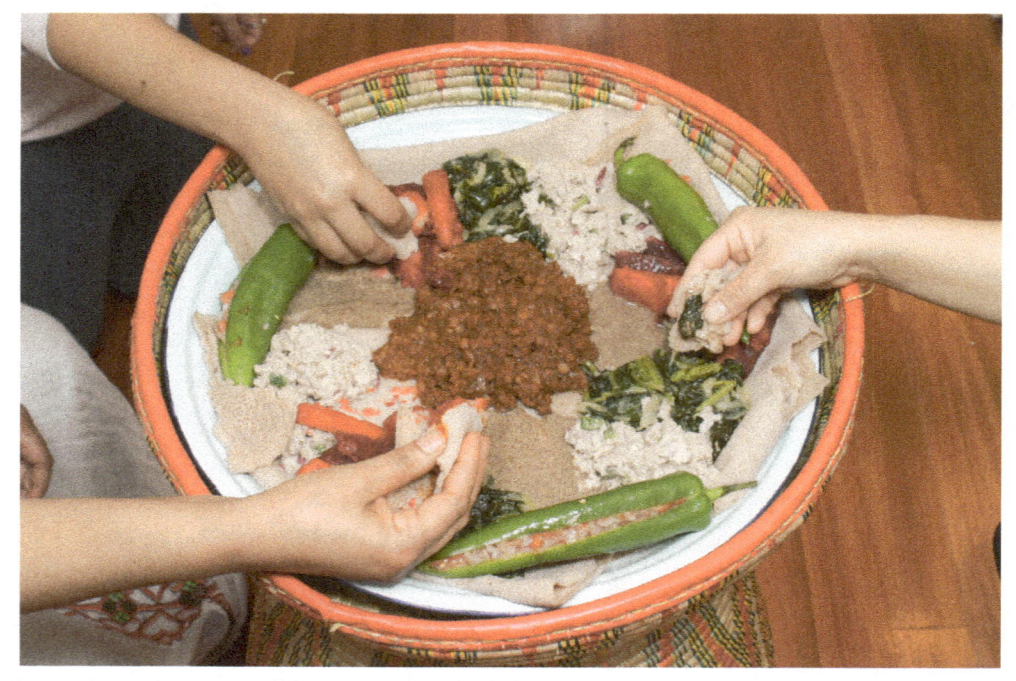

Above: Spicy Green Lentil Stew (p.129), Filled Peppers (p.167), Beets, Carrots and Potatoes (p.153), Safflower Fitfit (p.55), (Ethiopian Kale (p.161), on Injera (p. 33).

the rich, we have developed many excellent vegetable dishes. To help these people with with specialized diets to use the book, I have marked recipes as Gluten-Free, Vegetarian, Dairy Free and/or Vegan and with ingredient substitutions where necessary.

Ethiopian food is also becoming more popular in the United States as more families adopt Ethiopian children. I have met many wonderful families who have discovered our food because of their newest family members. And of course, the book is meant to help Ethiopians living away from Ethiopia - like my own children! - who would otherwise struggle to maintain their eating traditions.

I wrote this book to be a kind of Ethiopian culinary Bible. I included everything you need to know to create authentic Ethiopian cuisine in your home kitchen. You will find here my recipes for the best-known Ethiopian dishes, like the spicy chicken stew, Yedoro Wat or Doro Wat. I also share recipes for less well known but equally yummy dishes, including Dabbo, a savory artisan bread baked in a banana leaf, and Ayib Be Gomen, ground kale in homemade buttermilk cheese.

I live in the Pacific Northwest and like all chefs, I take in what's around me. I learn. I experiment. I love the local foods. So I also share here my Ethiopian styled recipes that feature the bountiful Pacific Northwest harvests of salmon, shrimp and mushrooms in Ethiopian fusion dishes. I hope you like them as much as my family, customers and I do!

Perhaps most important, in this book I will provide the Holy Grail of Ethiopian cooking: an easy-to-follow and reliable recipe for Injera, our famous leavened, spongy flatbread. You can benefit from my years of experimenting. I have developed a foolproof method for adjusting the Injera batter from whatever state it begins in – whether too thick, too thin, too fermented or too little fermented – into a batter that will produce perfect, leavened, sourdough rounds worthy of the finest restaurant in Addis Ababa. You will have to practice a little, but it can be done, if you learn my technique.

Our food is real food. You cannot buy it in a freezer or take it from a can. Our food must be made fresh, from scratch - get ready to peel potatoes and chop onions - as it has always been made. I can hardly wait to get you started!

Welcome to your Ethiopian Feast!

MY CULINARY JOURNEY

I was born in the small village of Gindeberet, Ethiopia. As the eldest girl of a family of eleven, I began helping my family at a very young age. My grandmother (my mother's mother) first taught me to cook and then my mother. They are my heroes. By age five, I was working with my mother daily to make the family meals. In my village, this was nothing special. I was just doing what I was supposed to do. I did not know it then, but this is where my journey as a chef began.

Cooking in Ethiopia is very different from cooking in America. Our family had three small buildings made of wood and mud, with dirt floors. One building was our house, where we slept. The other was a storage building. And the last was the kitchen hut in which we cooked over an open fire. It was also where the young cows lived. In our yard, we grew vegetables and there we also kept the full-grown cows that we girls milked. In the morning, I would run for half an hour to a small patch of forest to gather wood for the fire. I would tie it in a bundle, then tie it on my back and bring it home to my mother. Sometimes, you could get enough wood, but sometimes it was not enough. When we needed to, we also dried and burned cow dung. Using what we had, my mother made her cooking fire on the dirt floor of our cooking hut.

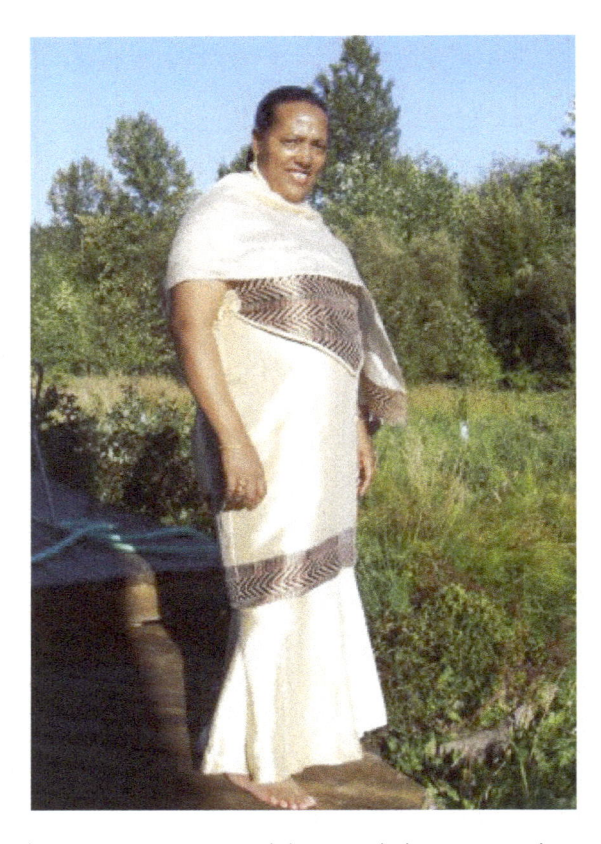

We also needed water to drink and cook. Every day I walked about ten minutes to reach the spring where I would fill a small jug with water. It had to be small because I was small! And you had to be careful - there were snakes that might bite you. After I filled my water jug, I used ropes to tie the jug to my back. Then I walked home. Sometimes one jug of water was not enough. Sometimes I had to go two, three, four times to get enough water. One time, I remember I went ten times. It sounds very difficult for a little girl, doesn't it? It's just what you do. I think it's like children having a cellphone today. Everyone just does it!

I met my husband Takele when we were both children in Gindeberet. After we married, we moved far from Ethiopia to South Africa. I never thought too much about how important my cooking and my food were to me until I was so far from home. In South Africa, Takele was studying for his Ph.D. in physics. We already had one daughter, Biftu, our eldest, and in South Africa, Bontu, our second daughter, was born. Of course I wanted to feed my family Ethiopian food, but I found that making Ethiopian food far from home was very difficult.

To eat Ethiopian food, you must make Injera - our pancake-like sourdough bread - and I found that I could not make Injera in South Africa! This is something many Ethiopian people discover when they leave the country, and so do non-Ethiopian people who try to make our foods. To begin to make Injera, you need a starter. Injera is like sourdough bread in this way. You use a little bit of your last Injera batter to start a new batch of Injera batter. In Ethiopia, I could always get a little bit of starter. Everyone makes Injera! But I had to begin from nothing in South Africa. I had to create my own starter.

But there were other hurdles. Outside Ethiopia, so many things were different. It used to be very hard to get the main ingredient, the special grain and flour called teff. In fact, when I lived in South Africa, it was not possible to buy teff anywhere in that country. I wanted to try to use barley flour but it was not possible to buy barley either. One day, my husband told me he had heard once of someone in Europe making Injera using rice flour. So I began to do my own experiments. I tried different grains and different combinations of different grains. I found the water, the air temperature, and so on were all different. Also, at home we always cooked our Injera on a flat clay plate. The plate was held up by large stones that sat around a wood fire on the floor of the cooking hut. A stove was so different! All these things can change how Injera will turn out.

I failed again and again. I was struggling. I tried again and again. I practiced and researched. This is what I always tell people: it is like when you go to school. You don't learn everything in one day. In school, some people learn faster. Some people are slower learners. Some people just give up. For me, it wasn't possible to give up. I wanted to learn. I wanted to play with it, to figure it out. I couldn't stop. I wanted to eat Injera. I love Injera! Then finally I got it. Now I want to share this with everyone.

It is so important to me to be able to make my people's food. I think it is hard to explain how important our food is to us Ethiopians. Maybe it is especially important for a woman. In Ethiopia, a woman has to know how to cook. Our most famous and special dish is Yedoro Wat or chicken stew. It takes all day long to make a pot of Yedoro Wat. Once a girl knows how to make Yedoro Wat, people say then she is ready to get married. And, they say, if you can't make Yedoro Wat, your man will eat it somewhere else. And no woman is going to let a man leave after she cooks him something that takes all day!

But Ethiopian food is special in another way. Our food is really about family and friends. It is about being together with people. That is why we eat all together, crowded together, around one plate. Today in Ethiopia, many people are beginning to eat food in the European way. Everyone has a separate plate with their own food on it. I remember a story about this from when I was a young girl. My father was a businessman and he brought special things to Gindeberet from Addis Ababa, the capital. He brought things like salt, coffee and clothing, and sold them in his shop that was near the market. And he took things from the village, like sheep and goat skins and teff, to sell in Addis. One day, my father had made enough money for us to leave the village and move to the town of Ambo. It was very fancy for us. We had electricity and running water. We had a house with wood floors that we polished every day. In Gindeberet, we always ate from one large plate, together, in our people's tradition. In Ambo, we children wanted to eat in the modern style, using separate plates. My father refused! Now I understand him better. I know how nice it is to eat, all together, from one family plate. A single plate for every person looks a little lonely. I think our traditional way of eating is very special. It is a little bit of the Ethiopian spirit, of sharing.

I want everyone in the world to be able to enjoy Ethiopian food. I am so proud of my people's food. I know many people have difficulty making Ethiopian food, American people, Europeans, even my own people when they leave Ethiopia. I had so much difficulty. But I think it is so important for young Ethiopians to keep their culture. I don't want them to lose their food.

In this book I will teach you how to make our most special dishes. We have special foods for celebrations. We have special foods for holy days. We have special foods to feed a woman after she has had a baby. We have special foods to eat while traveling. I will even show you how to make some foods that are specialties from my region of Ethiopia and that are not cooked anywhere else, not even other places in Ethiopia.

I am so lucky. My husband is now a physicist at Western Washington University in Bellingham, Washington, so today I live in this beautiful town that has so many kind people in it. There are so many good things that have happened to me in my life. But creating this book that makes it possible for everyone to make my people's food, this is my dream come true.

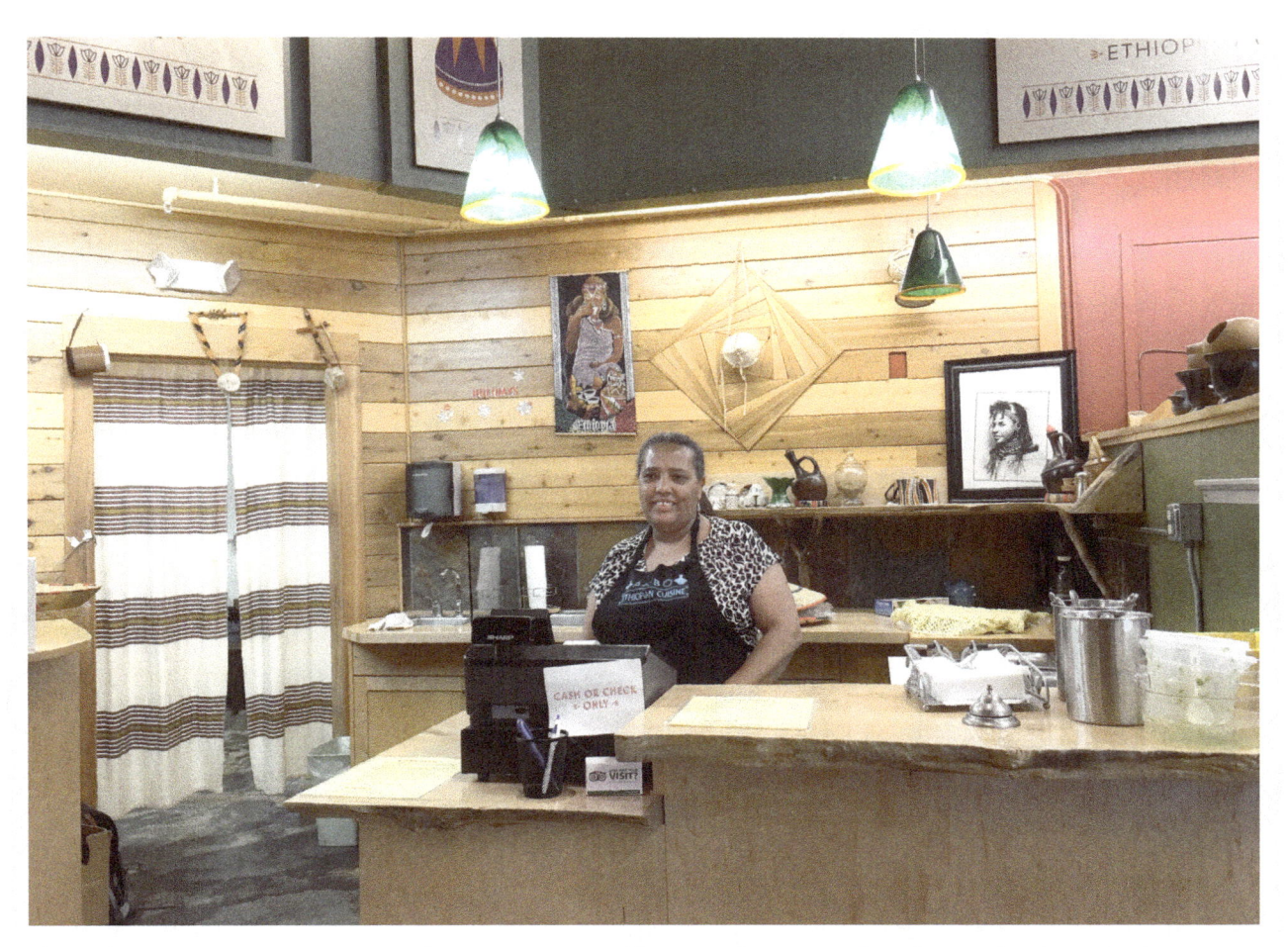

This is the restaurant where I serve Ethiopian cuisine and have made so many friends in Bellingham, Washington.

USEFUL EQUIPMENT

I have found that it is possible to make traditional Ethiopian food with the equipment most people already have at home - with one exception. I recommend that anyone who wants to cook Ethiopian food invest in an Injera pan or mitad.

Injera pans are similar to an electric skillet, but there are important differences. They both have temperature control of the cooking surface and a lid. But regular skillets have raised walls or edges. A true Injera pan is completely flat. This is important because when an Injera is done cooking, we have to slide something large and flat underneath the whole thing to remove it without breaking it. You cannot do this if the pan has walls! Also a regular electric skillet will have oils and scrapes if it is used for anything else. When you have an Injera pan, you do not oil or soap the pan to clean it. You only wipe it with a warm wet cloth. And you only use your Injera pan for cooking Injera. Nothing else! That will keep the nonstick surface perfect and clean, and your Injera will cook well and be easy to remove from the pan.

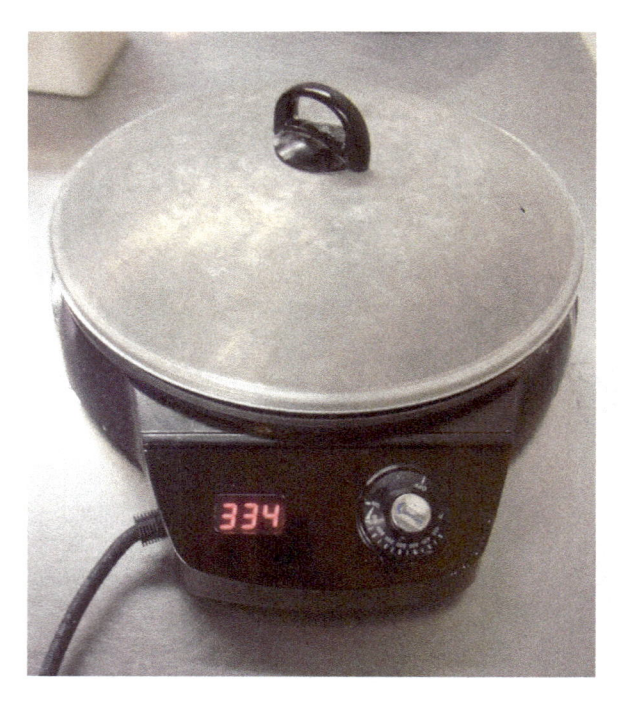

The Wass Injera Cooking Appliance, my current favorite.

I have bought several different Injera pans on the Internet and a simple search for "Injera pan" will turn up many possibilities. For many years, the only pan you could buy was the Silverstone Heritage Lefse Grill. It was designed to make a Norwegian pancake called Lefse and it works very well for Injera. I now use a Wass Injera Cooking Appliance called the Digital Mitad (see photo to left) and I like it very much. It is designed specially for Injera and works very well. I am sure new Injera pans will continue to become available.

ETHIOPIAN MEALS

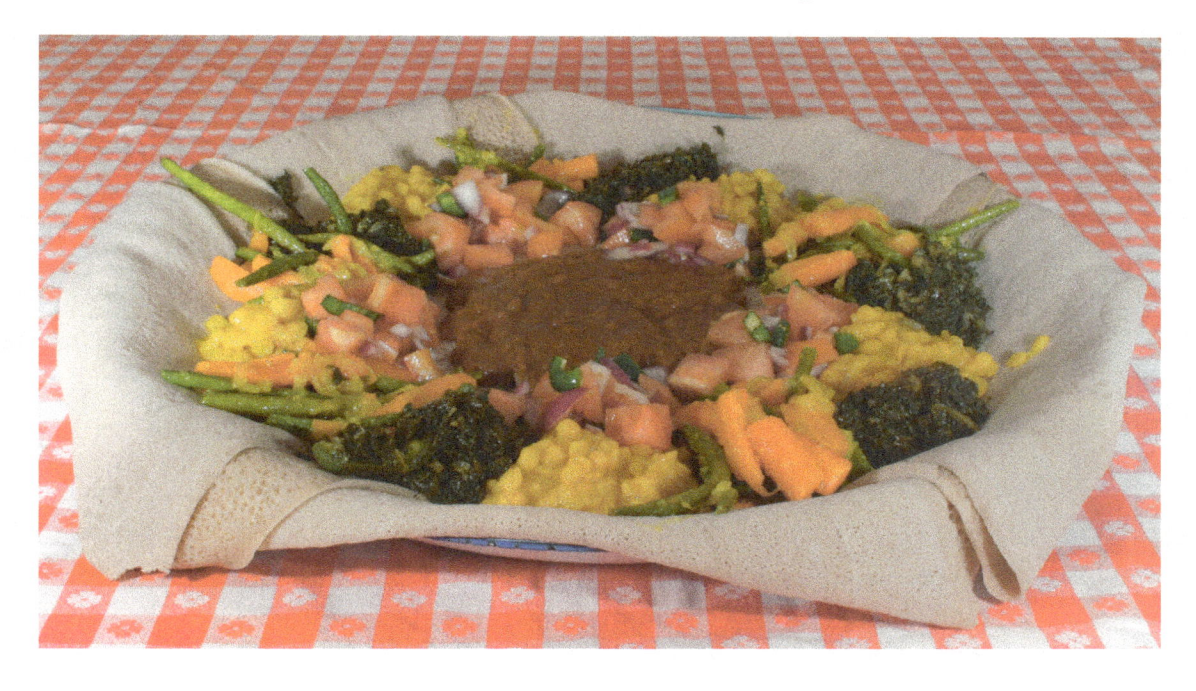

I think most people who are not Ethiopian first try Ethiopian food at a restaurant. From this they may get the idea that Ethiopians only eat dinner! Of course we eat breakfast, lunch and dinner like everyone else. In this book, I include recipes for foods eaten from morning until night and during different times and ceremonies in our lives.

Choosing dishes: This book is organized by ingredient type: seasonings, meats, veggies and so on. In Ethiopia, we value balance in our meals. First, we like to serve dishes of different color and texture together. Second, we balance between what we think of as hearty foods - the meats and legumes like lentils - and lighter vegetable fare. So we choose either a meat - Yedoro Wat is everyone's favorite - or a legume of some kind - meaning a lentil dish or perhaps shiro. To balance this meat or legume, we choose any non-lentil vegetable or homemade cottage cheese. We also always balance spicy with not spicy. You will notice that many of my recipes come in pairs of spicy and not spicy, with spiciness added in different ways, methods and amounts depending on the food. We have such pairs to allow us good variety of both types of food to create the balance that makes a meal feel truly complete.

Above: Ground Roasted Yellow Split Pea Stew (p. 137), Carrots and Green Beans (p. 157), Ethiopian Kale (p.161), Yellow Split Pea Stew (p. 135), and Fresh Tomato Salad (p. 171) on Injera (p. 33).

The Crown Jewel of African Cuisine

Ingredients and Spices: We Ethiopians cook using a number of handmade spice mixes, like Berberre or Q'imam. When you read recipes for dishes, you will see these spice mixes called for in the ingredients lists, marked with a page reference to the recipe for that spice mix. Some ingredients are marked with an asterisk. As explained in the recipes, these are special Ethiopian spices that you will need to buy at an Ethiopian market or from an online supplier. But do not fear! There are not too many, and they are easy to obtain and not very expensive. Once you have made or purchased just a few basic spice mixes, you can cook many different dishes.

Timing: Last but not least, you need to schedule time for your Injera batter to ferment. Choose a date for your feast and then plan to set up your Injera batter 6-7 days in advance. If you already have Injera starter from a previous feast, you can prepare a fresh batch of Injera batter 2-3 days in advance. Also please note: If you want to prepare a recipe using Berberre paste, please plan to prepare this spice mix 10-14 days in advance. See recipes for all details.

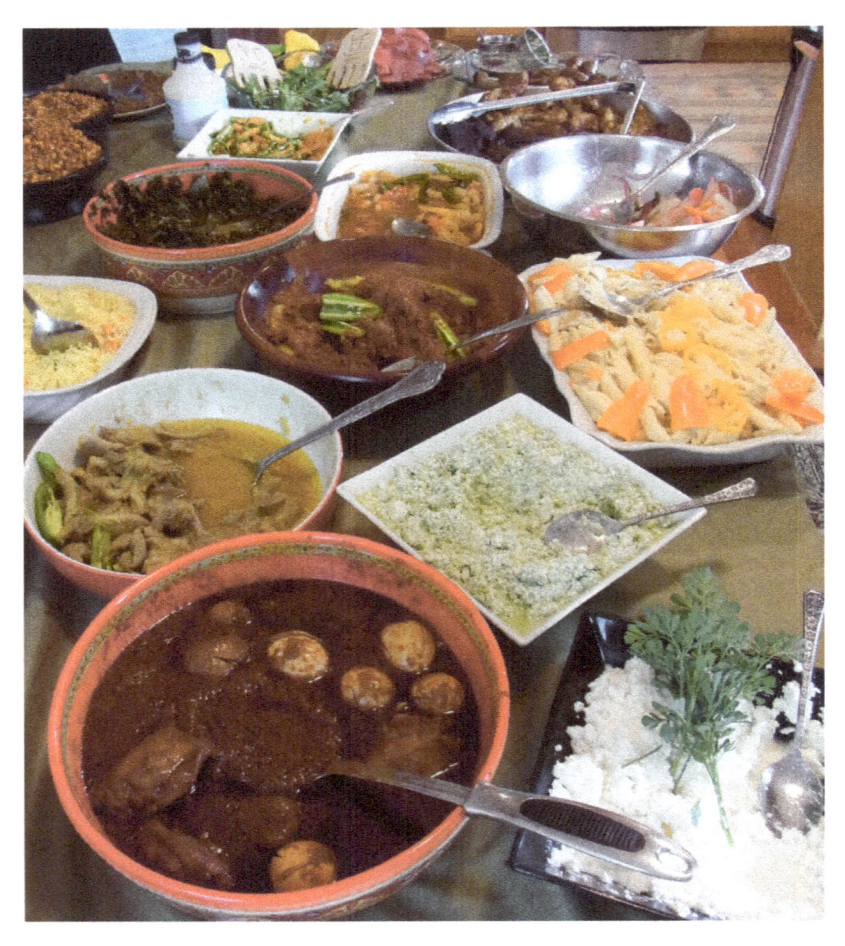

INGREDIENTS

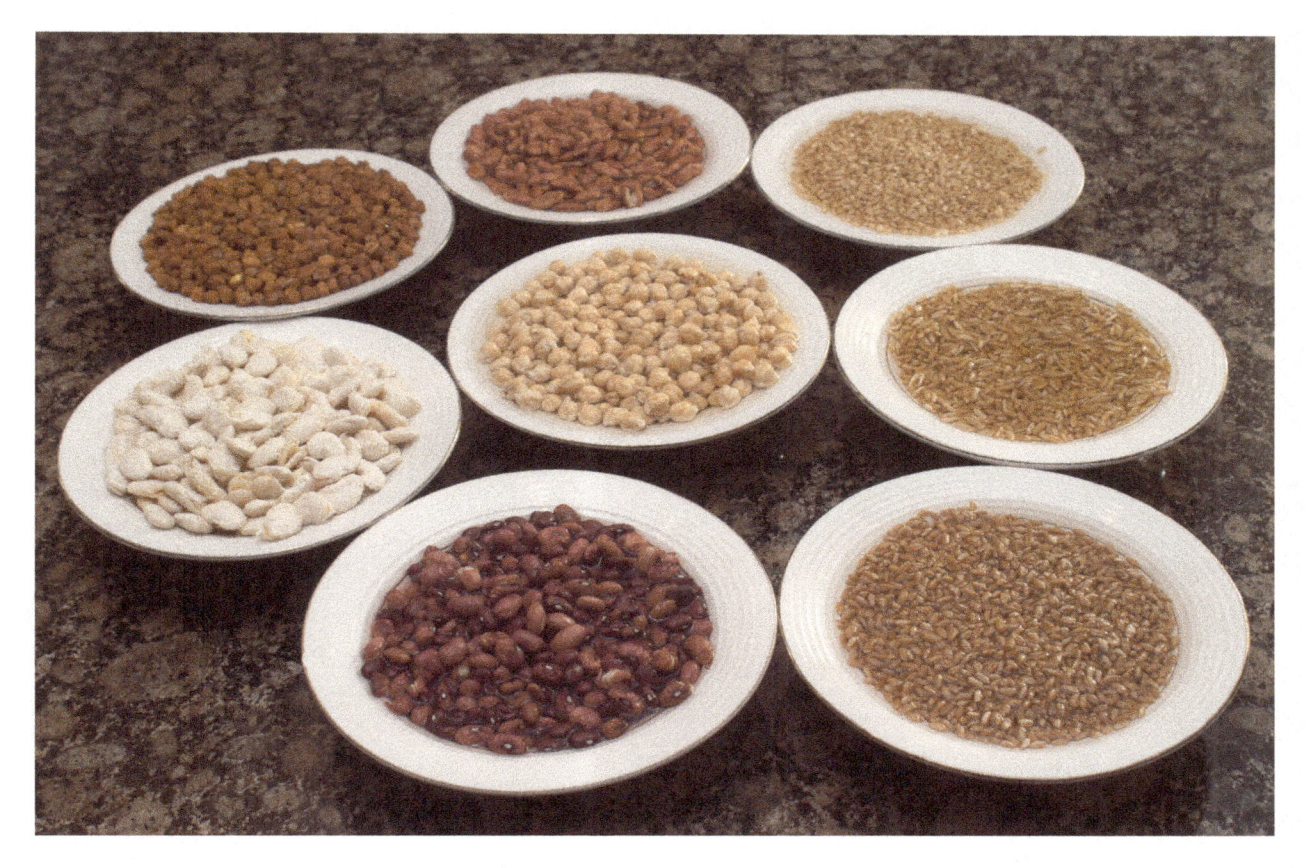

Some people think all Ethiopian ingredients must be very exotic and hard to get. But that is not true! Most ingredients in my recipes are things you can buy at any grocery store. You do not need special ingredients to begin. If you are lucky and live near a large city that has a "Little Addis" you can find everything you need. And many health food stores now carry these ingredients. But what if you don't have such places near you? That is okay because you can buy the short list of special Ethiopian ingredients that you need to make my recipes by going to the Internet. Below I list these special ingredient and where to purchase them online. Some online Ethiopian spice resources are: www.brundo.com, www.ethiopianspices.com, www.silkroadspices.ca. For details on specific items, see the following pages.

Above: Assorted beans and grains for Nifro (p. 181).

The Crown Jewel of African Cuisine

African long pepper: also "long pepper" or timiz. It is the seed head of a plant whose scientific name is Piper capense. Available at www.silkroadspices.ca.

Berberre: in this book, Berberre is used to add a spicy kick to foods and comes in two forms: powder or paste. The powder is the traditional form and must be bought in stores or online at www.ethiopianspices.com, www.brundo.com, or on amazon.com. I developed a recipe for Berberre paste (p. 29), which gives a thoroughly authentic taste but is much less expensive. The paste form is what I use in most of the recipes in this book.

Besobela: also called Ethiopian sacred basil. This sun-dried herb has a flavor that is distinct from Mediterranean or Thai basil. Mediterranean basil can be used as a substitute. Available at www.brundo.com or on amazon.com. In a pinch, one could substitute dried sweet basil, but the flavor will be less authentic.

Besso: powdered roasted barley. If you have a flour mill, you could make this yourself by dry roasting barley in a pan and then milling it. Or you can buy it online at www.brundo.com or on amazon.com by searching for Ethiopian besso.

Bishop's weed seeds: also called 'white caraway', nech azmud or ajwain. It can often be purchased at Indian or Asian Food Markets, or is available online at www.brundo.com.

California chili peppers, ground: These may be available in your grocery store. If not, it can be purchased on amazon.com.

Ground fenugreek: Known in Ethiopia as Abish. This spice is also a staple spice of Indian curries and can often be purchased at Indian or Asian Food Markets. Online it can be purchased from www.brundo.com or amazon.com.

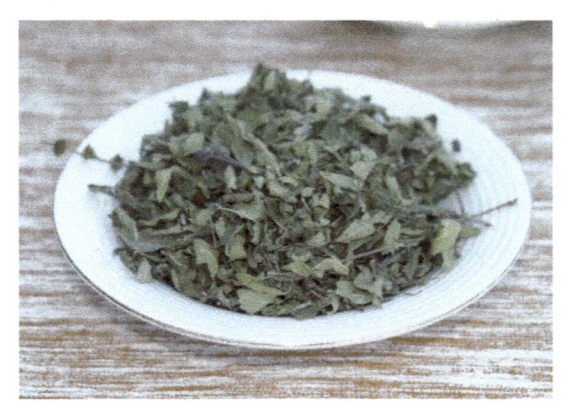

Koseret (Ethiopian "lemon bush").

Flax seed: These seeds are now readily available at most grocery stores. If yours doesn't carry these, you can try a health food store or find many venders selling it online at amazon.com.

Kamut berries: also called grain kamut. This is an ancient variety of wheat. Available at health food stores or online at amazon.com or bobsredmill.com.

Koseret: the dried leaves of the lemon bush plant

that is known by the scientific name Lippia javanica. Koseret can be purchased online at www.ethiopianspices.com or www.brundo.com. See illustration, facing page.

Mitmita: classic hot finishing spice for Ethiopian foods, containing red peppers and much more. Available online at brundo.com, www.ethiopianspices.com and via amazon.com.

Nigella seeds: also called Ethiopian black cumin, black caraway or tekur azmud. It can be bought online at www.ethiopianspices.com, www.brundo.com, or www.silkroadspices.ca

Rice flour (brown or white): It is carried by many grocers and health food stores. Also available on amazon.com.

Safflower seed: This is commonly sold in North America as bird food! Please do not use seeds sold for bird food as they are not food grade quality. You can buy safflower seeds for cooking with at www.brundo.com.

Shiro powder: finely ground roasted yellow split peas. Some Ethiopians use roasted chickpeas, or mixtures of different roasted legumes. If you have a flour mill, you could make this yourself by dry roasting yellow split peas (or other legumes) in a pan and then milling it. Or you can buy shiro powder online at www.brundo.com or www.ethiopianspices.com.

Teff flour (brown or white): the flour of this grain has traditionally been used to make Injera. It has become increasingly popular in recent years as a "super-food" or "super-grain" and can now be found in many grocery and health food stores. Also available from www.ethiopianspices.com, www.bobsredmill.com, or amazon.com.

Tenadam: the dried seed pods of the rue plant (traditionally Ruta chalepensis, but Ruta graveolens can be substituted). These are difficult to find for sale, so you may have to grow your own rue plants to have this ingredient.

Wheat berries: the entire wheat kernel except for the hull. Many grocery stores carry these as do most health food stores. Online you can purchase them at www.bobsredmill.com or through amazon.com.

Yirgacheffe or green unroasted Ethiopian coffee beans: used in our traditional coffee ceremony, in which it is roasted, ground, brewed and served. There are many varieties of green coffee bean available to use. Traditionally, Ethiopians use yirgacheffe beans specifically in their green state. Yirgacheffe is available online at www.brundo.com, www.ethiopianspices.com, or amazon.com.

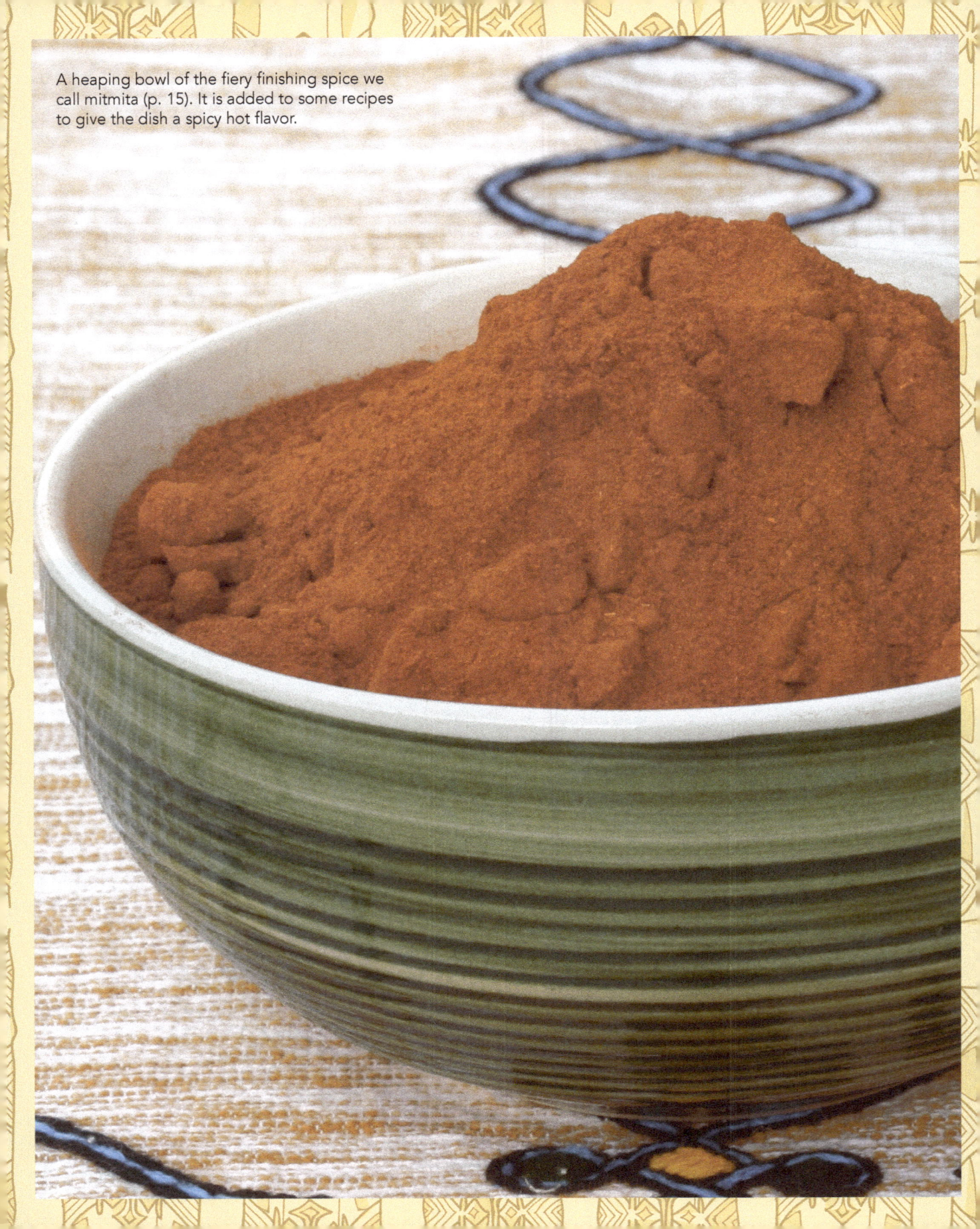

A heaping bowl of the fiery finishing spice we call mitmita (p. 15). It is added to some recipes to give the dish a spicy hot flavor.

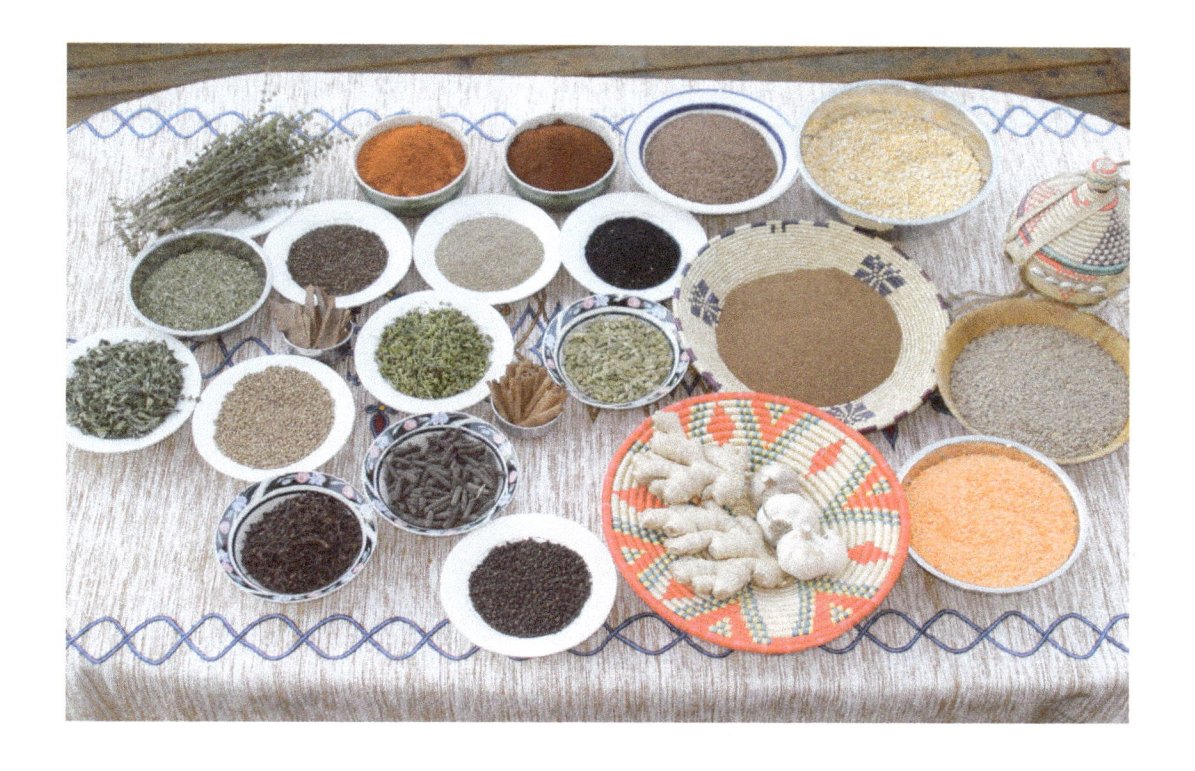

The Basics: Spices and Seasonings

    Look at our beautiful spices! What you see on this table in my backyard is the very big variety of spices and other ingredients that we use to make Ethiopian food so special and delicious! In Ethiopia we use many spices that will be familiar to you - like garlic and ginger - but we also use some special Ethiopian spices. It is the combination of the familiar and the exotic that creates the wonderful flavors that are unique to my country's food. In Ethiopia, we often use very special handmade spice mixes in our cooking. These mixes are simple to make and once you have made a few, you will be ready to cook nearly any Ethiopian dish! Our most famous spice mix is Berberre, the rich, spicy specialty that gives the beautiful color and taste to our most famous dish, Yedoro Wat, or Chicken Stew (p. 59).

Above: An array of many of the spices used in Ethiopian cooking.

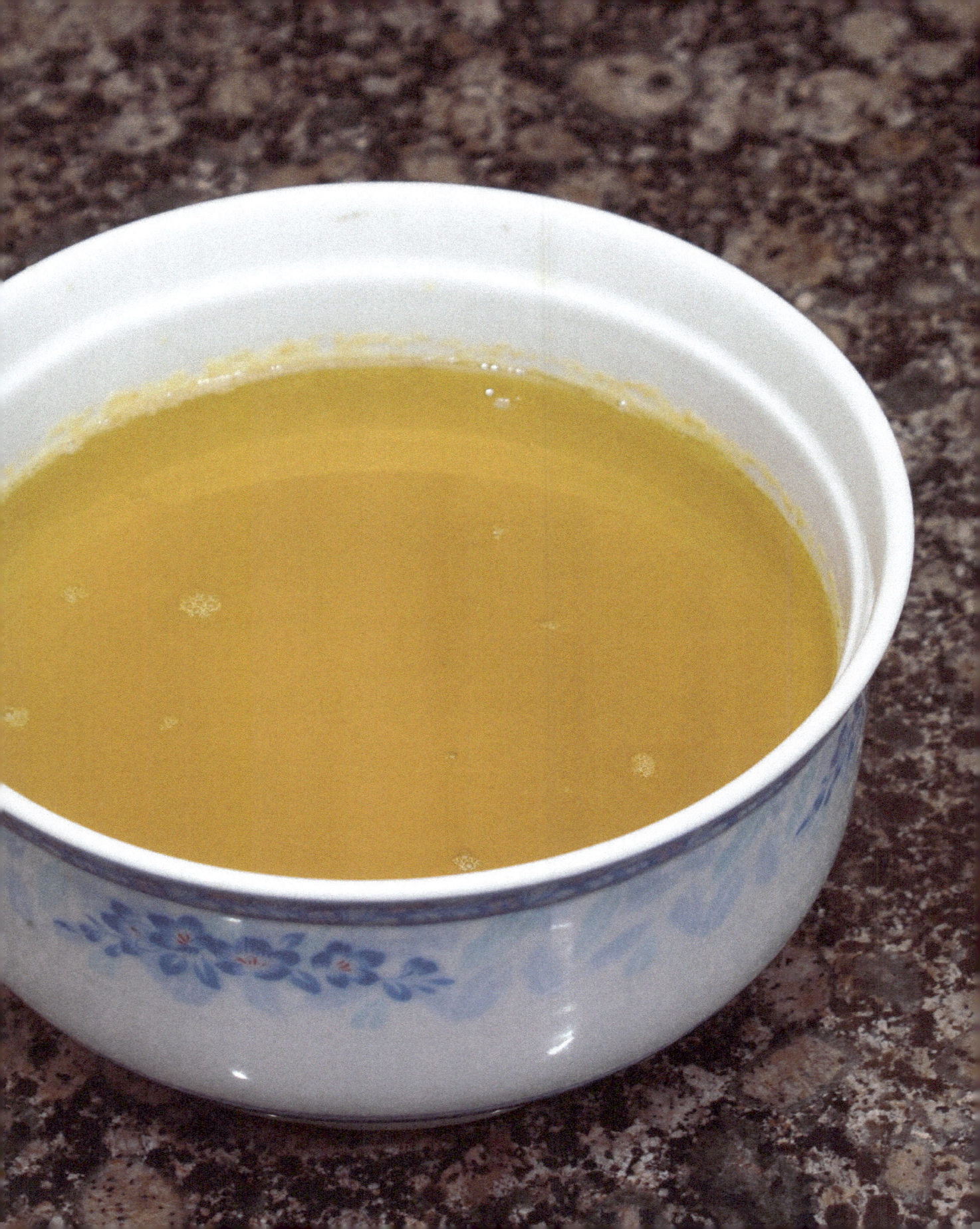

Spiced Clarified Butter
ንጥር ቅቤ
(Niter Kibe) (V) (VG) (GF) (DF)

Time: 2–3 days
Makes: 3 cups
Difficulty: ●●○○○

This seasoning, essential to so many Ethiopian recipes, is purified by clarifying the butter in a process that also allows the full flavors of the spices to develop.

Ingredients:

Unsalted butter (or vegan butter substitute), 2 lb, softened
Koseret*, ½ cup
Q'imam, ½ tsp (p. 25)
Turmeric, ½ tsp
Ground fenugreek*, 1 Tbsp

*available at specialty stores and online, see p. 16

Directions:

1. With your hands, knead the butter (or vegan butter substitute - we recommend Earth Balance, as its flavor produces the most authentic Niter Kibe) and all other ingredients. Let the mixture sit 2–3 days in a large covered pot at room temperature.

2. After it has sat for 2–3 days, place the pot over medium-high heat for 10–15 min, stirring twice.

3. Remove the pot from the heat, let it cool and settle for ~30 min, and then pour through a fine strainer into clean jar or other storage container, removing the spices and milk solids from the clarified butter.

4. Discard the spices and milk solids, and refrigerate the clarified butter in a clean, sealed container until needed. Niter Kibe will keep for at least 1 month in the refrigerator.

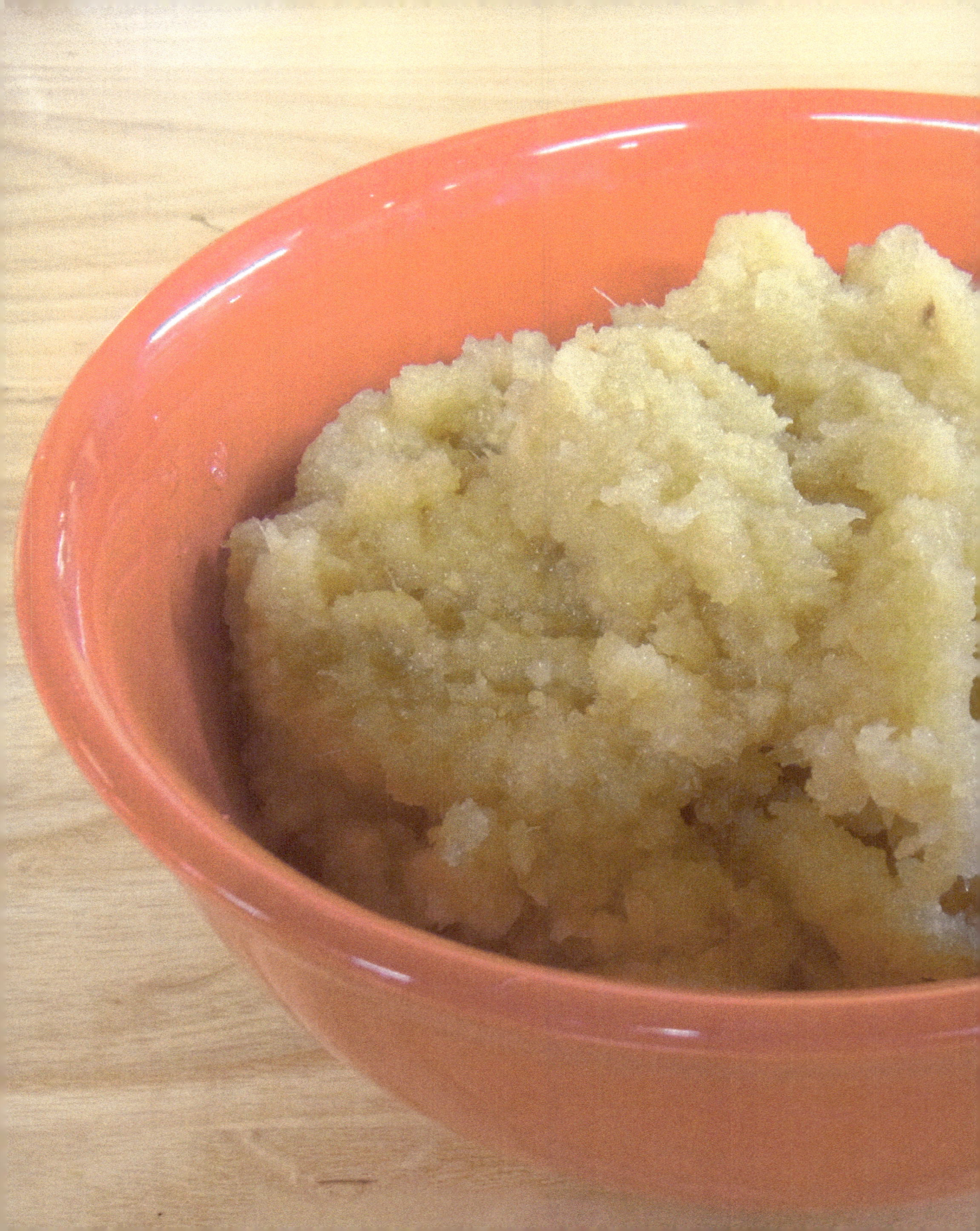

Spices & Seasonings

Ginger-Garlic Paste
ዝንጅብል እና ነጭ ሽንኩርት
(Zingibel Inna Nach Shinkurt) (V) (VG) (GF) (DF)

Time: 7 min
Makes: 1 quart
Difficulty: 🌶

This mixture is used in many Ethiopian recipes, both spicy and mild, particularly for seasoning meats and vegetables. It is quick to make, and can be made on the day that you are cooking an Ethiopian dinner.

Ingredients:

Garlic cloves, peeled, 2 lb
Ginger root, washed (unpeeled), 1⅔ lb, coarsely chopped

Directions:

1. Place garlic and ginger into a food processer and process 4–5 min, until it forms a smooth paste, scraping the sides once or twice during this time.
2. Place in a sealed container and refrigerate until use. Keeps in the refrigerator for at least 1 month, if you make sure always to use a clean utensil each time you remove some from the container.

Note: if you plan on cooking Ethiopian meals infrequently, you can make smaller amounts of this paste, using approximately the same ratio of garlic to ginger root.

The Crown Jewel of African Cuisine

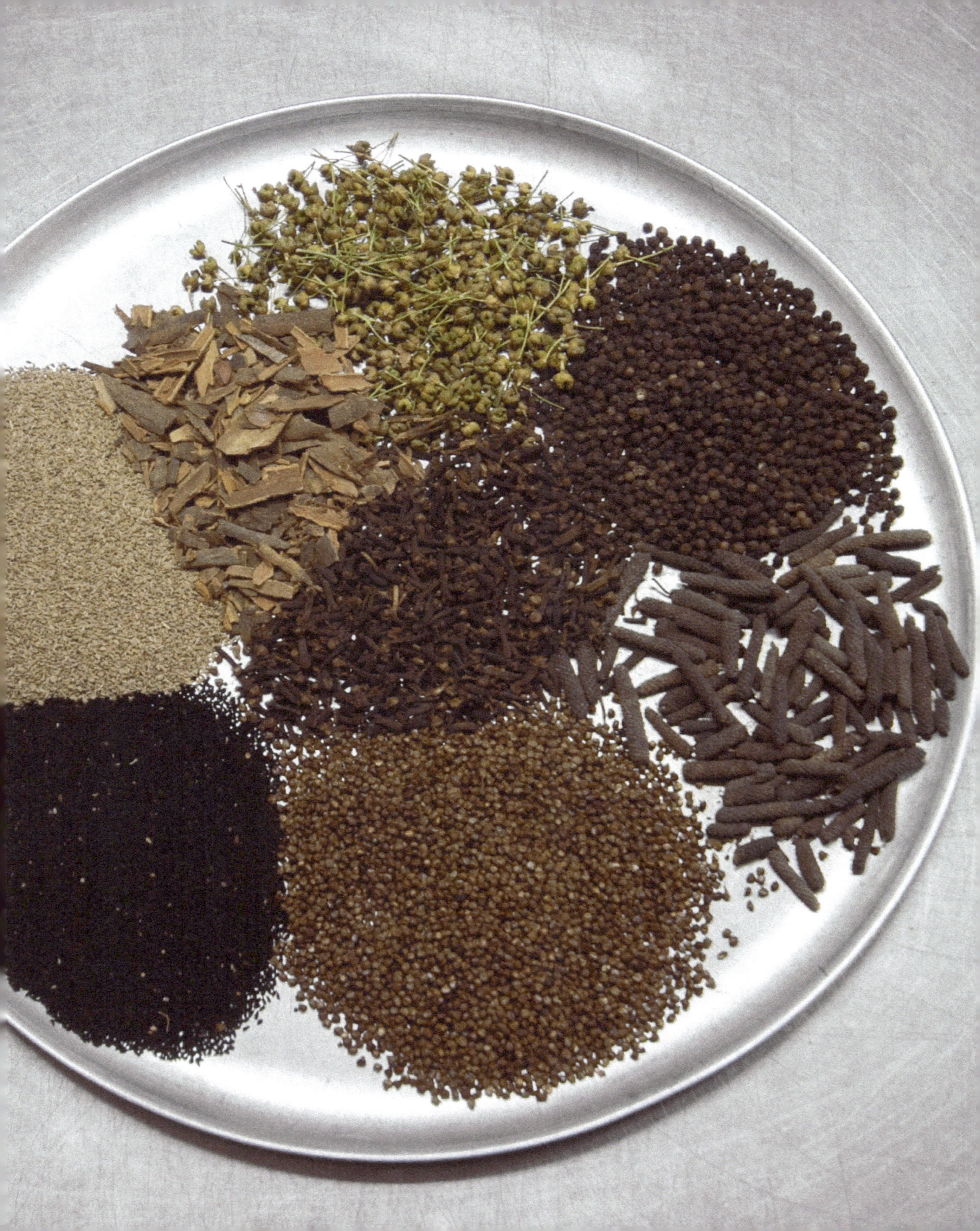

Spices & Seasonings

Q'imam
ቅመም

(Q'imam) (V) (VG) (GF) (DF)

Time: 10 min
Makes: 2 cups
Difficulty:

This spice mix is used as a finishing spice in Ethiopian recipes, similar to how garam masala is used in Indian recipes. Some of the spices that are used in this recipe can be difficult to find in stores, but they are readily available online through Ethiopian spice vendors. Please see page 15 for details.

Ingredients:

Cardamom seeds, ½ cup
Nigella seeds*, ½ cup
Bishop's weed seeds*, ½ cup
African long pepper*, whole, ½ cup
Tenadam**, ½ cup (optional)
Black peppercorns, whole, ½ cup
Whole cloves, ½ cup
Cinnamon sticks, broken into 1 inch pieces, ½ cup

*available at specialty stores and online, see p. 16
**difficult to find, see p. 17

Directions:

1. Heat oven to 300°.
2. Place all ingredients on a baking sheet and warm in the oven for 5 min. After this time, the spices should be fragrant.
3. With a spice grinder, grind the spices together in batches, until it forms a fine powder. This should take about 45 seconds per batch.
4. Combine all of the ground spices in a bowl and mix thoroughly. Place it in a jar and store with your other dried spices until needed for use. This mixture will keep for several months.

The Crown Jewel of African Cuisine

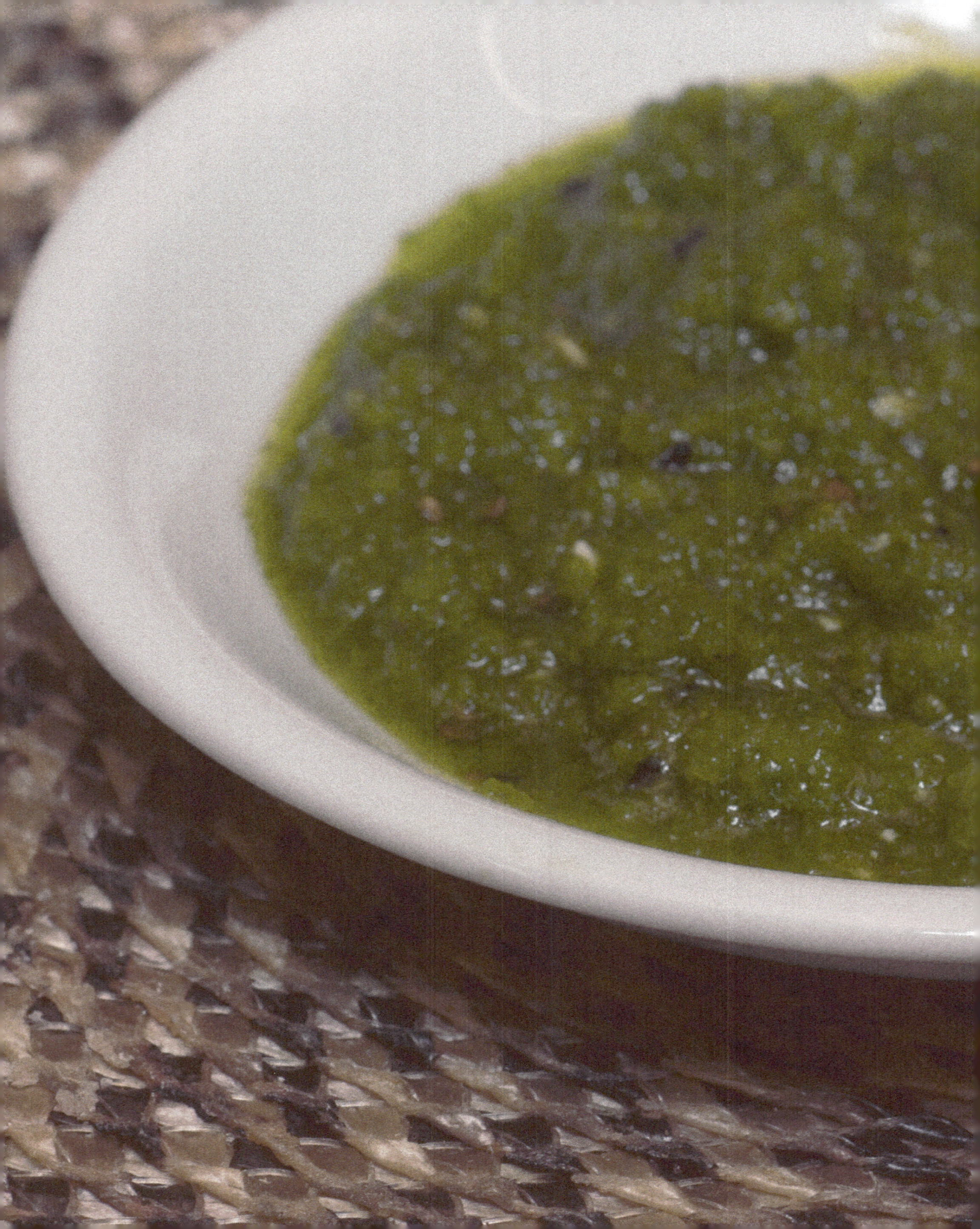

Jalapeño Relish

ቆጭ ቆጫ

(Q'och Q'ocha) (V) (VG) (GF) (DF)

This spicy and refreshing relish can be used on all savory foods.

Time: 5 min
Servings: many
Difficulty: 🌶🌶🌶🌶

Ingredients:

Cilantro, 1 large bunch, bottom part of stems removed
Bishop's weed seeds*, 2 tsp
Nigella seeds*, 2 tsp
Ginger-Garlic Paste, ½ cup (p. 23)
Salt, 2 Tbsp
Jalapeños, 2 lb, stems removed, not seeds

*available at specialty stores and online, see p. 16 and 17

Directions:

1. Combine all ingredients—except jalapeños—in bowl of food processor. Blend for 30 seconds and remove to a large bowl.
2. Put jalapeños in bowl of food processor. Blend for 15 seconds or until finely chopped.
3. Add jalapeños to bowl with other ingredients and mix thoroughly.
4. Return mixture to bowl of food processor. Blend for 2 min or until smooth.
5. Place in airtight container and refrigerate until use.

Note: For smaller batches, one can combine all of the ingredients (including the jalapeños) in the processor and blend for 2 ½ min.

The Crown Jewel of African Cuisine

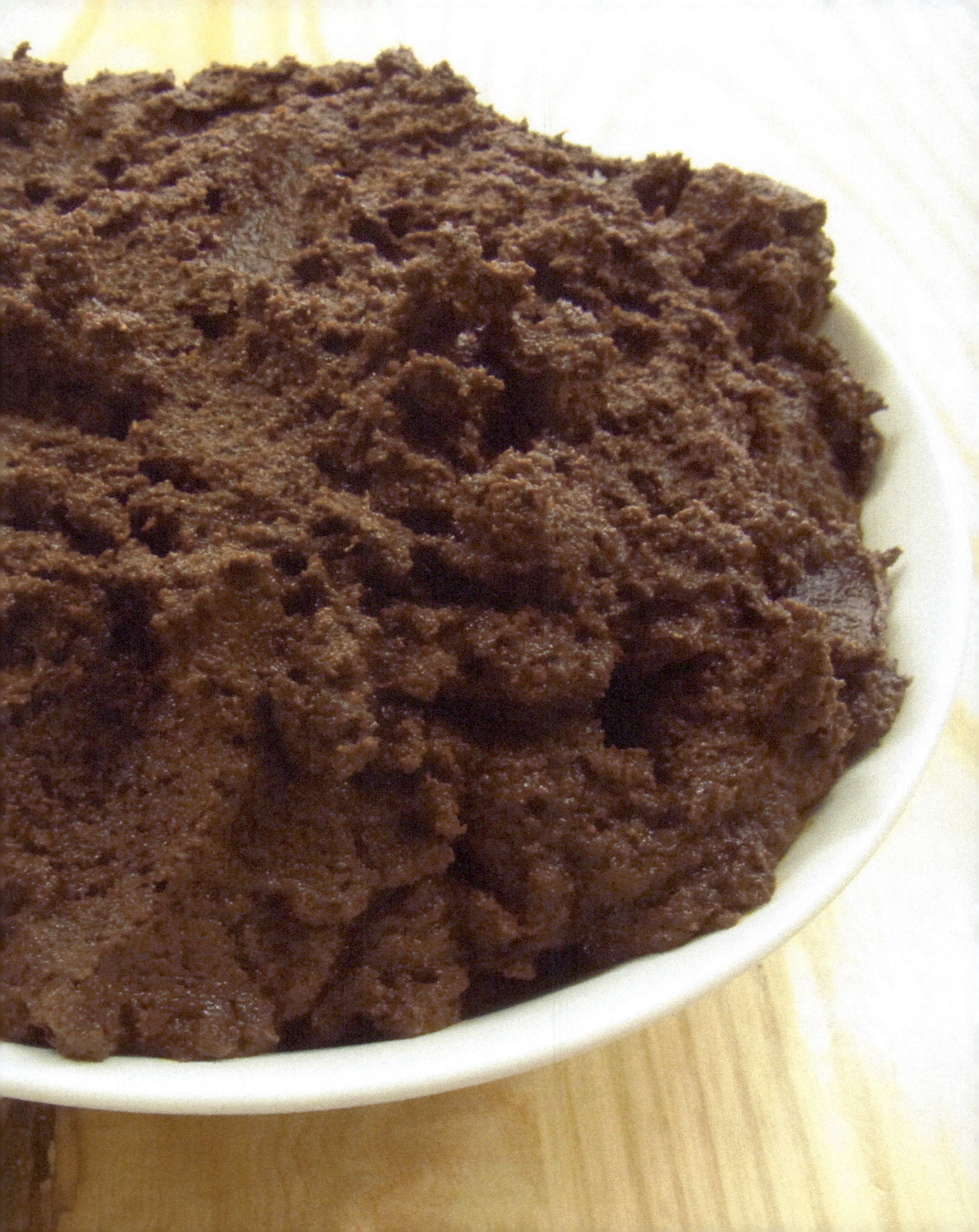

Spices & Seasonings

Berberre Paste
በርበሬ
(Berberre) (V) (VG) (GF) (DF)

Time: 10–14 days
Makes: 12 cups
Difficulty:

Berberre is an essential ingredient for spicy Ethiopian recipes. I developed the recipe for this essential spice mix as an adaptation to working in an American kitchen. The flavors develop over time, so be sure to let it sit in the refrigerator for the suggested amount of time. In Ethiopia, this spice mix is normally used as a dry powder, made by sun-drying the peppers and spices, grinding them together, roasting them, and then grinding them again into a fine powder.

Ingredients:
Ginger-Garlic Paste, 1 cup (p. 23)
Q'imam, 1 Tbsp (p. 25)
Salt, 1 Tbsp
Ground California chili peppers*, 3 cups
Ground chili powder, 3 cups
Ground paprika, 3 cups
Ground cayenne pepper, 2 Tbsp (more if you like your food spicy)
Water, 8 cups

*available at specialty stores and online, see p. 16

Directions:
1. Place all ingredients in a large bowl. Mix with a rubber spatula to combine thoroughly into a smooth paste.
2. Put the paste into a sealed container and refrigerate for 10–14 days before using it in recipes.
3. Berberre paste will keep for at least a month in the refrigerator, especially if you are careful to use clean utensils each time use take some from the container, avoid mixing other foods into the paste, and limit its time out of the refrigerator.

The Crown Jewel of African Cuisine

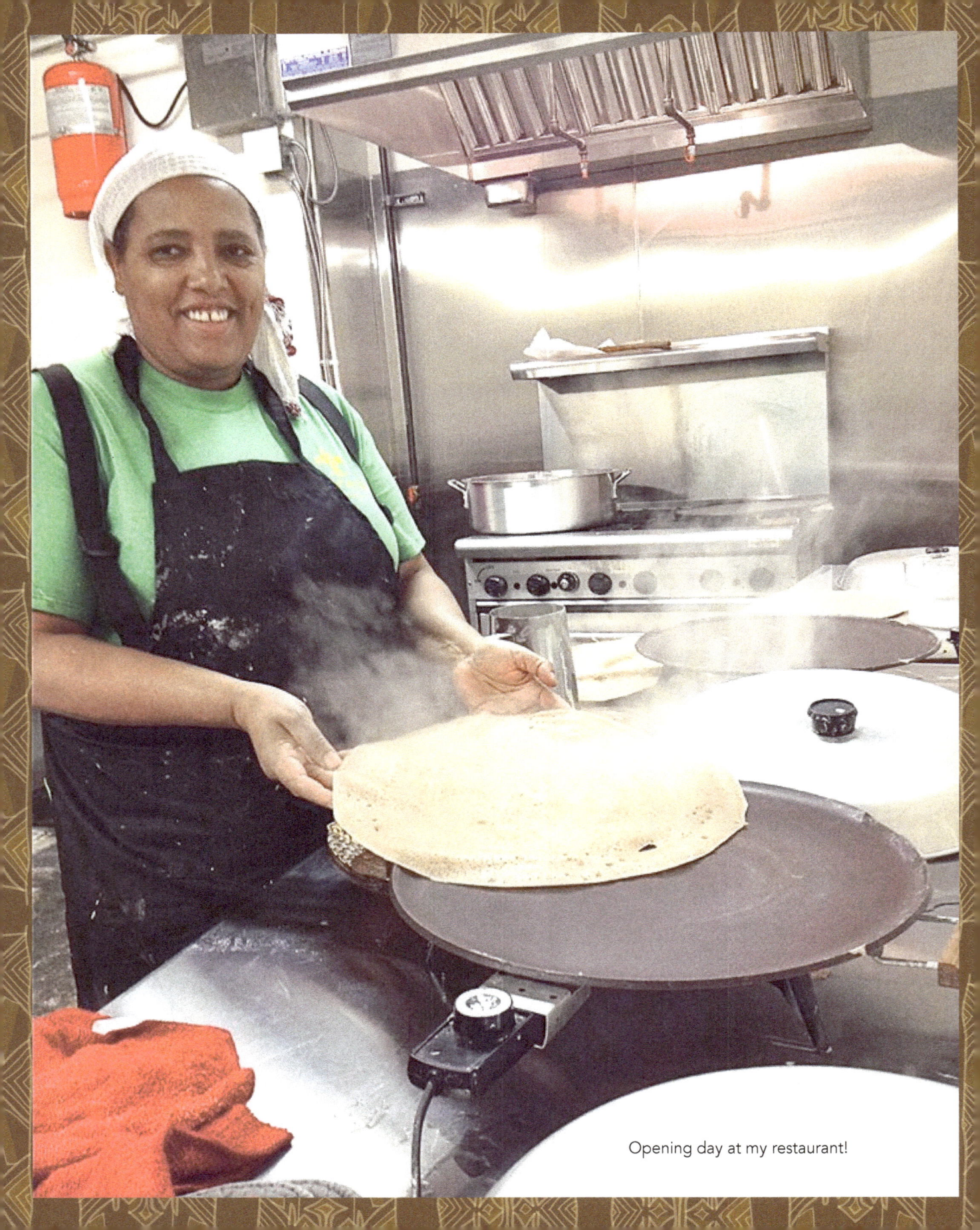

Opening day at my restaurant!

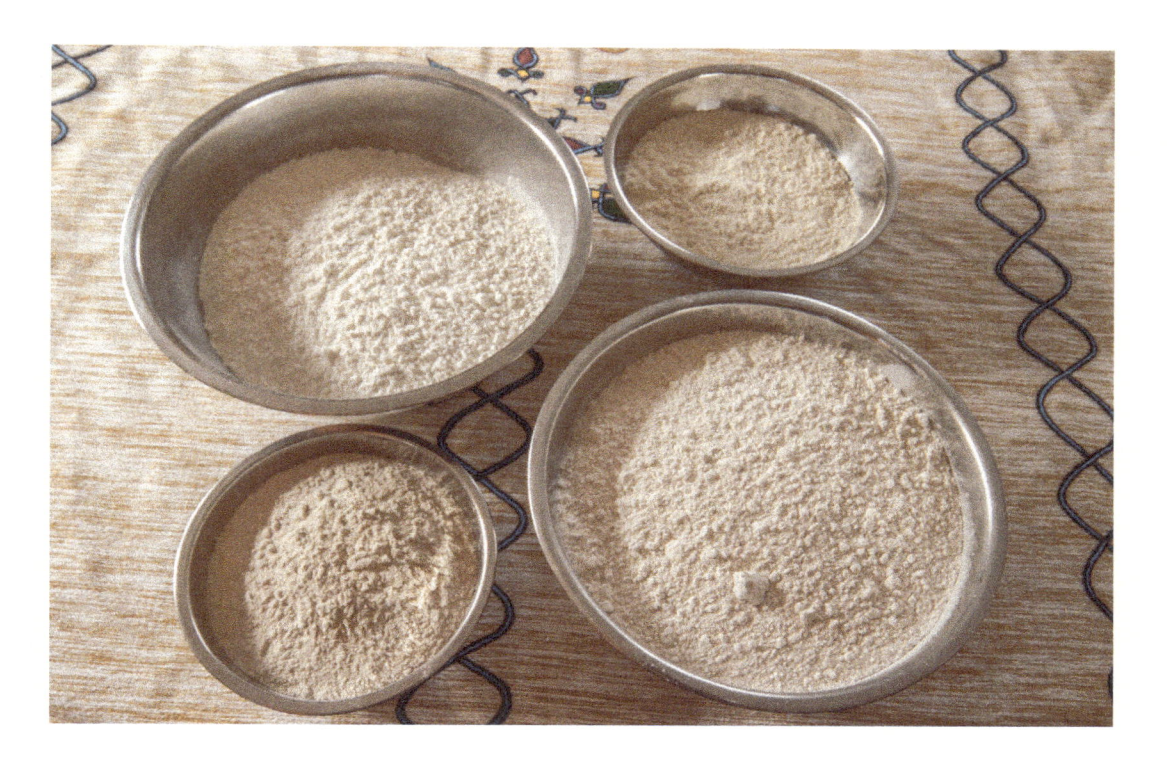

The Staff of Life:
Injera and other Breads and Grains

    Our very special steamed sourdough bread round - which you can see me pulling off the mitad on the left - is the heart of Ethiopian cooking. We eat Injera at every meal, with every kind of food and in many different ways. In this chapter, you will learn how to make the famously difficult Injera using a recipe that took me many years of experimenting to create. Every day at my restaurant I prepare stacks of fresh Injera and every day they are gobbled up! While we love Injera every day, we also do have some baked breads that we cook for special occasions. I have included a few of those recipes here including the recipe for Dabbo, a beautiful loaf baked in banana leaves. I gave out Dabbo in honor of the opening day of my restaurant. Also, be sure to try the spicy breakfast cake Genfo (p. 51) - it is my children's favorite!

Above: ingredients for Traditional spicy breakfast cake called Genfo (p. 51).

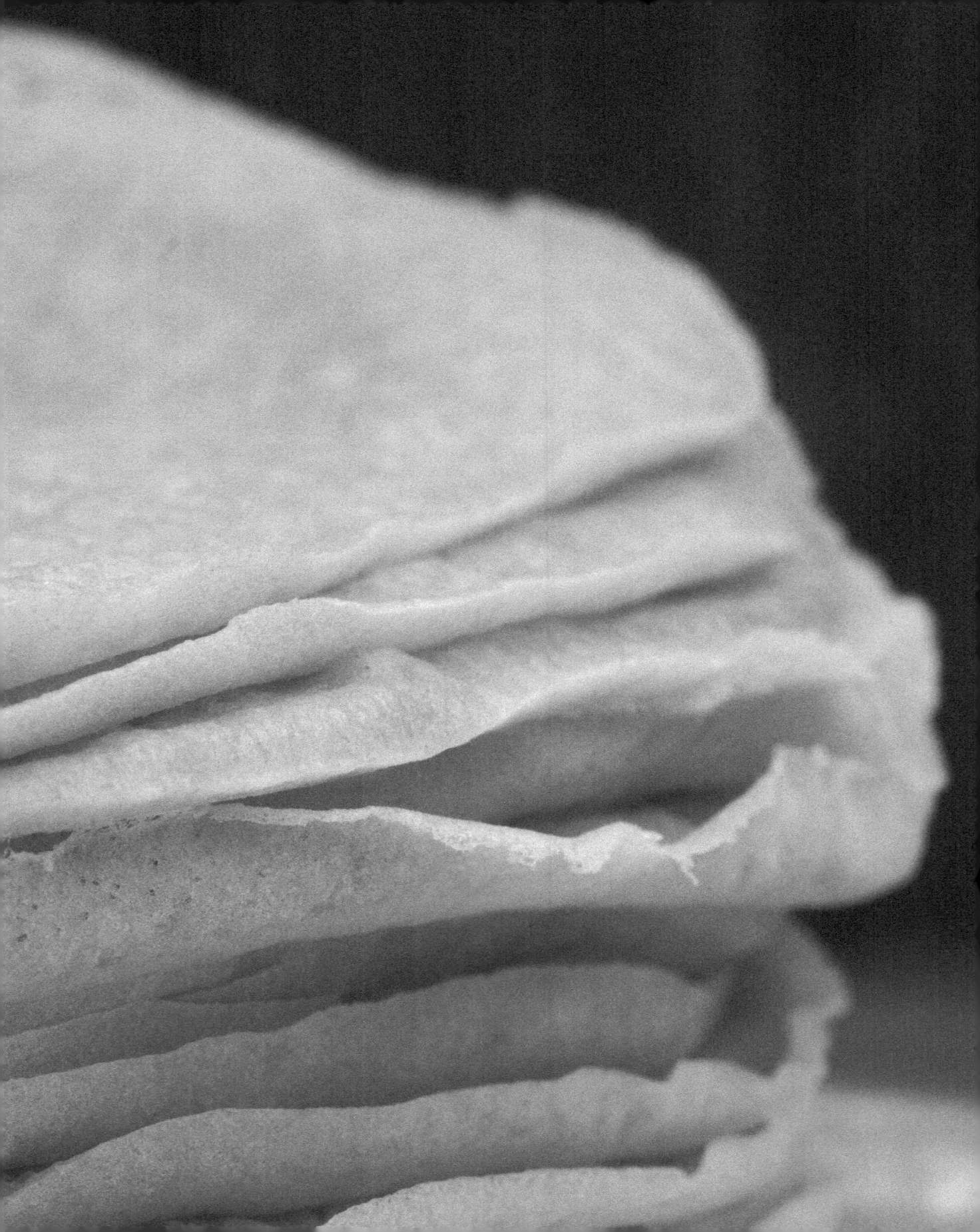

Injera, Breads & Grains

Ethiopian Flatbread
እንጀራ
(Injera) V VG GF DF

Time: 2 weeks if starting from scratch, or 2–3 days if you have Injera starter
Serves: 6–8
Difficulty: 🌶🌶🌶🌶🌶

Injera is the heart of almost every Ethiopian meal. A good Injera has many "eyes" - which we call ayin - meaning the little holes that soak up the flavors of the food. We serve the Injera on a platter on top of a basket called the mesob. Everyone shares one dish and you use your hands to pick up bite-sized pieces of food wrapped in Injera. We don't need a fork, knife or spoon because we have Injera! But if you like to eat it with utensils, that is good too.

Like sourdough bread, Injera is made from a live starter culture. The fermentation done by the culture gives Injera its slightly sour flavor. Because it involves fermentation, Injera can be somewhat temperamental, so please follow the instructions carefully.

In traditional Ethiopian cooking, Injera is made with the flour made from the grain known as teff, which is gluten-free. Injera can also be made with flours made from wheat, corn, barley, rice, and sorghum, or a combination of these flours. Here I combine teff and rice flours to make a gluten-free Injera that is both spongy and flavorful.

In the traditional Ethiopian cookhouse, Injera is cooked over a fire on a clay pan called a mitad. In more modern kitchens, cooks can use specially made electric mitads.

Ingredients:

For Injera starter:
Active dry yeast, 1 Tbsp
Non-chlorinated water, 2 cups
Rice flour* (brown or white), 1 cup
Teff flour* (brown or white), ¾ cup

For the batter:
Rice flour (brown or white), 1 lb
Teff flour (brown or white), 1 lb
Injera starter, ½ cup
Non-chlorinated water, ~6 cups

*available at specialty stores and online, see p. 17

Directions:

Step 1: Make the starter *(start this process 7–8 days before you want to eat the Injera, unless you already have starter, in which case you can start making the Injera 2–3 days before you want to eat it)*

1. In a large ceramic or glass bowl, combine 1 package (~1 Tbsp) active dry yeast with 2 cups lukewarm non-chlorinated water. (Chlorine reduces the activity of the yeast, making it difficult to produce a sufficiently active culture. If your water supply contains chlorine, boil it for 5 min to remove the chlorine and let it cool prior to using. Alternatively, use bottled spring water.) Stir until the yeast is dissolved.

2. In a separate bowl, thoroughly combine 1 cup rice flour and ¾ cup teff flour.

3. Pour the flour mix into the bowl with the yeast-water mix and stir with a whisk until it is smooth (a few small lumps are ok).

4. Pour the starter into a container that has sufficient room for the starter to expand (it may expand up to 4x in volume). Cover securely with a cloth, place in a warm location, and stir it daily for 5 days. At the end of the 5th day, pour the starter

Injera, Breads & Grains

into a clean, sealable jar (canning jars work well for this) and refrigerate. This starter can remain in the refrigerator for 2 weeks before using. If you need to keep it longer, see the note in the box at right.

Step 2: Prepare the Injera dough *(2–3 days before eating)*:

1. In a large bowl, thoroughly combine 1 lb brown or white rice flour, and 1 lb teff flour.
2. Add ½ cup of starter culture (before doing this, be sure to pour off any fluid that may have accumulated on top of the culture).
3. Add 2 cups lukewarm non-chlorinated water and work the mixture with your hands until it forms a firm ball of dough. Add more water ¼ cup at a time, if needed, to get the dough to form a ball.
4. Using the heel of your hand, knead the dough for 5–7 min.
5. Break approximately ⅓ of the dough into small pieces, and put the pieces in a blender with 2 cups non-chlorinated water. Blend 30 sec, or until smooth, and pour into a large (~2 gal) plastic sealable container. This step can be done by hand if you do not have a blender, but be sure to break up all of the small lumps.
6. Repeat with the rest of the dough until it is all blended, adding the blended mix to the large plastic container.
7. Seal the container, place it in a warm location, and leave it for approximately 36 to 60 hours, until the batter has a layer of separated fluid on top and is slowly releasing bubbles. The amount of time it takes to get to this point depends on various factors, including temperature, freshness of your culture, and the variety of yeast in your culture. Be sure to check the batter every 12 hours after the first day has passed, to catch it at the proper point. If you wait too long you may miss the bubbly stage, and the fermentation will begin to produce too much alcohol, diminishing

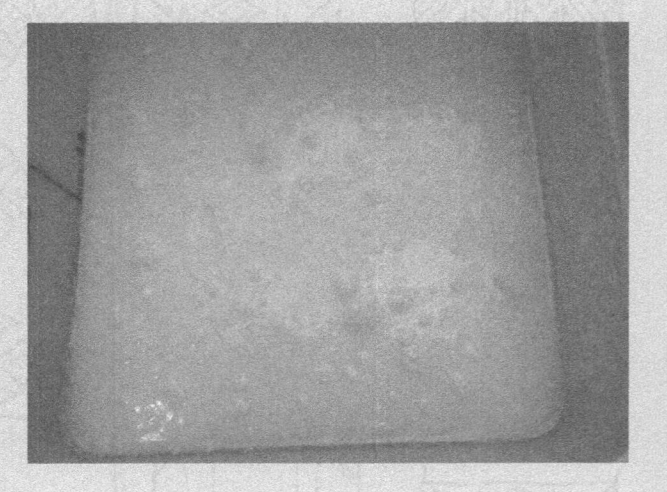

> **Important Note:** Before cooking your first Injera, reserve 1 cup of the batter in a clean, sealable jar (place this in the refrigerator). This supply will serve as the starter the next time you make Injera, saving you a lot of time by allowing you to start with Step 2 the next time you make Injera. To keep the reserved starter active, feed it every 2 weeks. If you do not do this, the starter culture will weaken.
>
> To feed the starter, pour off any fluid that has accumulated on the top of the batter, add 4 Tbsp rice flour, 4 Tbsp teff flour, and ¼ cup non-chlorinated water. Stir to mix, reseal the jar, and return it to the refrigerator. If you keep a culture for many weeks without cooking Injera, it is a good idea to periodically transfer the culture to a new, clean jar to reduce the risk of mold.

Injera, Breads & Grains

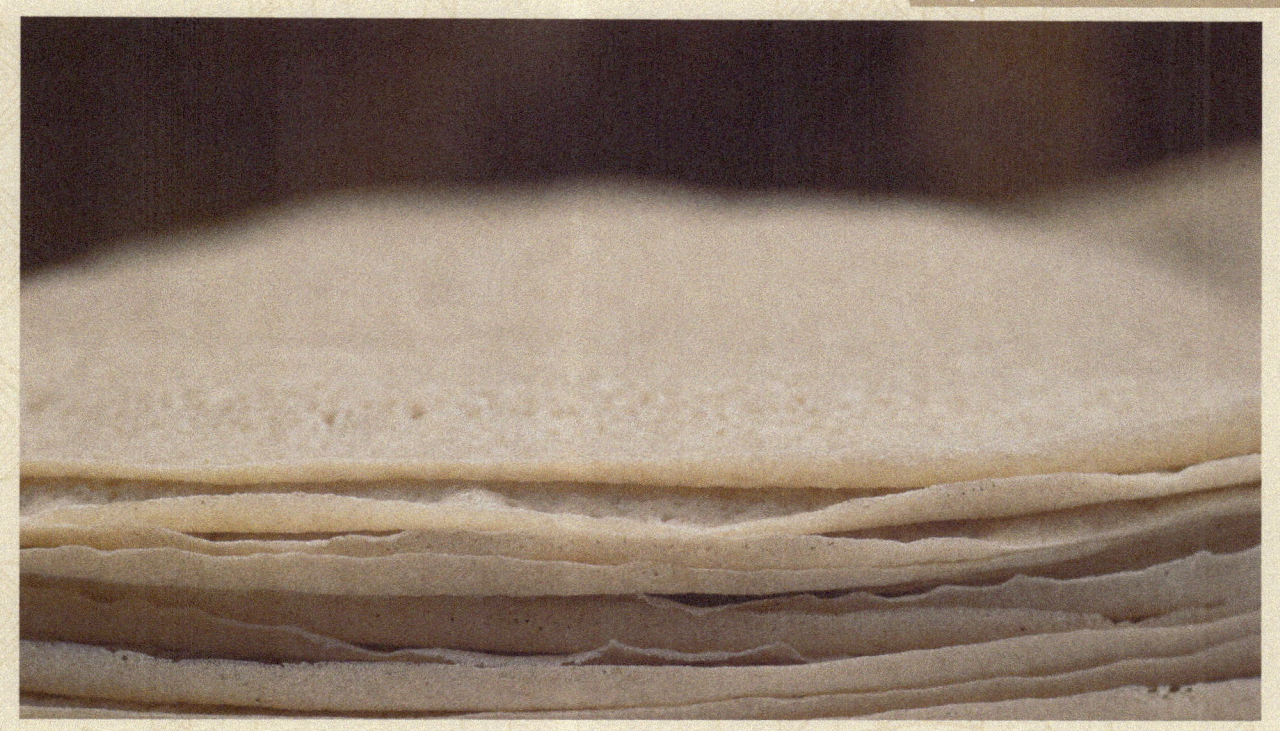

yeast activity (and bubbles).

8. At the point when the batter is releasing bubbles, pour the fluid off of the top of the batter.

9. In a small saucepan over high heat, bring 1½ cups non-chlorinated water to a boil, add ½ cup of the batter, and cook 1 min, stirring continuously. The batter will thicken to a sticky porridge (*absit*) during this time.

10. Remove the saucepan from the heat and let the absit cool to a temperature at which it is not hot to the touch (~30 min).

11. Once the absit has cooled, return it to the container with the rest of the batter, and stir to combine.

12. In 2–3 batches, blend the batter–absit mix for about 30 sec per batch until smooth. Return it to the fermentation container and let it sit until many bubbles have formed in the batter (1–12 hours). Before proceeding past this step, it is important that the batter have many bubbles suspended in it, since those bubbles will form the 'eyes' (*ayin*) that give Injera its porous texture. How long it takes for these bubbles to develop can vary considerably, depending on how active your yeast culture is.

13. Once the batter is bubbly, stir 2 cups lukewarm non-chlorinated water into the batter. The batter should reach the consistency of cream or very thin cake batter. To test the consistency, put your hand in the batter and remove it. Most of the batter should easily pour off of your hand, leaving just a thin, somewhat transparent coating. Another way to test

The Crown Jewel of African Cuisine

Injera, Breads & Grains

the consistency is to pour 1 tsp of the batter onto a plate from a height of 1 inch. It should spread to form a round area about 1¾ inches across. If you need to thin the batter more, stir in additional water, ¼ cup at a time.

Step 3: Cook the Injera (do this the day before or the morning of the day on which you want to eat the Injera):

1. Heat a non-stick electric griddle to 450°F.
2. To make your first Injera, place 1½ cups of the Injera batter into a pitcher. From about 12 inches above the pan surface, pour this batter onto the pan, using a swift, smooth, circular motion, starting from the outside edge, and spiraling toward the middle. Try to evenly cover the entire pan surface. Once the batter is poured, do not tip the pan, unless it is necessary to move the batter from a place where it was poured on too thickly. The batter will set quickly, so if you do need to tip the pan, do so right away.
3. After about 25 sec, you should start to see many small holes form and set in the batter (see lower right above). At this point, cover the pan with a lid.
4. Cook 1–2 min more, until the edge of the Injera starts to lift off of the pan, the surface of the Injera is somewhat dull, and the sizzling sounds have subsided. If your Injera is quite thin, you may need to cook it covered for as little as 30 sec.
5. With a quick motion, lift the edge of the Injera with one hand (careful – the Injera and the pan are quite hot!) and slide a wicker spatula (*sefede*) or large piece of cardboard (a pizza box cover works well for this) under the entire Injera.
6. Transfer the Injera to a large plate that is covered with a clean cloth, laying it flat on the cloth.
7. At this point, examine your first Injera to see if has cooked to your liking.

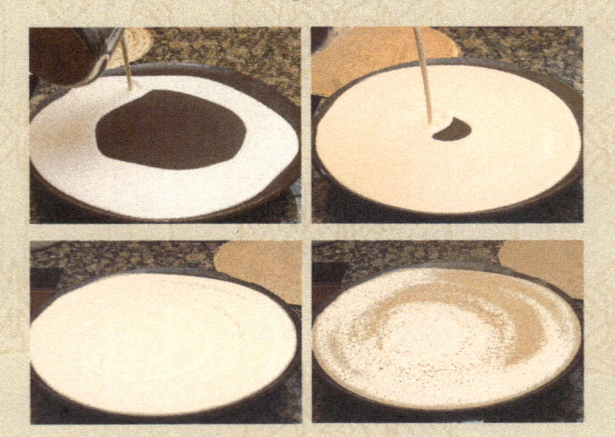

   - If the Injera is too thick and dry, stir ¼ cup water into the batter and make another Injera.

   - If the Injera is too soft and sticky, add ¼ cup flour (rice or teff) to a blender along with enough batter so that it can blend smoothly, stir the blended mix into the rest of the batter, wait 20–30 min, and make another Injera.
8. Once the batter is producing Injera that you like, reserve 1 cup of the batter in a clean jar (refrigerated), to serve as the starter for the next time you cook Injera

Facing page: Removing a freshly cooked Injera (top), and a meal of Injera (p. 33), Yedoro Wat (p. 59), Cottage Cheese (p. 117), Lettuce, Pepper and Tomato Salad (p. 169) and Potatoes with Carrots (p. 149) (bottom).

(see box on p. 34). Then, cook the remaining Injera one at a time until the batter has been used up, stacking the Injera on top of each other.

9. After the stack of Injera has cooled to near room temperature, cover it with plastic wrap and let it sit until you are ready to eat. If it sits for few hours to 1 day, the Injera will soften a bit and become more spongy, making it even better than when it is fresh off of the pan.

Leftover cooked Injera can be kept at room temperature for 1–2 days. If you want to store it longer, fold it into a large, sealable plastic bag and store in the freezer (defrost for 3–4 hours at room temperature prior to eating).

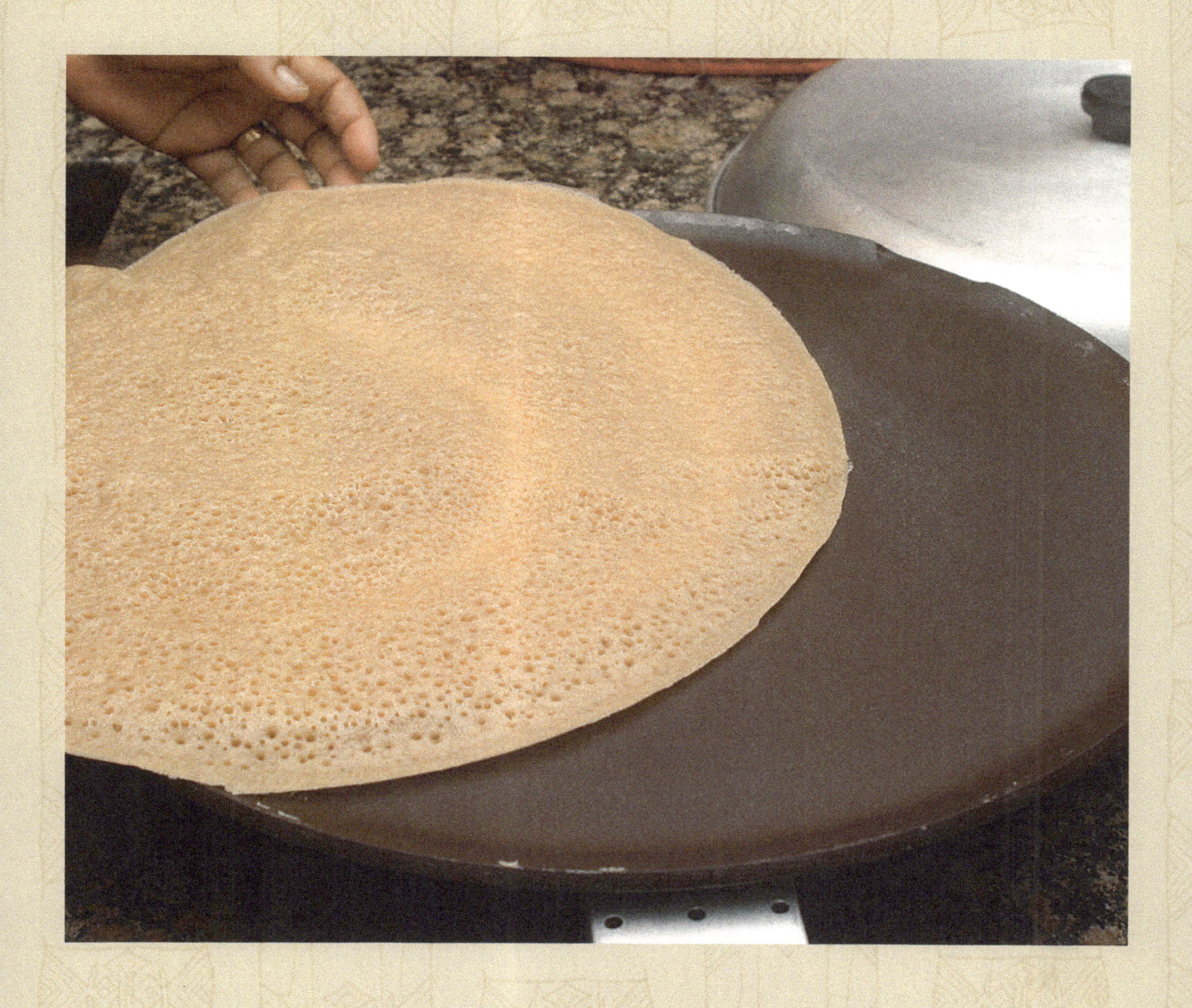

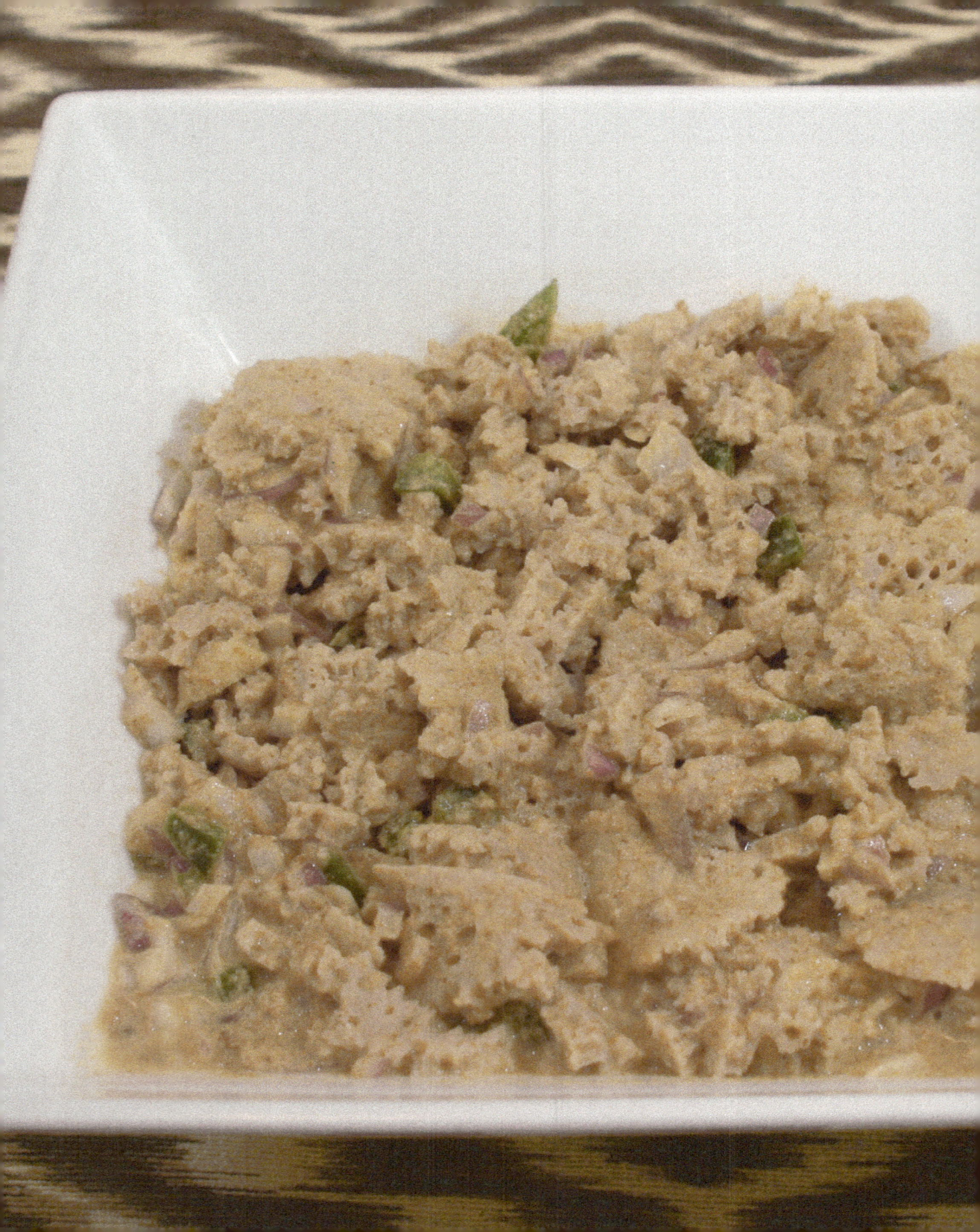

Injera, Breads & Grains

Sesame Stew
የሰልጥ ፍትፍት
(Yeselit Fitfit) Ⓥ ⓋⒼ ⒼⒻ ⒹⒻ

Time: 20 min
Serves: 5
Difficulty: ♦♦◊◊◊

This side dish is one of the many ways we make use of leftover Injera (p. 33).

Ingredients:

Raw sesame seeds, 1 cup
Red onion, ½ medium, finely diced
Jalapeño, 1, seeds and stem removed, finely diced
Salt, 1 tsp
Water, 1 cup
Injera, ½ round

Directions:

1. Heat Injera pan or other nonstick fry pan or electric skillet to 450° F.
2. Pour sesame seeds onto pan and stir constantly for 3-4 min until browned. They will sizzle and jump during this time.
3. Remove from heat and set aside to cool.
4. Once cooled, grind the sesame seeds in a spice grinder (or coffee grinder) in batches (15 seconds per batch) using short pulses.
5. Combine onion, jalapeño, salt and water in a medium serving bowl.
6. Add 1 cup powdered sesame seeds to the bowl and mix thoroughly.
7. Break up the Injera into bite-sized pieces and mix into the bowl.

The Crown Jewel of African Cuisine

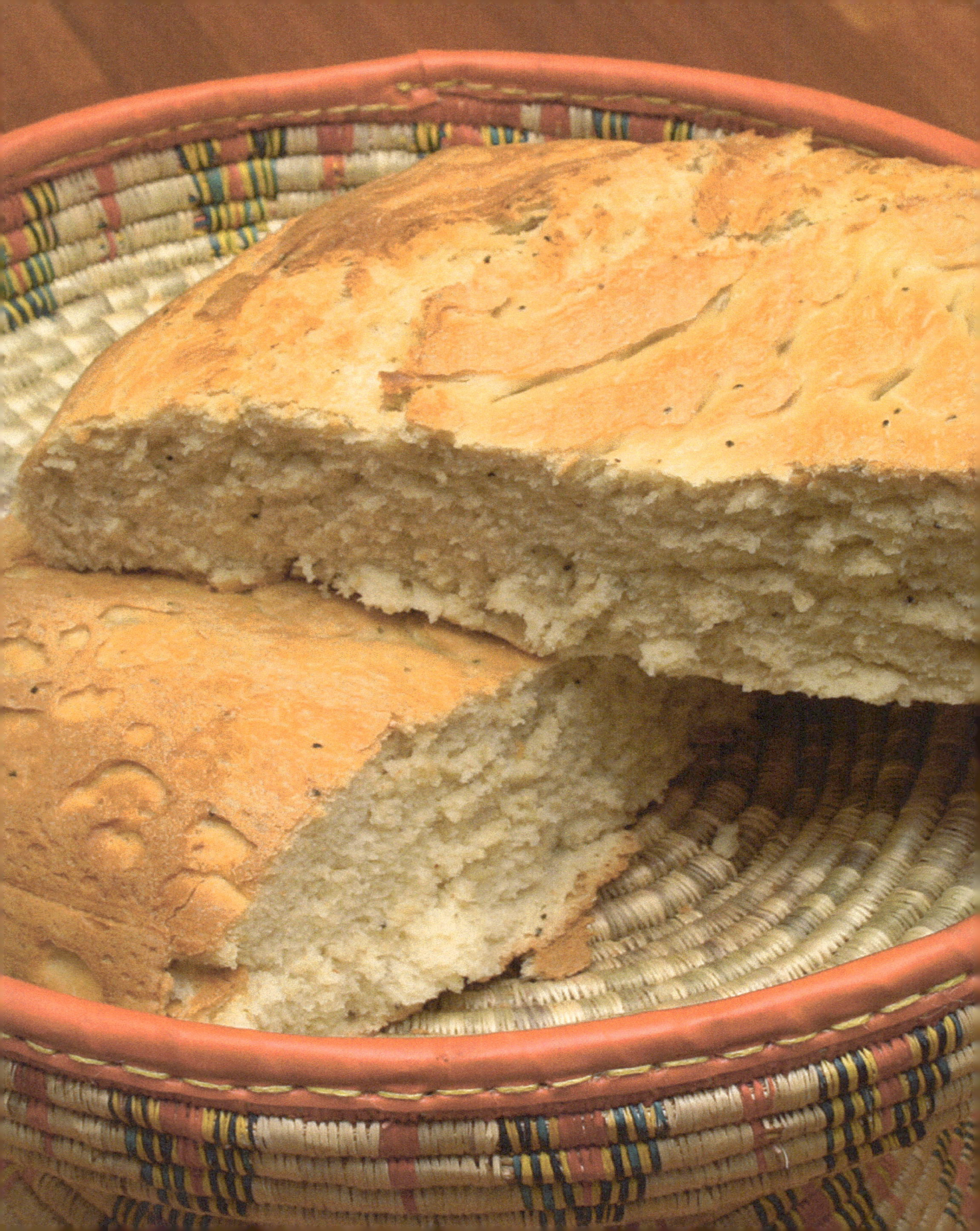

Injera, Breads & Grains

Bread Baked in Banana Leaves
ዳቦ
(Dabbo) Ⓥ ⓋⒼ ⒹⒻ

Time: 4 hr 15 min
Serves: 12–15
Difficulty: ♦♦♦◊◊

This bread is usually eaten either as a snack or with tea in the morning, for breakfast. It can be eaten plain or with spiced clarified butter (Niter Kibe, p. 21). I served it at my restaurant's grand opening!

Ingredients:
Dry activated yeast, 1 Tbsp
Water, 6 cups lukewarm
Sugar, ½ cup
Nigella seeds*, 1½ tsp
Bishop's weed seeds*, 1½ tsp
Vegetable oil, ⅔ cup
Salt, 1 tsp
Unbleached wheat flour, 20 cups (5 lb)

*available at specialty stores and online, see p. 16 and 17

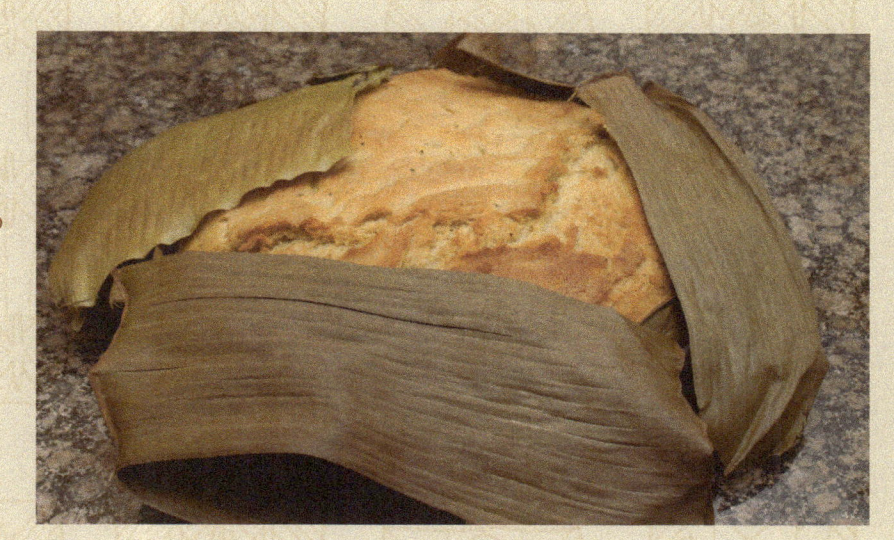

Directions:
1. Combine yeast and water in a bowl and let sit 1 min.
2. Place the other ingredients in a large bowl, add yeast mix, and knead for 3 min.
3. Cover and leave the bowl in a warm place for 1 hour.
4. Punch down the dough with about 10 quick strokes, folding the outer edge over the middle after each stroke. Let it rise again for 1 hour.
5. Punch down the dough once more, again with about 10 quick strokes, folding the outer edge over the middle after each stroke, and let it rise for 1 more hour.
6. Preheat an oven to 400°F.
7. Line a round cake pan (15 inch diameter, with 2 inch flat sides) with banana leaves (allow the leaves to extend far out of the pan, as you will be folding them over the top of the bread).
8. Punch the dough down once more and turn it out into the pan, over the leaves. Spread the dough gently with your fingertips to fill the pan, then fold the leaves over it to completely cover the dough.
9. Place pan in oven and cook 1 hour, or until top leaf is thoroughly browned.
10. Remove from oven, let the bread cool ~10 min, remove the leaves, and cut the bread into serving sizes.

The Crown Jewel of African Cuisine

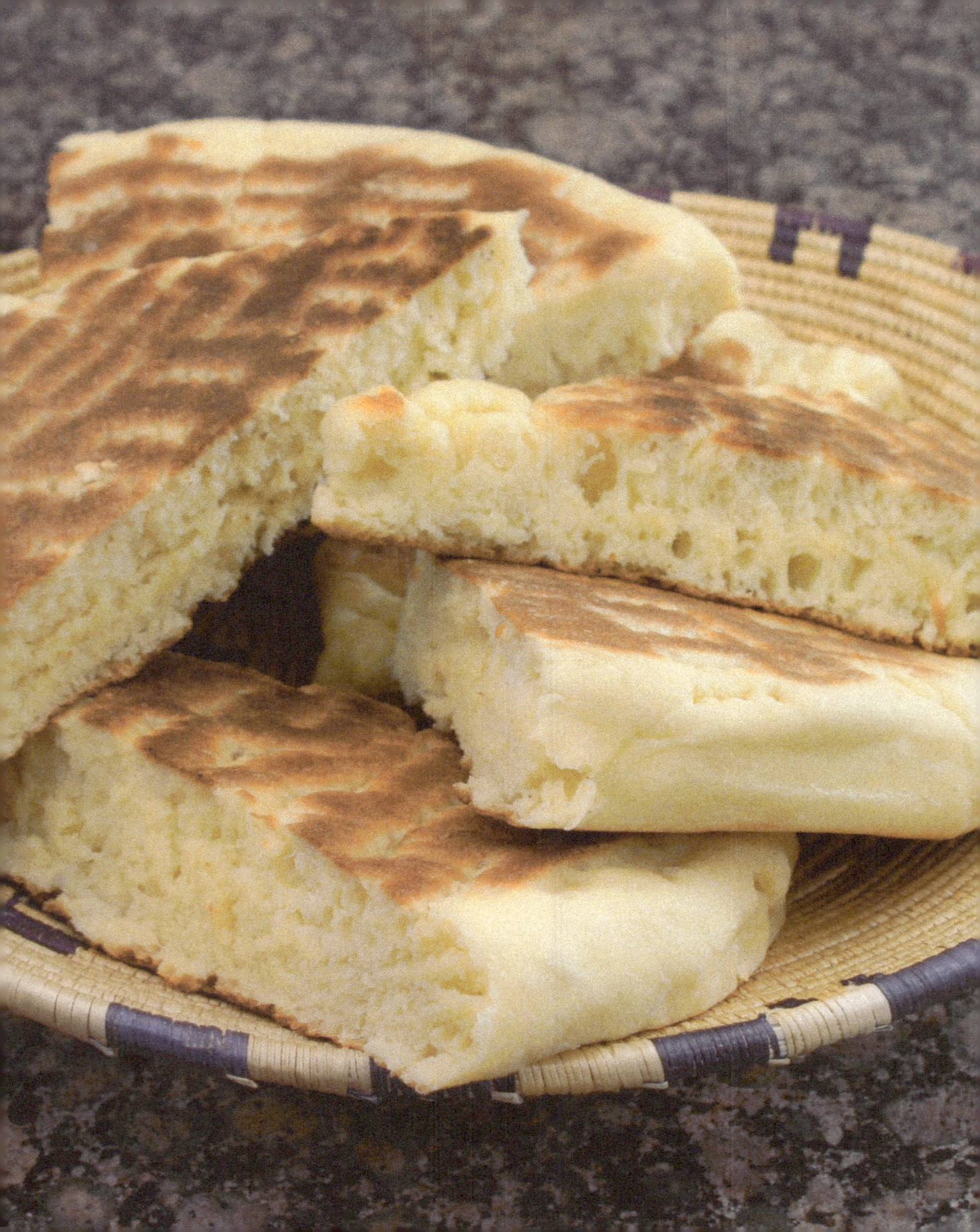

Injera, Breads & Grains

Decorated Bread
አምባሻ
(Ambasha) V VG DF

Time: 3 hr 25 min
Serves: 8
Difficulty: ●●●○○

This Ethiopian version of an Eritrean bread is eaten for many reasons and in many different circumstances. It is a favorite for grandparents to make for their grandchildren. Parents give it to teenagers to keep them full. And men eat it because they think it makes them strong. This bread can be served with tea.

Ingredients:

Dry activated yeast, ½ tsp
Water, 4 cups lukewarm
Unbleached all purpose flour, 8 cups
Salt, ½ tsp
Sugar, ¼ cup
Vegetable oil, ⅓ cup plus 2 tsp

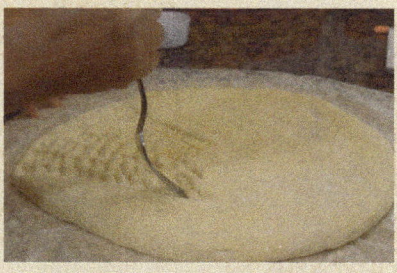

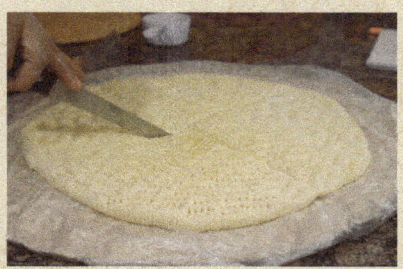

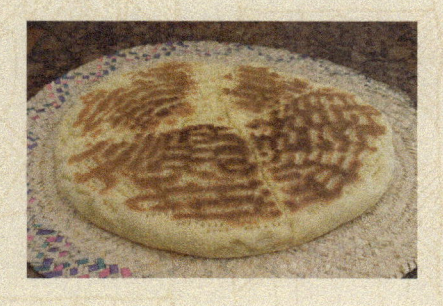

Directions:

1. Combine yeast and water in a bowl and let sit 1 min.
2. Combine remaining ingredients (except 2 tsp oil) in a large mixing bowl. Add water-yeast mixture and mix until ingredients begin to form a ball.
3. Turn dough out onto a floured surface and knead by hand for 7-10 min.
4. Return dough to mixing bowl and leave uncovered in warm place for 3 hours, punching dough down after 1 hour, again after 2 hours, and again after 3 hours.
5. Turn dough out onto a floured surface and spread into a circle about 15 inches in diameter. It should be about ½ inch thick.
6. Moisten your hands with oil and gently rub the top surface and outer edges to coat with oil.
7. Pour 2 tsp oil into a shallow dish.
8. Dip a fork into the oil and use the fork to poke decorative rows of holes on the upper surface of the dough, starting at the middle and radiating outward. Alternatively, you can dip a butter knife into the oil and use the knife to cut decorative lines.
9. Heat an electric Injera pan to 400 degrees (or heat a large flat skillet over medium heat).
10. Place the dough in the pan, cover, and cook 7 min. The bottom should be browned, but not burned.
11. Flip the bread in the pan, cover again, and cook 3 min.
12. Flip the bread again, reduce the heat to low. Cook, uncovered, for 5 min.

The Crown Jewel of African Cuisine

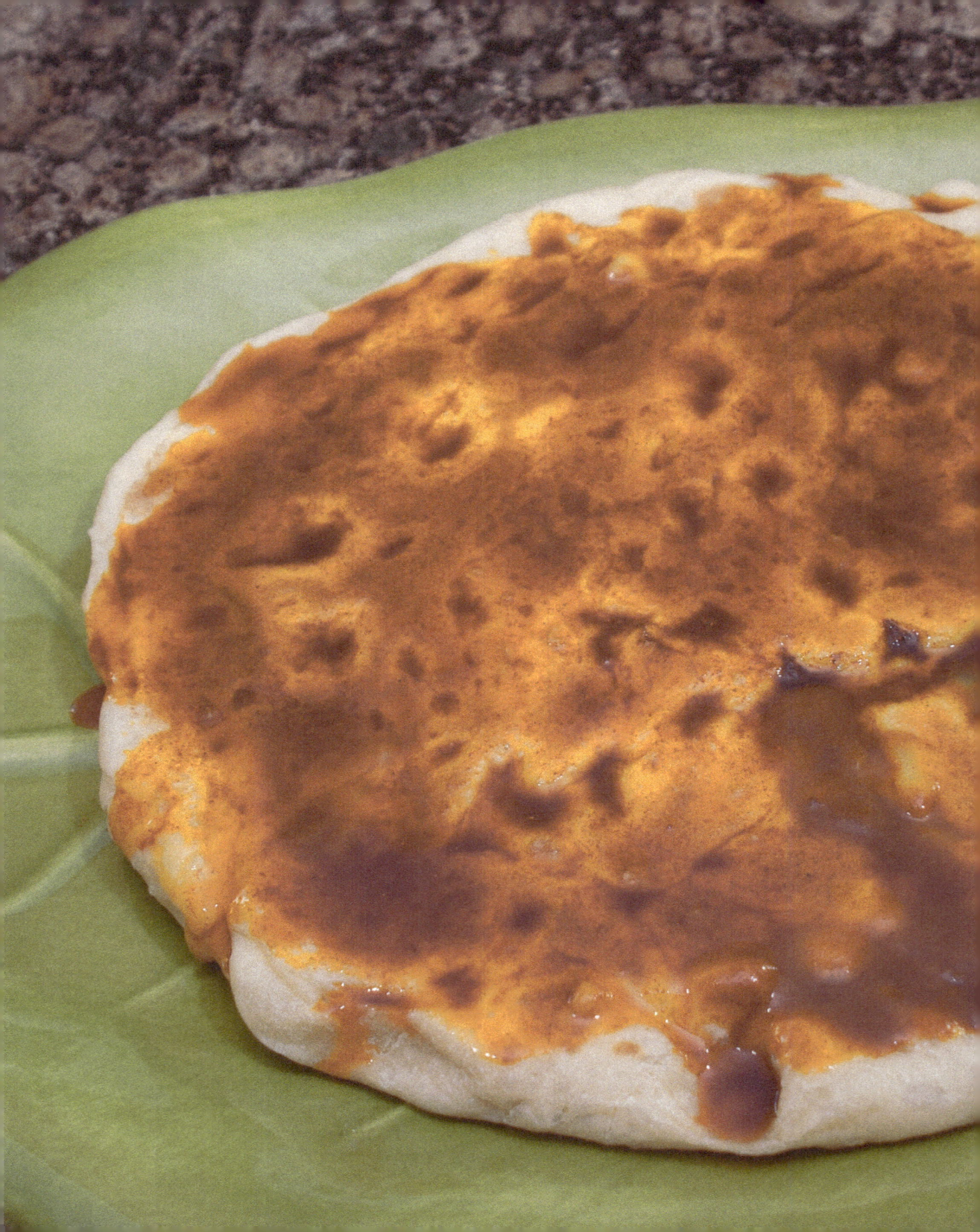

Injera, Breads & Grains

Breakfast Bread
ቂጣ
(Qix'a) Ⓥ ⓋⒼ ⒹⒻ

Time: 2 hr 15 min
Serves: 6–8
Difficulty: ♦♦◊◊◊

This bread is typically eaten in the morning as breakfast.

Ingredients:

Dry activated yeast, 1½ tsp
Water, 1 cup lukewarm
Unbleached all purpose flour, 1½ cups
Vegetable oil, 2 Tbsp plus 1½ tsp
Sugar, 2 Tbsp
Salt, pinch

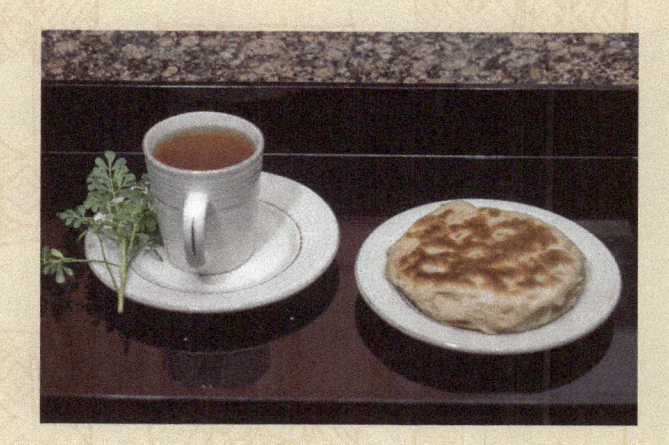

Directions:

1. Combine yeast and water in a bowl and let sit 1 min.
2. Combine remaining ingredients in a large mixing bowl. Add water-yeast mixture and mix to form a thick batter.
3. Cover bowl and set aside at room temperature to rise.
4. Punch down or flip batter after first hour and again after a second hour.
5. Heat an Injera pan to 450 degrees.
6. Pour the batter into the pan, spreading it to ¾ inch thickness.
7. Use your fingers to poke many dimples into the upper surface.
8. Cover and cook 7 min.
9. Flip the bread and cook 7 min, uncovered.

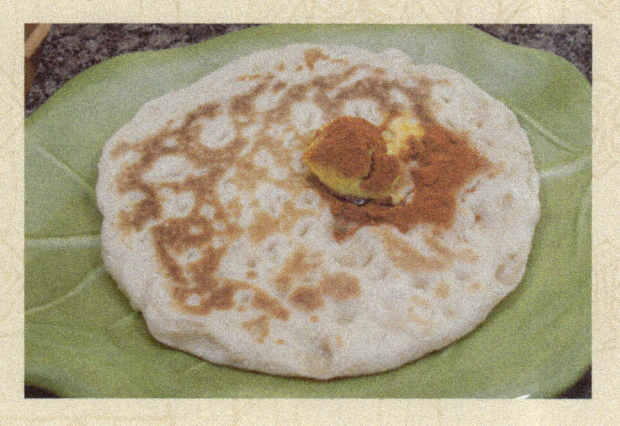

Note: This bread can be served as is. It can also be decorated and seasoned with a combination of ¼ cup melted Niter Kibe (p. 21) and 1-2 Tbsp Berberre powder (p. 16). Alternatively, instead of cooking the dough as one large round, this bread can be made as many smaller rounds by pouring 1½ cups of batter at a time onto the Injera pan and cooking as above. This bread can also be broken into pieces for use in Chachabsa (p. 47).

The Crown Jewel of African Cuisine

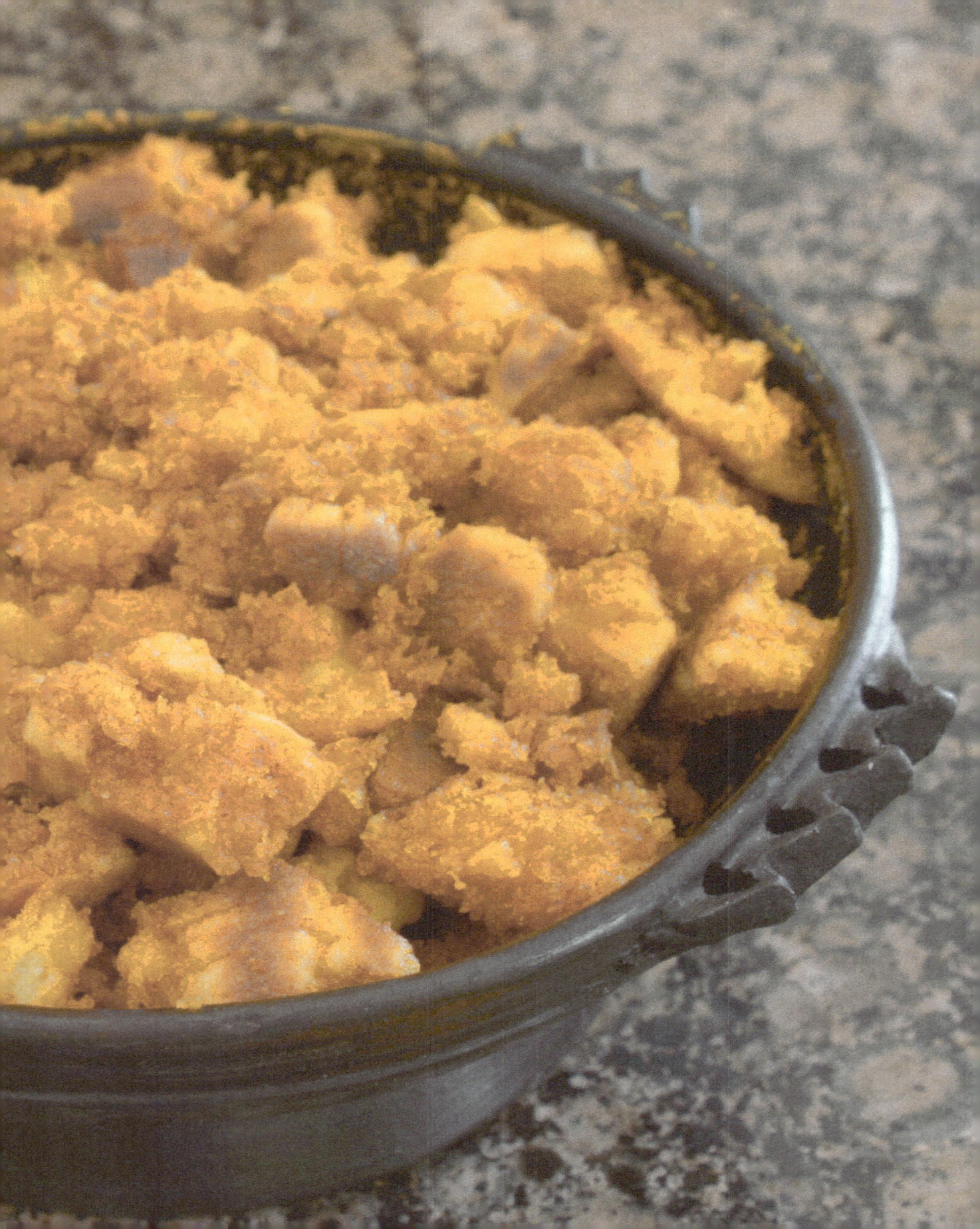

Spicy Torn Bread
ጨጨብሳ
Chachabsa (V) (VG) (DF)

This is a tasty dish to make if you have leftover Breakfast Bread (p. 45) or Decorated Bread (p. 43).

Time: 5 min
Serves: 3–4
Difficulty:

Ingredients:

Breakfast bread (p. 45), ½ loaf or decorated bread (p. 43), ¼ loaf
Berberre powder*, 1 Tbsp
Niter Kibe, ½ cup, melted (p. 21)

*available at specialty stores and online, see p. 16

Directions:

1. Break bread into bite-sized pieces and place into medium sized bowl.
2. Add Niter Kibe and Berberre powder and mix thoroughly with hands to combine.

Injera, Breads & Grains

The Crown Jewel of African Cuisine

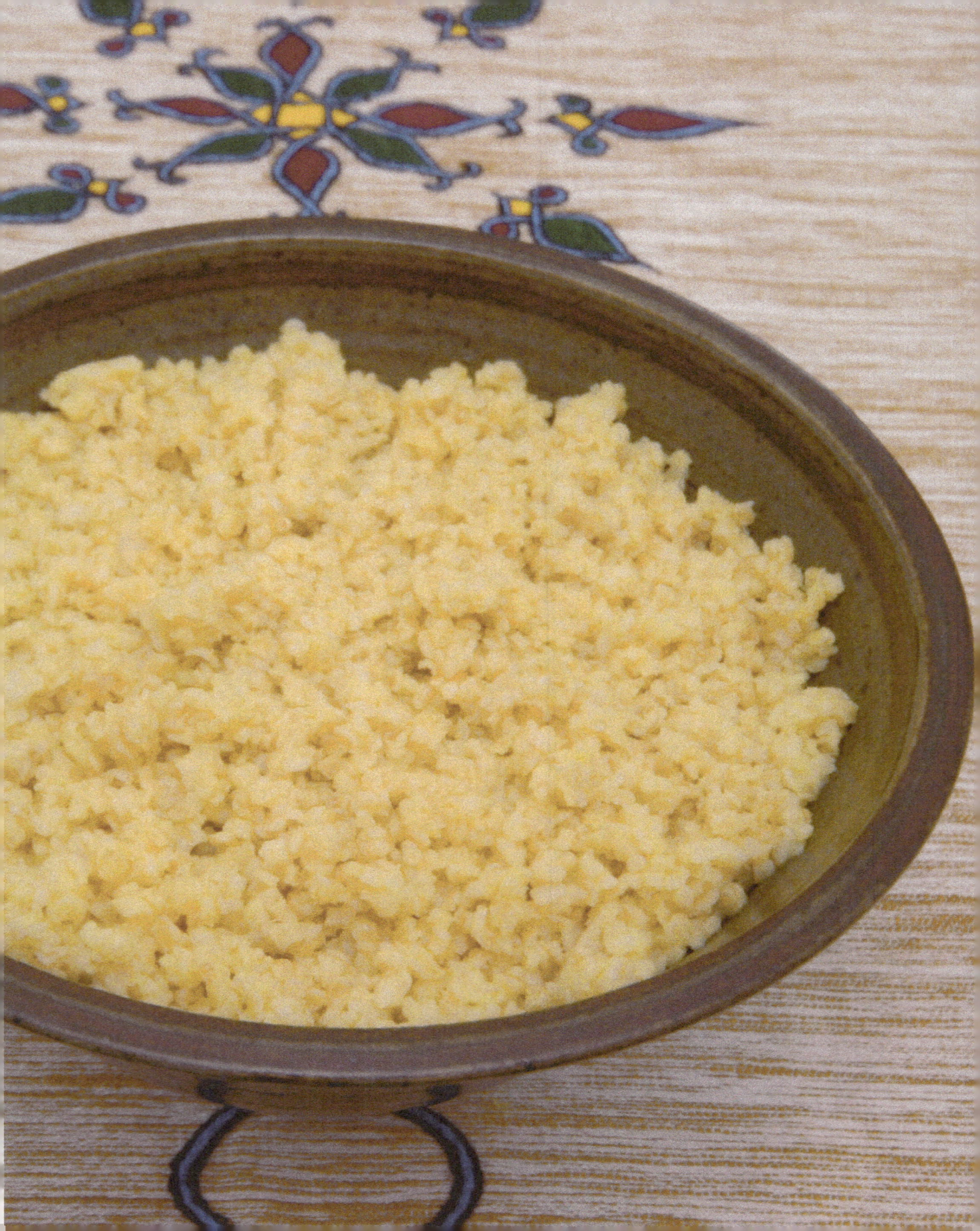

Injera, Breads & Grains

Breakfast Bulgur
ቂንጬ

Q'inche (V) (VG) (DF)

This is such a warm and filling breakfast!

Time: 1 hr
Serves: 5–6
Difficulty: ♦♦♢♢♢

Ingredients:

Water, 8 cups, plus more for rinsing
Salt, 2 tsp
Cracked wheat bulgur, 2 cups
Niter Kibe, 1 cup, plus a small amount to butter the serving bowl (p. 21)

Directions:

1. Bring 8 cups water and the salt to a boil in a medium saucepan.
2. While the salted water is heating, pour bulgur into a bowl, add enough cold water to rinse it, pour off the rinse water, and repeat a few times, until the rinse water runs clear. Pour off the excess water.
3. Add rinsed bulgur to boiling water, reduce heat, and simmer (uncovered) for 30 min, stirring every 10 min or so.
4. Reduce heat to low, cover, cook 5 min, remove from heat, pour bulgur into a bowl, and refrigerate for 20–30 min.
5. Heat a pot over high heat, add Niter Kibe and the cooled bulgur, and cook 5 min, stirring constantly to thoroughly mix, breaking up any clumps that may form.
6. Remove pot from heat.
7. Melt 1–2 tsp Niter Kibe and use it to evenly cover the inside of a serving bowl.
8. Tip the cooked bulgur into the bowl, break up the last clumps, and serve.

The Crown Jewel of African Cuisine

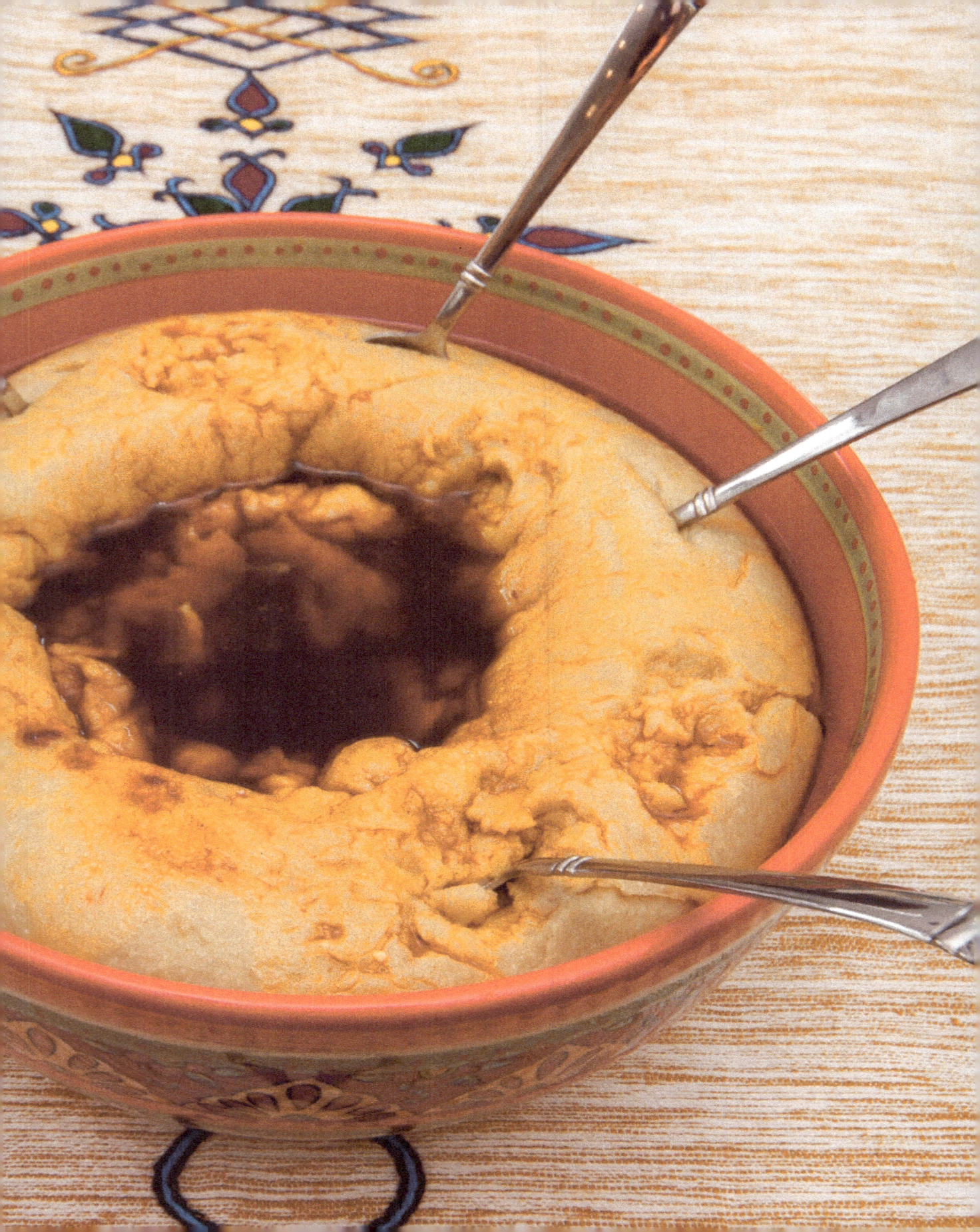

Injera, Breads & Grains

Traditional Spicy Breakfast Cake
ገንፎ / ማርቃ
(Genfo/Marqaa) Ⓥ ⓋⒼ ⒹⒻ

Time: 1 hr
Serves: 8–10
Difficulty: ♨♨♨♨♨

This hearty breakfast cake is a favorite treat. My children love this on a weekend morning. It is so fortifying that it also served as a restorative meal for women who have recently given birth.

Ingredients:
Unbleached all purpose flour, 1 cup
White teff flour, 1 cup
White corn flour, 1 cup
Barley flour*, 1 cup
Water, 14 cups
Salt, 1 teaspoon
Niter Kibe, 1 Tbsp plus enough to coat a large bowl plus 1 cup for serving (p. 21)
Berberre powder* (or if you want it even spicier, use mitmita* instead), 2 Tbsp

*available at specialty stores and online, see p. 16

Directions:

Dry Roasting the Flours

1. Combine the 4 kinds of flour in a large bowl. Mix thoroughly.
2. Heat a nonstick griddle or electric fry pan to 300 degrees.
3. Pour half of the flour mix onto the griddle to dry roast, stirring constantly to prevent burning. After 8 min, the mixture should be fragrant and about the color of white teff flour.
4. Remove mixture from pan. Repeat dry roasting with second half of flour mix.

Preparing the Batter

1. Combine water and salt in a large saucepan. Cover and bring to a boil.

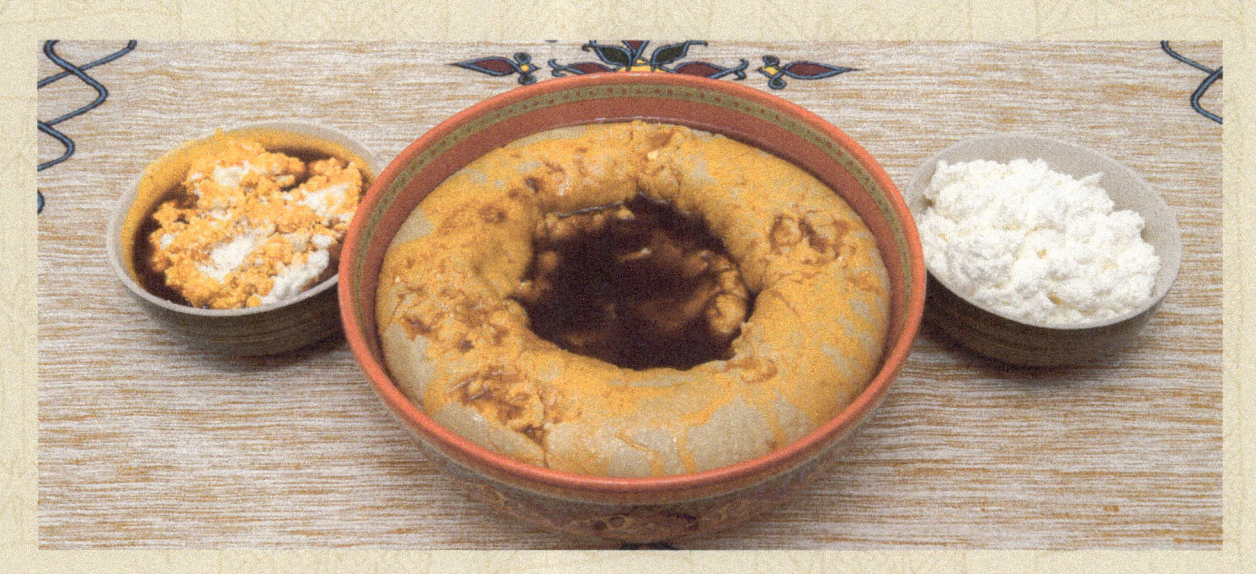

Genfo can be served with Basic or Spicy Cottage Cheese (p. 117).

The Crown Jewel of African Cuisine

Meat & Seafood

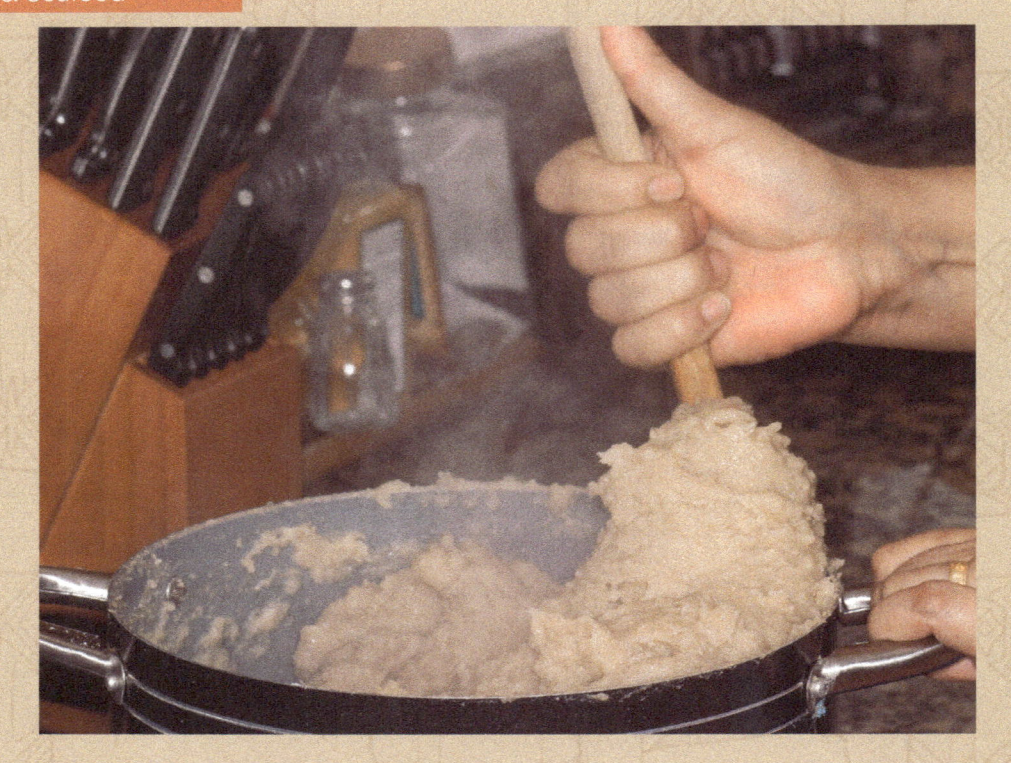

2. While waiting for the water to boil, sift cooled flour to remove clumps. Discard clumps.
3. Reduce to low heat to maintain water at a simmer.
4. Remove approximately half of the water from pot and set aside.
5. Add roasted flour mixture to the pot with remaining water. Stir mixture constantly with a spatula or wooden spoon as it thickens, adding ¼ cup of reserved water every 2 min.
6. After 6 min on low heat (1½ cups of the reserved water will have been added), increase the heat to high, cover, and cook 2 min.
7. Reduce heat to medium, keeping saucepan covered. Stir every 1–2 min and add ¼ cup water every 2–3 min. After around 7 min, the batter should form a thick paste.
8. Stir in 1 Tbsp Niter Kibe and cook 2 min.
9. Turn off heat.
10. Coat a large bowl with Niter Kibe and turn the batter from the saucepan into the bowl.
11. Flip the batter to coat both sides with Niter Kibe.
12. Make a cup-like indentation in the middle of the upper surface. Place 1 cup Niter Kibe into the indentation and sprinkle 2 Tbsp Berberre powder or mitmita onto the Niter Kibe. Once the Niter Kibe has melted, stir the Berberre powder or mitmita into it.

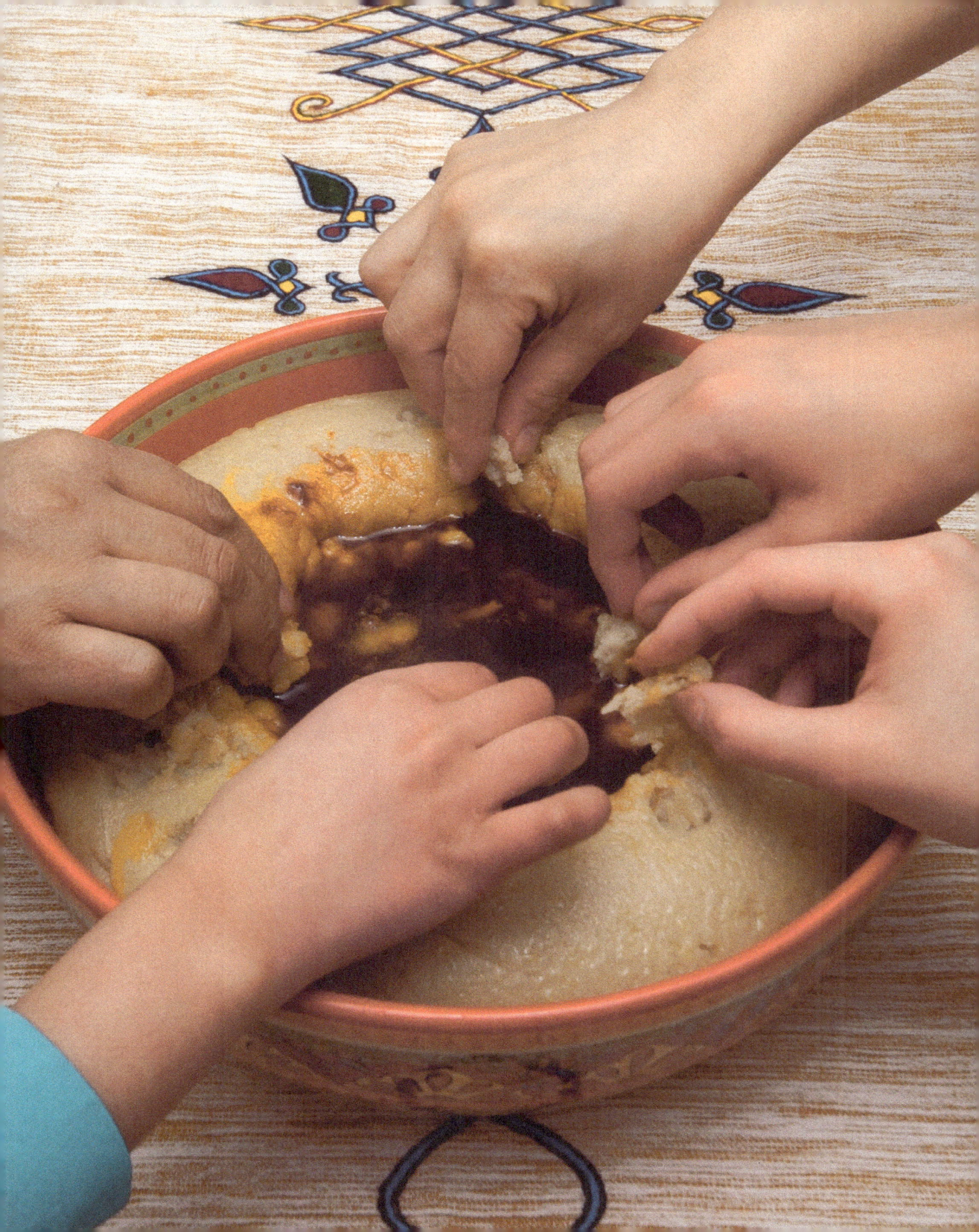

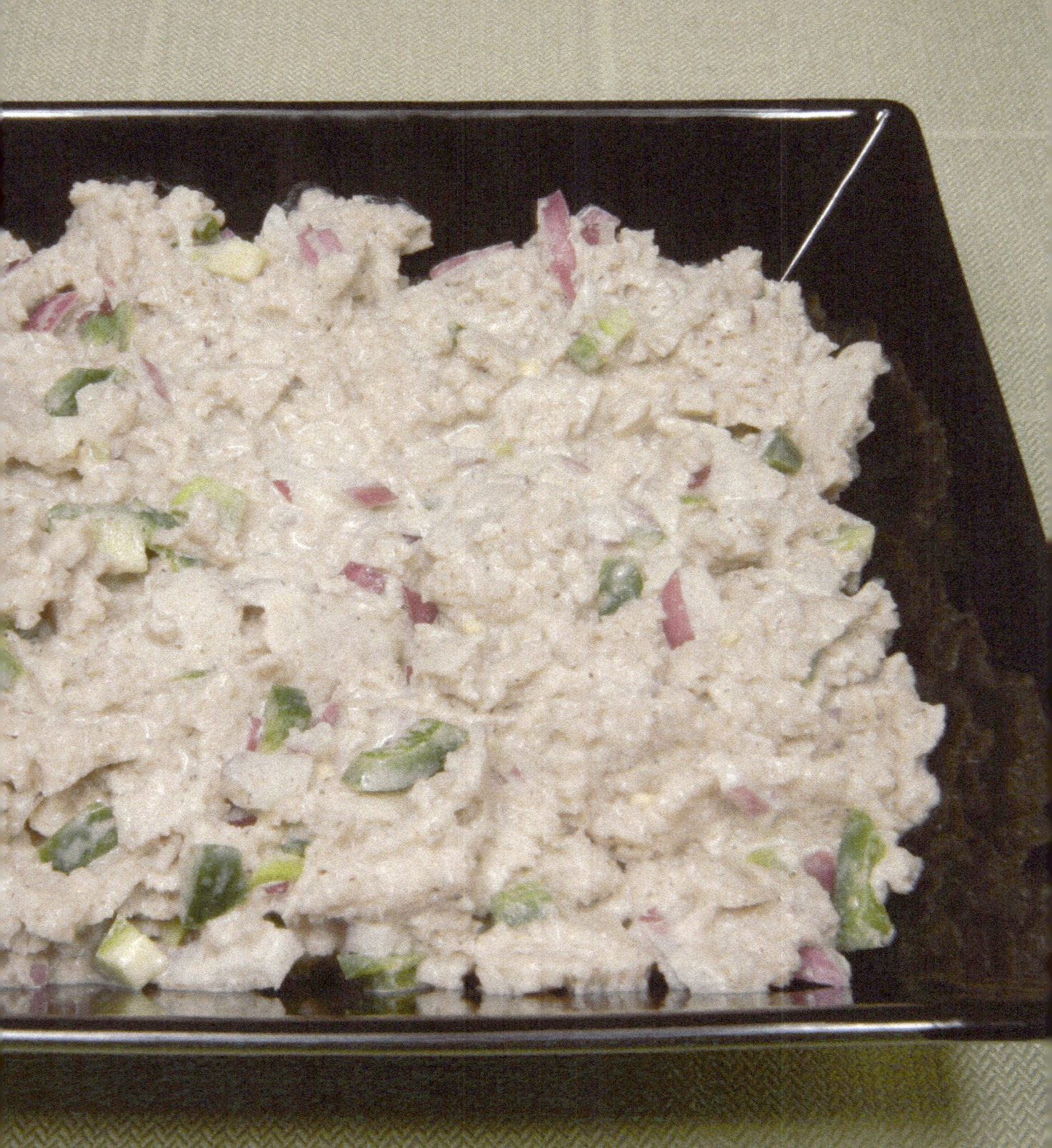

Injera, Breads & Grains

Safflower Fitfit
ሱፍ
(Suf) Ⓥ ⓋⒼ ⒼⒻ ⒹⒻ

Time: 1 hr 30 min
Serves: 6–8
Difficulty: ♦♦♢♢♢

This is another yummy way to eat leftover Injera (p. 33). and make it special with safflower.

Ingredients:

Safflower seeds*, whole, hulled, 1 cup (Caution: do not use safflower seeds that are marketed as bird seeds, as these may not meet safe human consumption standards)

Water, 5½ cups total

Red onion, ½ medium, finely diced

Jalapeño, 1, stemmed and finely diced

Salt, 1 tsp

Injera, 1½ rounds, torn into small pieces

*available at specialty stores and online, see p. 17

Directions:

1. Add safflower seeds and 3 cups water to a medium saucepan, place over high heat (uncovered), bring to a boil.
2. Reduce heat and simmer for 35 min.
3. Strain the safflower seeds in a colander and rinse with cold water until cool.
4. Combine the drained seeds with ½ cup water in the bowl of a food processor fitted with a blade, and process 3-4 min until it forms a smooth paste.
5. Remove paste to a small bowl, add 2 cups water, and work the paste with your hands until it is evenly mixed with the water, forming a milky mixture.
6. Strain the mixture over a bowl to remove and discard any small bits of safflower seed that did not get adequately processed, then cover the bowl and refrigerate at least 30 min to cool.
7. Add onion, jalapeño, salt, and Injera pieces to the milky safflower mixture, stir to combine, and serve.

The Crown Jewel of African Cuisine

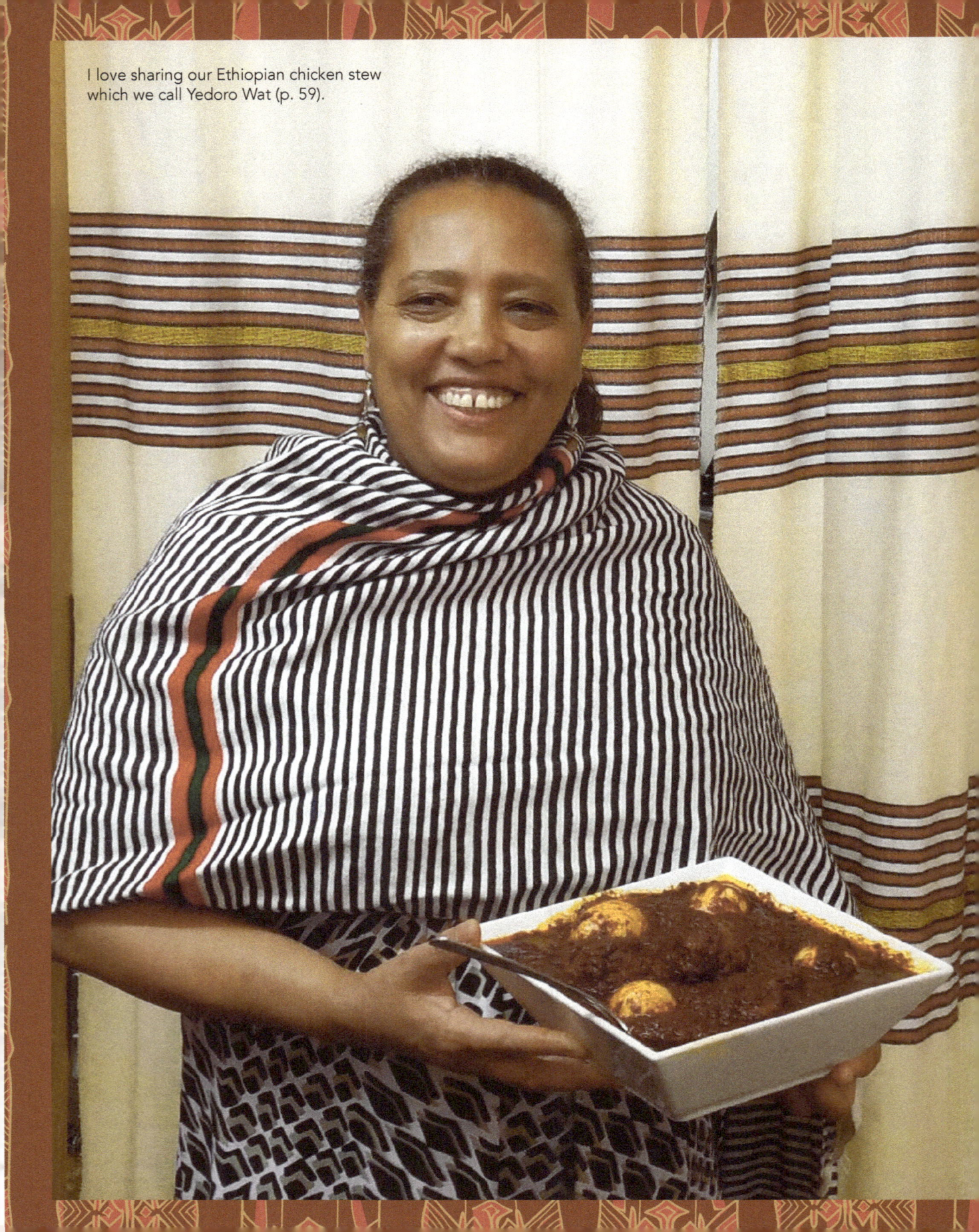

I love sharing our Ethiopian chicken stew which we call Yedoro Wat (p. 59).

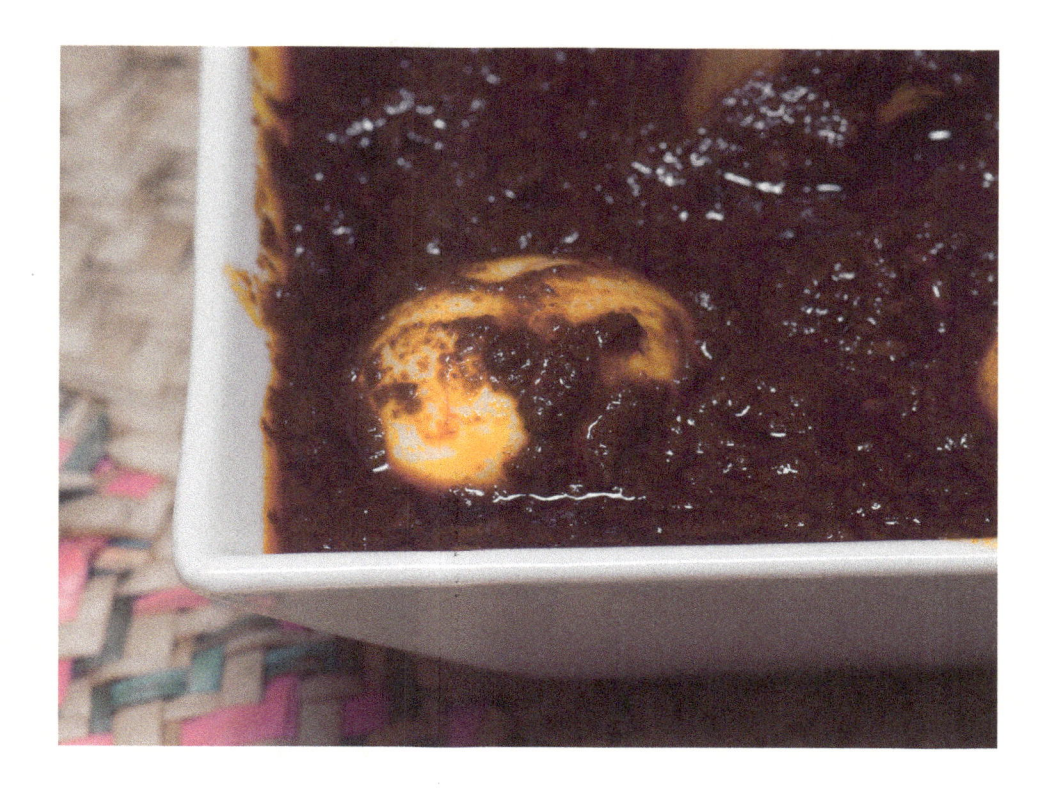

The Most Admired of Foods: Meat and Seafood Main Dishes

In Ethiopia, meat dishes have a very high status. They are served on the most important and special occasions; a wedding isn't a wedding without Yedoro Wat, our famous Ethiopian chicken stew. Growing up in a village, we didn't buy meat as we do here at the grocery store. We had our own animals that lived on our property. So unlike most other American chefs, but like most Ethiopians, I have long known how to slaughter and prepare all the different parts of an animal for a delicious dinner. At my restaurant, it is the meat dishes that are the most popular. Everyone always wants to eat my Yedoro Wat. My lamb dishes are also very popular and often sell out. So you can come to my restaurant early or you can use this book to learn how to make everything you want anytime for yourself!

Above: Close-up of one of the hard boiled eggs in the rich Yedoro Wat stew.

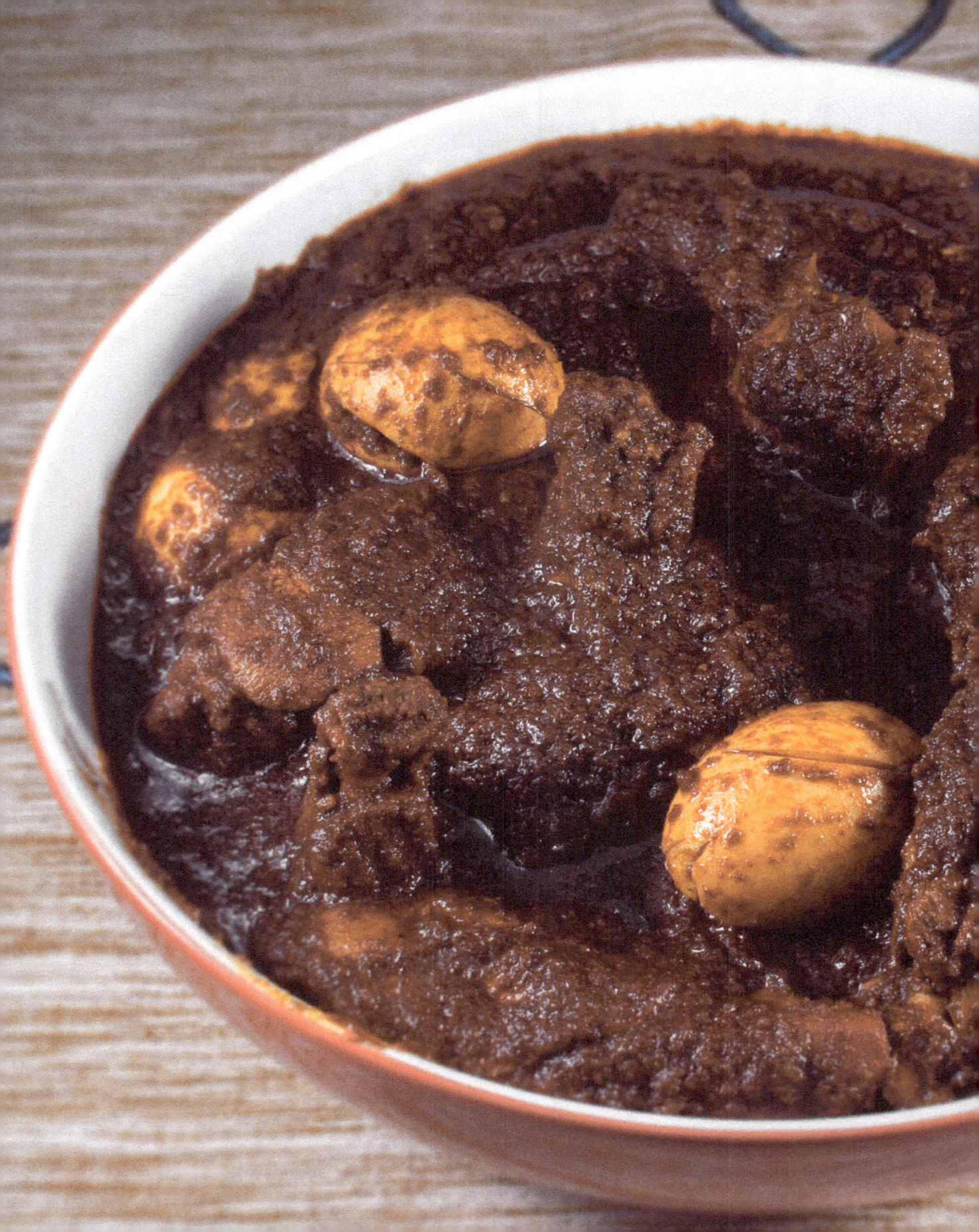

Meat & Seafood

Chicken Stew
የዶሮ ወጥ
(Yedoro Wat) GF DF

Time: 3 hr
Serves: 6–8
Difficulty: 4/5

Any Ethiopian person will be flattered and impressed if you serve them this delicacy, also called *Doro Wat*. It marks a meal as a special occasion. This is the most beloved dish in Ethiopia, and is served in most restaurants there, despite the fact that it takes a long time to prepare.

Ingredients:

Whole chicken (~2 lb), separated into pieces (see p. 60), or 8–10 drumsticks
Yellow onions, 6 large (~4½ lb)
Vegetable oil, 1 cup
Berberre paste, 2 cups (p. 29)
Ginger-Garlic Paste, 2 Tbsp (p. 23)
Salt, 3 tsp plus 4–5 Tbsp for brining the chicken
Water, 1½ cups
Lime, 1
Q'imam, 2 tsp, (p. 25)
Niter Kibe, 1 cup (p. 21)
Eggs, 10

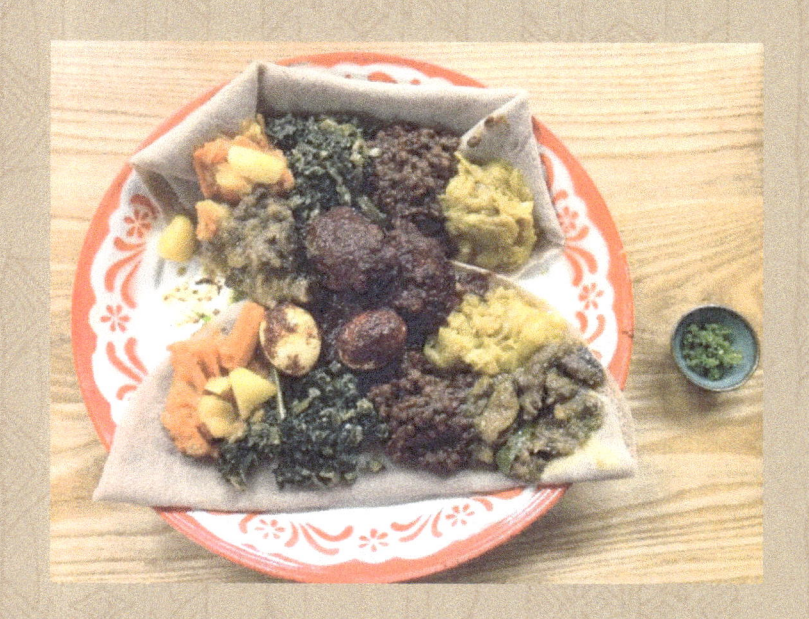

Directions:

1. Coarsely chop onions, put in food processor, and purée to a smooth paste.
2. Pour onion purée into large (~12 qt) pot and cook partly covered for 25 min on medium-high heat, stirring every 2–3 min to prevent sticking.
3. Add vegetable oil, stir, reduce heat to medium, and cook 20 min more, or until onion purée has turned yellow, stirring every 2–3 min. During this time, begin separating and brining the chicken (see p. 60).
4. Add beribere and Ginger-Garlic Paste and stir to mix. Cook 25 min, stirring every 2–3 min. Reduce heat to low and cook 25 min, stirring every 5 min. During this time, finish separating and brining the chicken.
5. Add salt and chicken pieces to the pot, stir, and increase heat to medium, stirring occasionally. After 10 min, add 1 cup water and cover. Cook 5 min, stirring twice.
6. Add ½ cup water and the Q'imam, increase heat to high, bring to a boil, reduce heat to

The Crown Jewel of African Cuisine

Meat & Seafood

simmer, and then add Niter Kibe.

7. Gently simmer for 45 min, stirring every few min to prevent sticking.
8. While the rest is simmering, place eggs in a small saucepan and cover with cold water. Place on high heat, cook 15–20 min, then rinse in cold water and let stand in cold water until cool enough to peel. Peel the eggs, score each with 3–4 parallel slices (¼ inch deep) on each side, add to the chicken, stir gently to mix, and turn off heat. Serve on Injera.

To separate and brine a whole chicken:

1. Reserve the neck and liver.
2. With kitchen shears, remove and discard wing portion beyond the drumette.
3. Remove skin from chicken (except the drumettes), starting at the head end. It may help to use a paring knife to separate the skin from the meat. Discard skin.
4. Trim fat from chicken.
5. Remove legs and separate the thighs and drumsticks.
6. With chicken breast side up, remove the drumettes. Then, cutting diagonally, remove the breast meat from the sides of the breast on each side, leaving some meat attached to the breastbone.
7. Remove the central portion of the breast (traditionally in Ethiopia, this portion is reserved for the male head of the household).
8. Cut the back into quarters.
9. Trim any remaining fat from the pieces.
10. Place neck, drumettes, leg pieces, breast pieces, and back pieces in a large bowl, cover with warm water, add 2–3 Tbsp salt, and stir thoroughly. Pour off water.
11. Squeeze the juice of 1 lime over the chicken pieces, add the squeezed lime halves, mix thoroughly, and soak 8–10 min. After this time, you may find that additional fat becomes apparent. Remove this fat.
12. Add 2 Tbsp salt and enough warm water to just cover the chicken, mix thoroughly, and let soak 8–10 more min.
13. Remove lime halves, pour off liquid, and rinse pieces several times with warm water until water runs clear.
14. Place pieces on clean cutting board and cut off the ends of the bones of the large pieces to expose the marrow. Remove wishbone from central breast piece.
15. Cut breast pieces in half lengthwise, and make a few slices (½ inch deep) across the grain on these pieces and the other large pieces. The chicken is now ready to cook.

Meat & Seafood

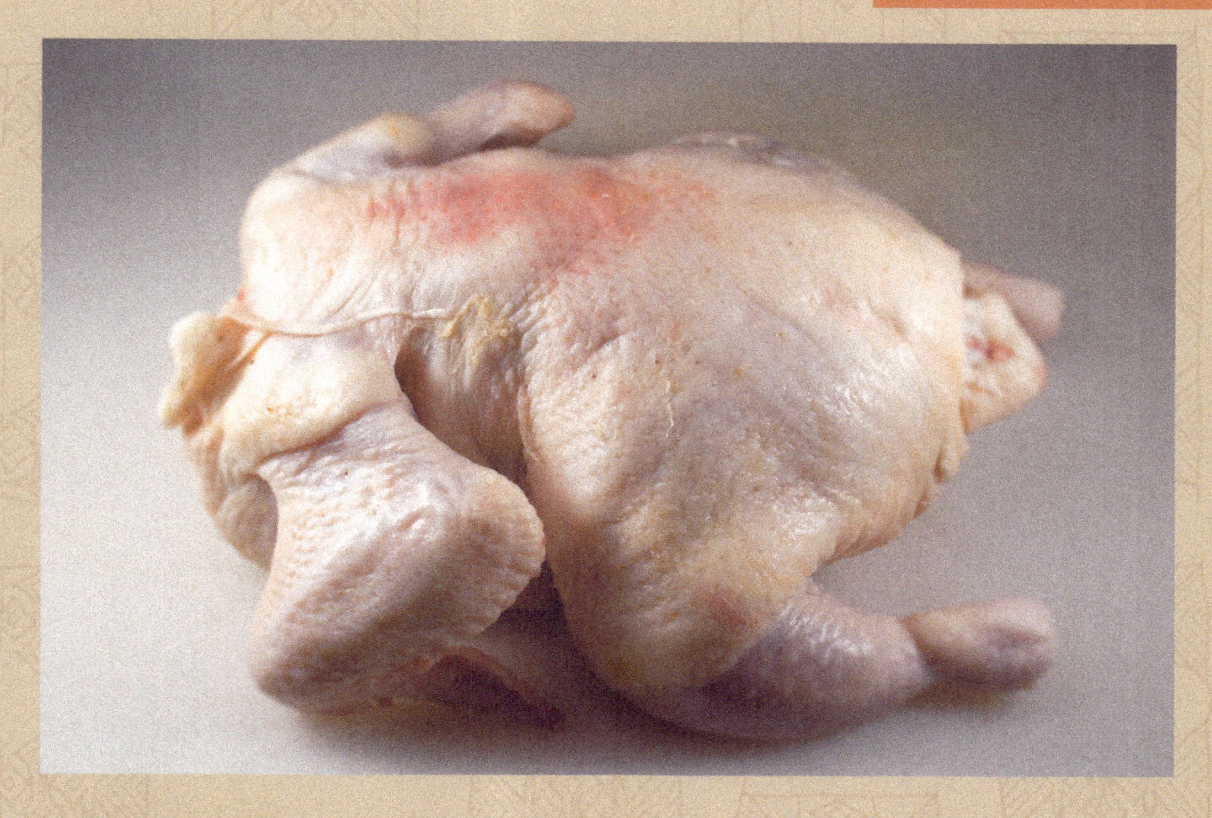

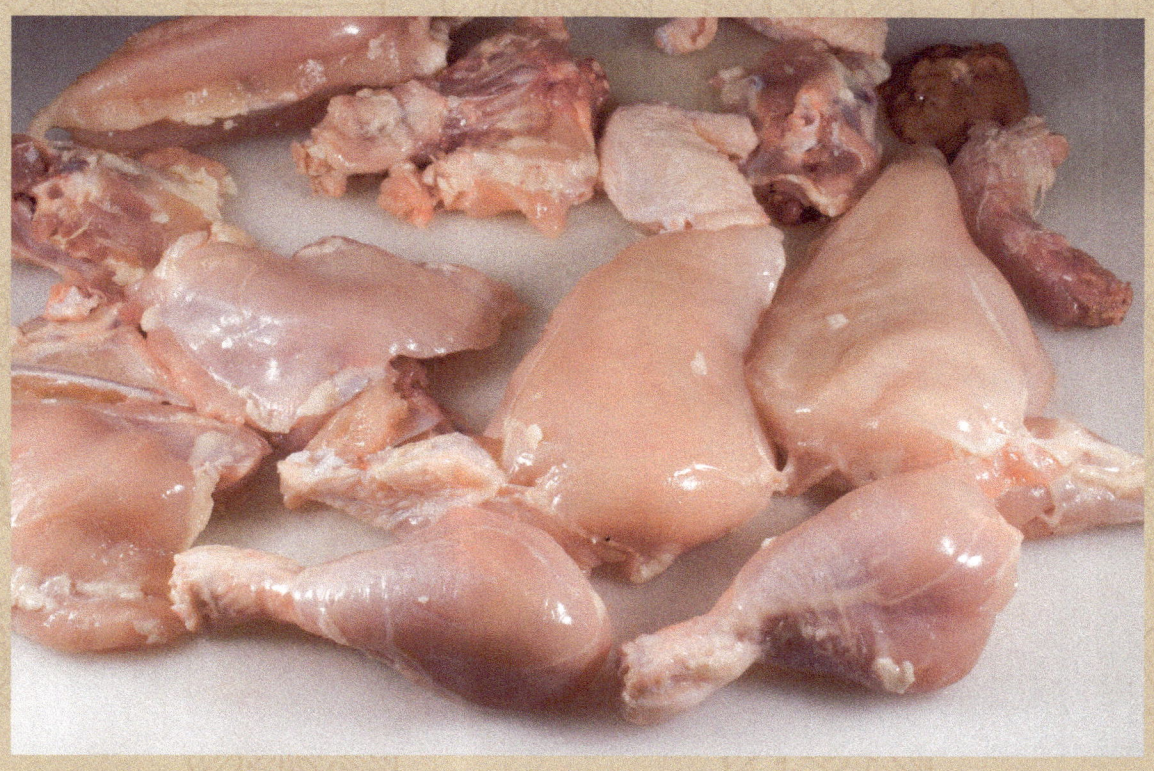

The Crown Jewel of African Cuisine

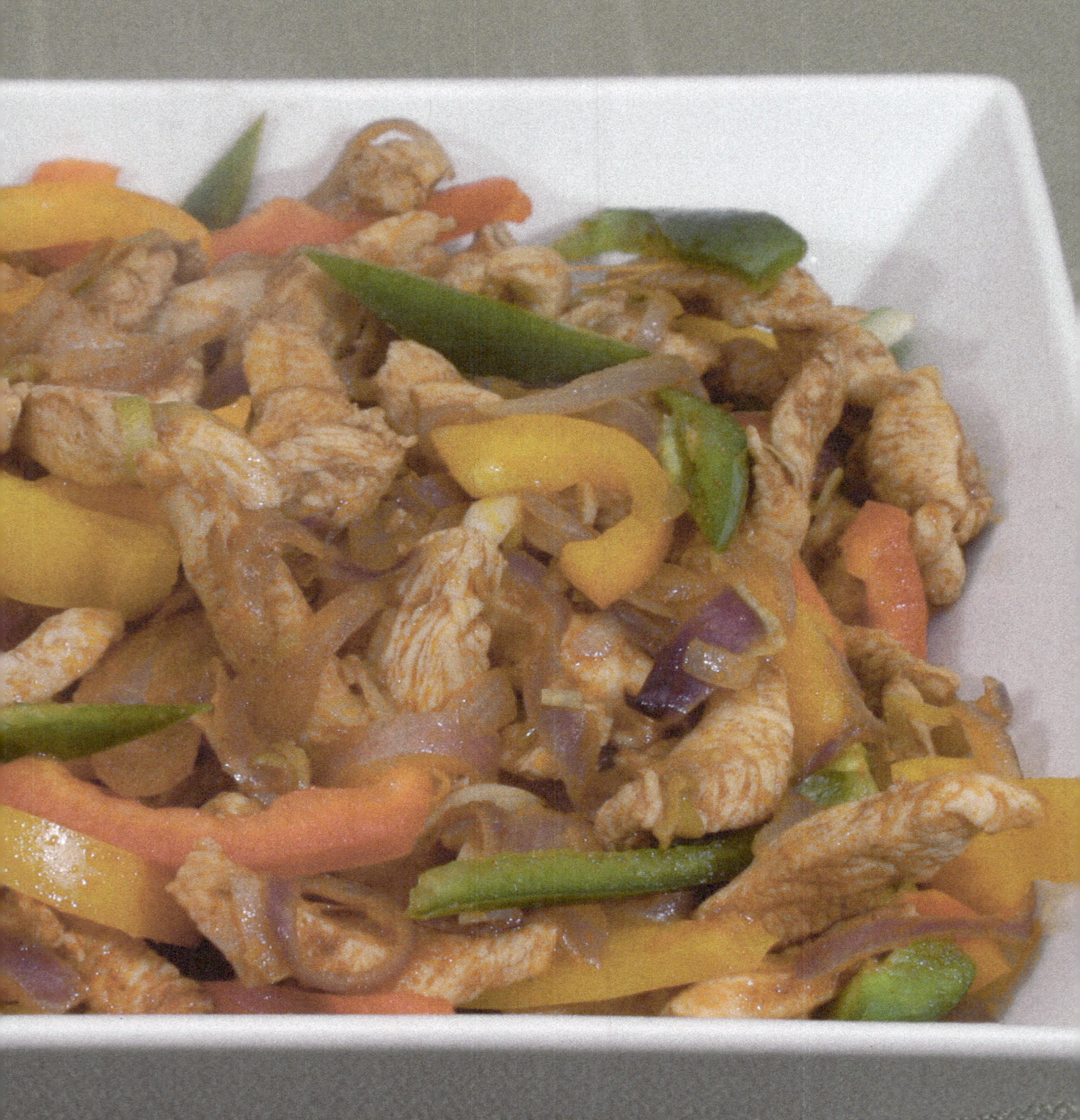

Meat & Seafood

Sautéed Chicken
የዶሮ ጥብስ
(Yedoro Tibbs) GF DF

Time: 20 min
Serves: 5
Difficulty: ●●○○○

A delicious chicken alternative to other Tibbs dishes.

Ingredients:

Leek, 1, removing all but bottom 4 inches
Chicken breast fillets, 2 lb
Vegetable oil, ⅓ cup
Red onion, 1 medium, cut in half, then into ¼ inch thick wedges
Garlic cloves, 5, coarsely chopped
Niter Kibe, 1 tsp (p. 21)
Salt, 1 tsp
Berberre paste, 1 Tbsp (p. 29)
Jalapeño, 1, stemmed, seeded, julienned into ¼ inch by 3 inch pieces
Red, yellow and orange bell pepper, ⅓ of each, cut into ¼ inch wide strips

Directions:

1. Cut leek in half lengthwise, then slice crosswise into ⅛ inch wide slices.
2. Rinse chicken fillets in cold water and pat dry.
3. Cut fillets crosswise into ¼ inch wide strips.
4. Heat oil in a large frypan on high.
5. Add leek, onion, garlic, Niter Kibe, salt, Berberre paste and chicken to pan then stir to mix.
6. Cook 10 min, stirring constantly.
7. Remove to serving dish and garnish with raw jalapeño and bell peppers.

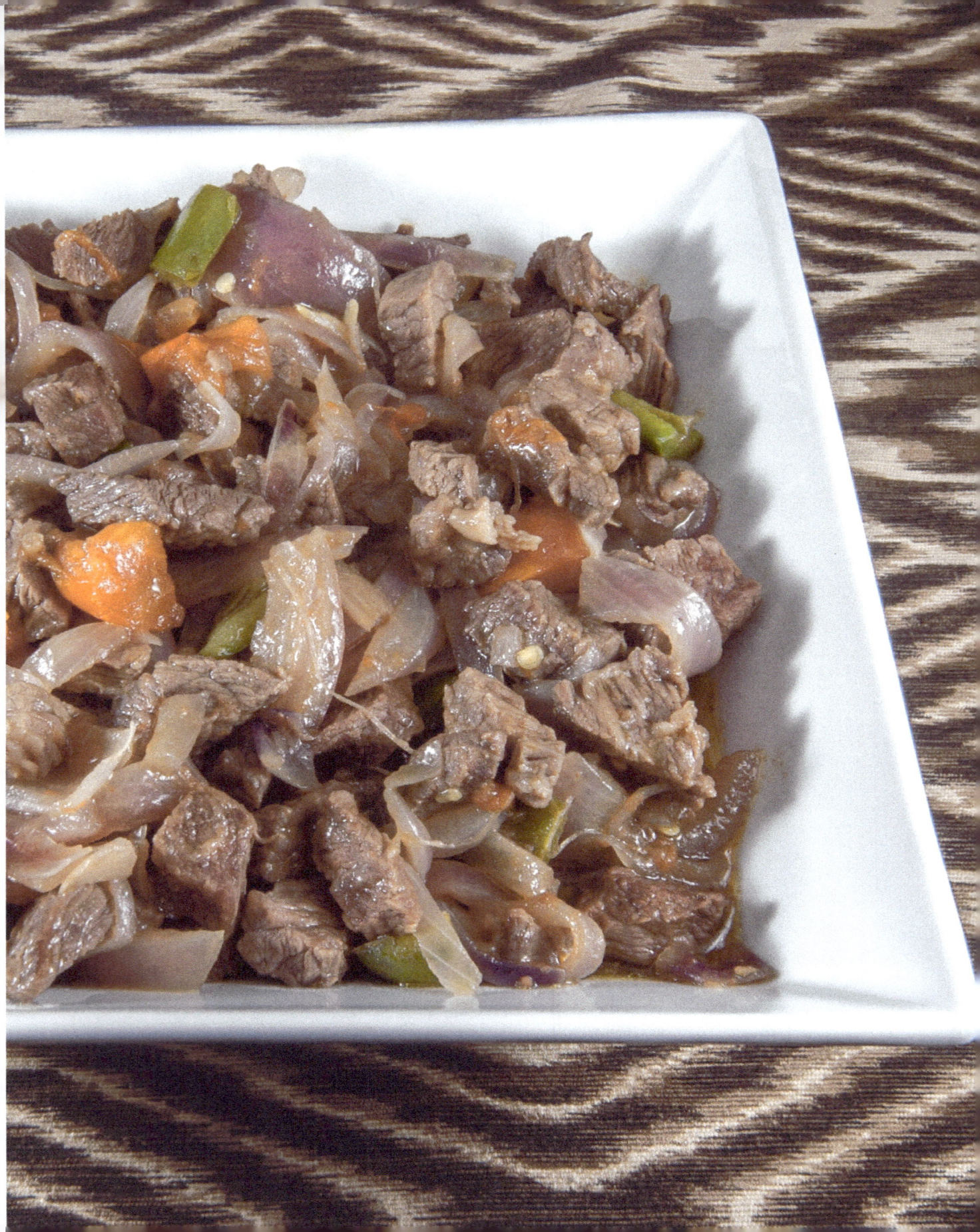

Sautéed Beef
የሥጋ ጥብስ
(Yesiga Tibbs) GF DF

Time: 25 min
Serves: 6–8
Difficulty: ♨♨

Tibbs is our version of stir-fry. It is quick to prepare and can be so colorful. In this recipe I use beef, but other Tibbs recipes in this cookbook feature different meats. Tibbs can be served for any occasion and is found on menus of most Ethiopian restaurants.

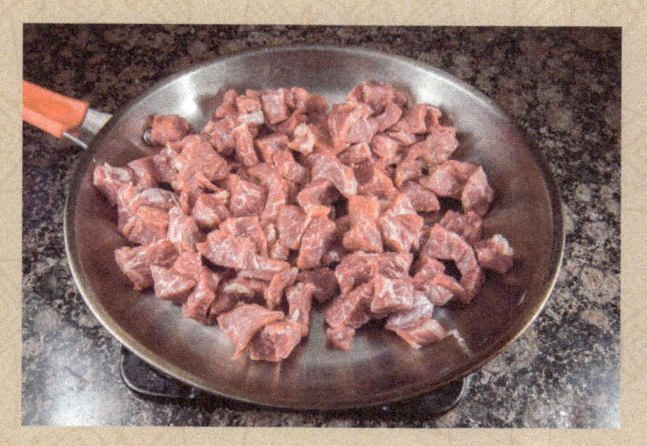

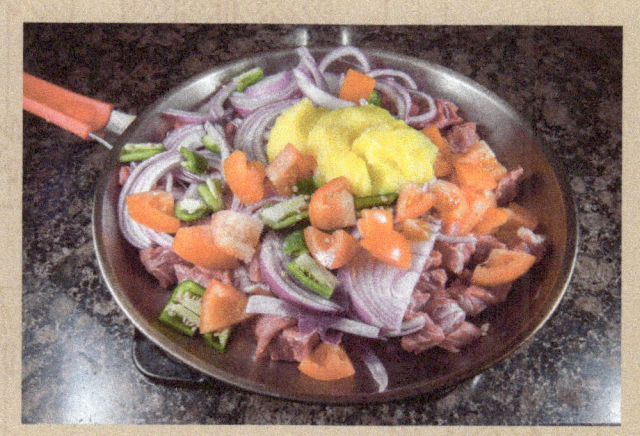

Meat & Seafood

Ingredients:

Beef cross-rib or other boneless roast, 2 lb

Red onion, 1 medium, cut lengthwise in half, and then sliced ¼ inch thick.

Plum tomatoes (optional), 2, cut into ½ inch dice

Jalapeños, 2, coarsely chopped, stemmed but not seeded

Niter Kibe, 1 cup (p. 21)

Salt, 1 ½ tsp

Directions:

1. Trim excess fat from roast, including ribbons that run through it. Cut meat into ¾ inch dice.

2. Place meat and all other ingredients in a large frying pan, and stir to combine. Cook 3 min over high heat, uncovered, stirring frequently to prevent sticking.

3. Reduce heat to medium-high, and cook approximately 10 min, stirring occasionally until the juices are reduced to a thick sauce. Serve.

The Crown Jewel of African Cuisine

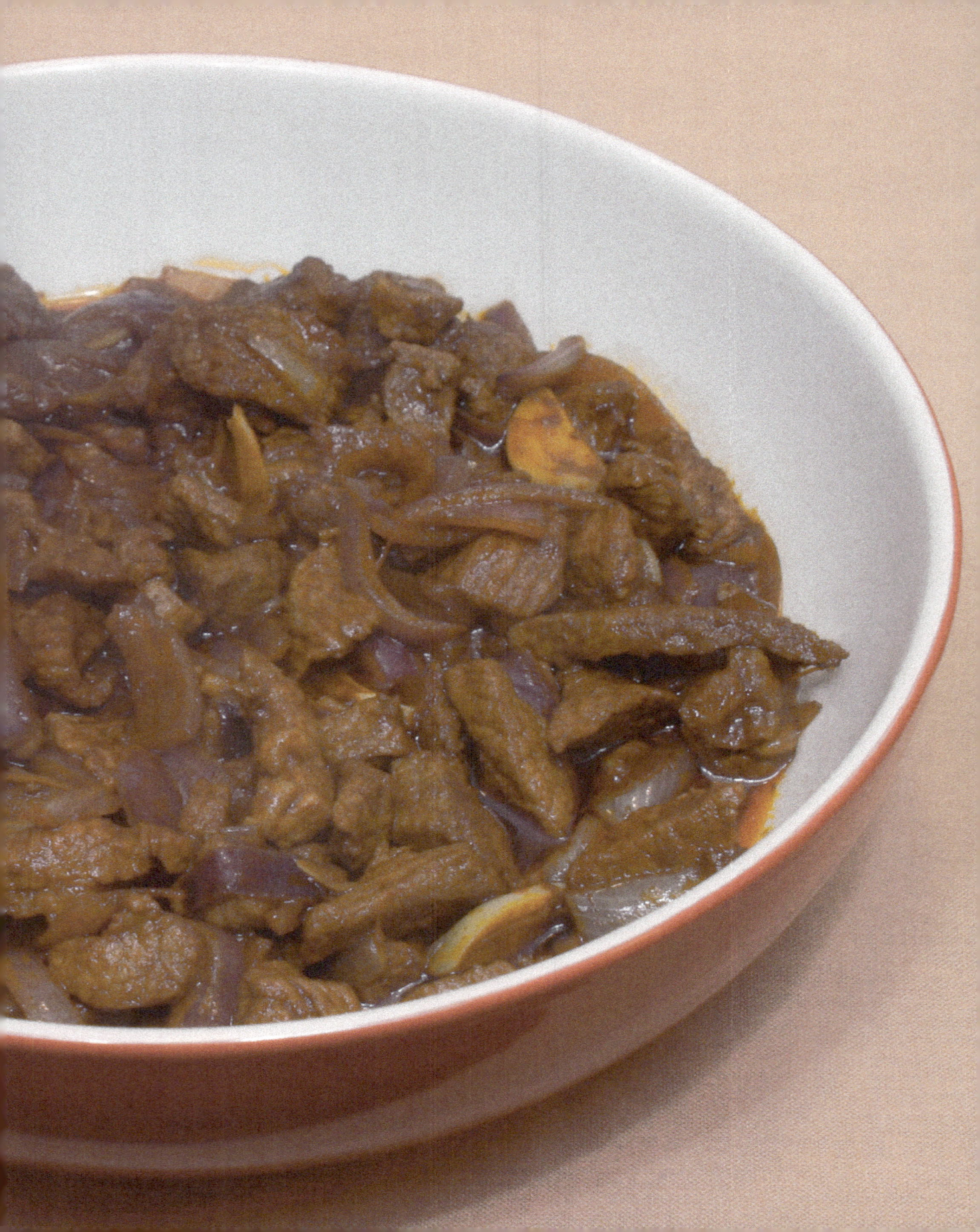

Meat & Seafood

Spicy Sautéed Beef
ዝልዝል ጥብስ
(Zilzil Tibbs) GF DF

A spicy version of Yesiga Tibbs (p. 65).

Time: 25 min
Serves: 5
Difficulty:

Ingredients:

Eye of round roast, 1 lb
Vegetable oil, ⅓ cup
Red onion, 1 large, cut in half lengthwise and sliced into ¼ inch wedges
Garlic, 3 cloves, finely sliced
Salt, 1 tsp
Niter Kibe, ⅓ cup (p. 21)
Berberre paste, ¼ cup (p. 29)

Directions:

1. Slice beef into bite sized pieces (~1½ inches by ½ inch by ¼ inch).
2. Heat oil in frying pan over medium-high heat.
3. Once pan is hot, combine all ingredients in pan and stir thoroughly to mix.
4. Cook, uncovered, for 15 min, stirring every few min so that it cooks evenly.

The Crown Jewel of African Cuisine

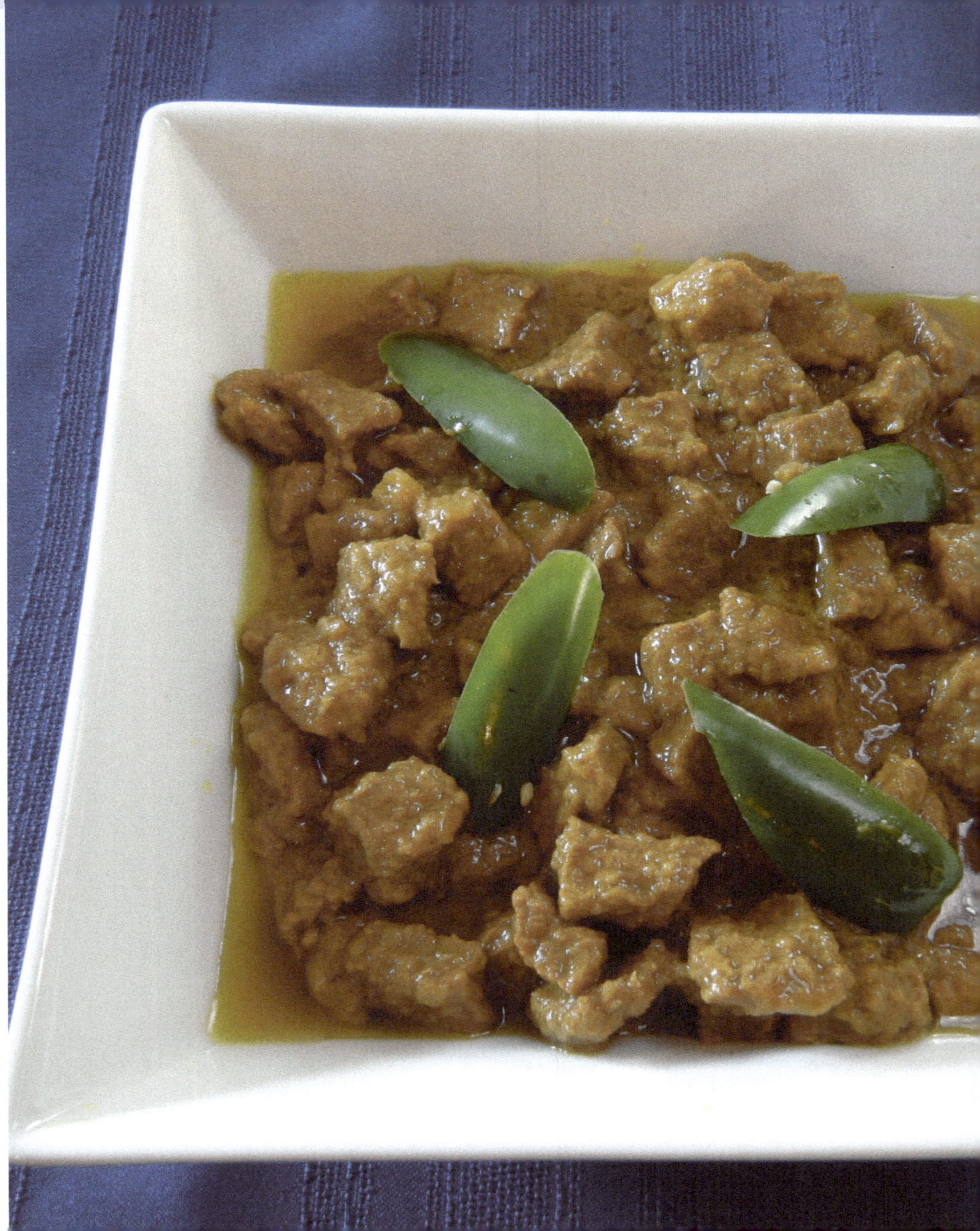

Meat & Seafood

Beef Stew
የስጋ አልጫ
(Yesiga Alicha) GF DF

Hearty and delicious. The sauce is so good on Injera (p. 33)..

Time: 1 hr 15 min
Serves: 5
Difficulty:

Ingredients:

Beef stew meat, 2½ lb
Yellow onion, 1 large, finely chopped
Vegetable oil, ½ cup
Turmeric, 1 tsp
Ginger-Garlic Paste, 2 Tbsp (p. 23)
Water, 2 cups
Salt, 1 tsp
Niter Kibe, 1 Tbsp (p. 21)
Besobela*, several flowerheads
Jalapeño, 1, stemmed, seeded, and quartered lengthwise

*available at specialty stores and online, see p. 16

Directions:

1. Dice beef into ½ inch square pieces.
2. Place onions in small nonstick pot over high heat. Cook 7 min, covered, stirring occasionally.
3. Add oil. Cook 6 min, stirring occasionally, then reduce heat to medium.
4. Add turmeric, Ginger-Garlic Paste, diced beef and a few Tbsp water. Cover, bring to a simmer over medium-high heat, and cook 25 min.
5. Add remainder of the water and salt and continue to simmer for another 25 min.
6. Add Niter Kibe and besobela. Cook 2 min.
7. Remove to a serving dish and garnish with jalapeños.

The Crown Jewel of African Cuisine

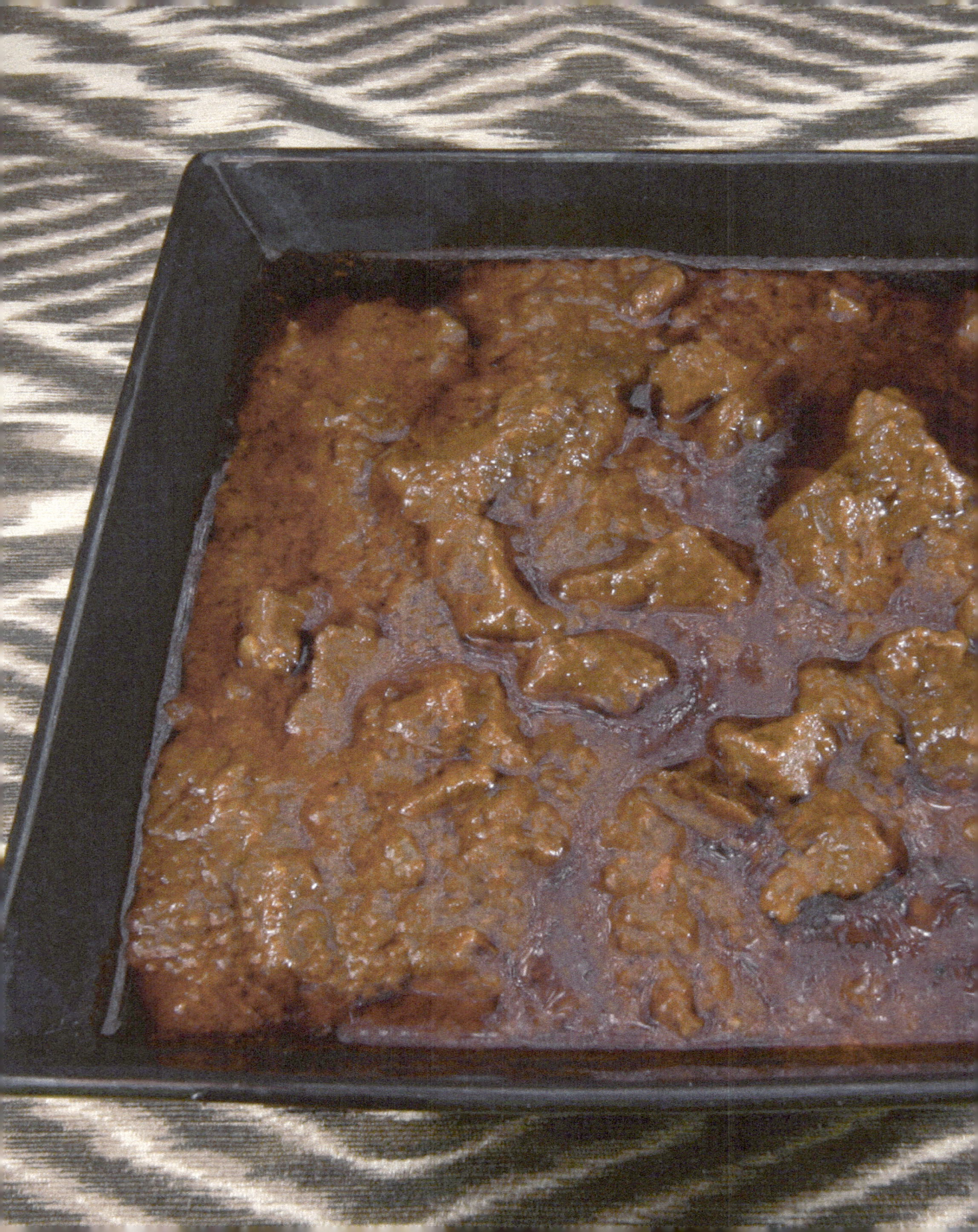

Spicy Beef Stew
ዝልዝል ወጥ

(Zilzil Wat) GF DF

Time: 1 hr 30 min
Serves: 5
Difficulty:

A very spicy stew for those who love fiery dishes. Not for the faint of heart!

Ingredients:

Red onions, 4 medium, finely chopped
Water, 2 cups total
Cross rib beef roast, 2 lb, boneless (can substitute other roast cuts)
Vegetable oil, ½ cup
Berberre paste, 1½ cups, (p. 29)
Ginger-Garlic Paste 1½ Tbsp, (p. 23)
Salt, 2 tsp
Niter Kibe, ½ cup, (p. 21)
Q'imam, 1 tsp. (p. 25)

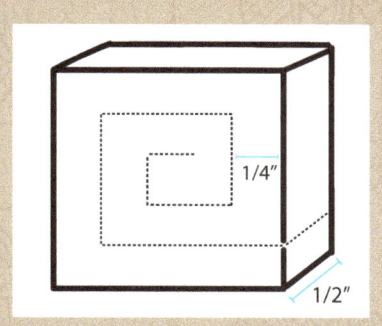

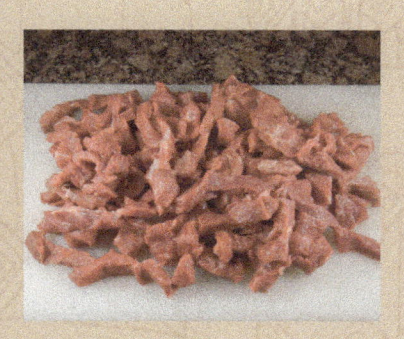

Directions:

1. Place onions and ½ cup water in medium pot over medium-high heat. Cover and cook 25 min, stirring every 10-15 min. While the onions are cooking, prepare the beef.
2. Trim excess fat from the roast, then slice across the grain into ½ inch thick pieces. Next cut each of these slices to form a ribbon that is about ¼ inch thick and ½ inch wide, using the unusual technique shown in the illustration (left).
3. Cut ribbons into 4 inch lengths and set aside.
4. Once the onions have begun to dry out (after ~25 minutes), add oil and cook another 5 min, uncovered. Stir occasionally to prevent sticking.
5. Add Berberre paste, Ginger-Garlic Paste and salt, and stir thoroughly to mix. Cook 7 min, stirring frequently to prevent sticking.
6. Add ½ cup water, stir, reduce heat to medium, and cook 3 min.
7. Ball up the beef ribbons together and squeeze them firmly to get rid of excess juices.
8. Add beef to onions, stir thoroughly, and increase heat to medium-high. Cook uncovered for 5 min, stirring occasionally to prevent sticking.
9. Reduce heat to medium. Cover and cook 5 min.
10. Stir in ½ cup water, Niter Kibe, Q'imam, and cook 8 min.
11. Reduce heat to medium and add ½ cup water. Cover and cook 10 min at a vigorous simmer, stirring occasionally.
12. Lower heat to a gentle simmer, and cook 15 min.

The Crown Jewel of African Cuisine

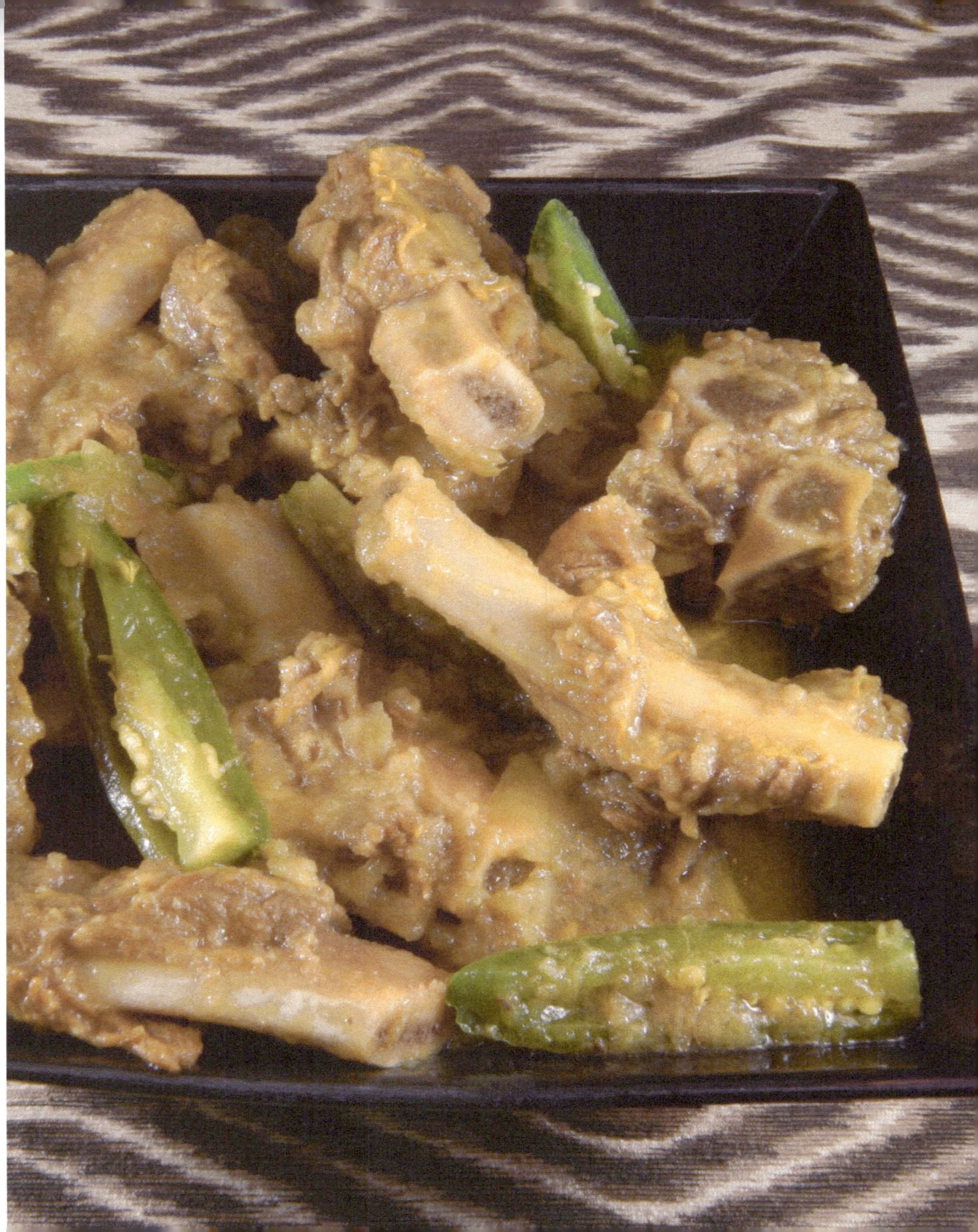

Meat & Seafood

Beef Back Ribs
ቅቅል ወጥ
(Kikil Wat) GF DF

Time: 1 hr 30 min
Serves: 6
Difficulty:

Every country has its way to cook ribs. This is my country's version. It is very rich and fun to eat.

Ingredients:

Beef back ribs, 4 lb
Yellow onions, 2 large, coarsely chopped
Salt, 2 tsp
Turmeric, ½ tsp
Ginger-Garlic Paste, 1 Tbsp (p. 23)
Water, cold, 10 cups
Niter Kibe, ½ cup (p. 21)
Jalapeño, ½, stemmed but not seeded, quartered lengthwise

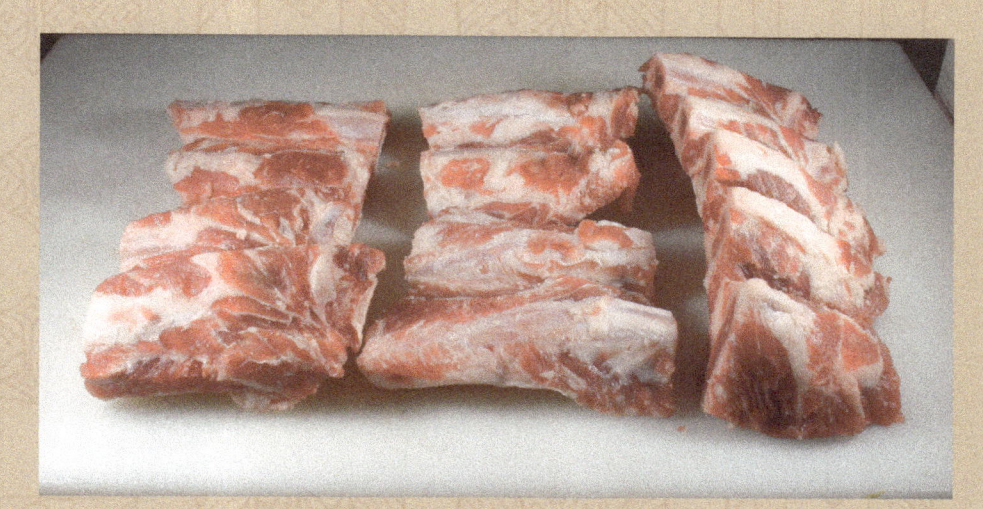

Directions:

1. Separate the ribs into pieces by cutting between each bone. Trim excess fat and membrane from each piece.
2. Rinse the ribs.
3. Place chopped onions in the bottom of a large pot, lay ribs on top of onions and, without stirring, add salt, turmeric, Ginger-Garlic Paste, and water. Cover and cook over high heat for 12 min.
4. Stir thoroughly, reduce heat to medium-high, return cover, and cook 1 hour, stirring every 10-15 min.
5. Stir in the Niter Kibe and cook 15 min.
6. Add jalapeño pieces, remove from heat, and serve.

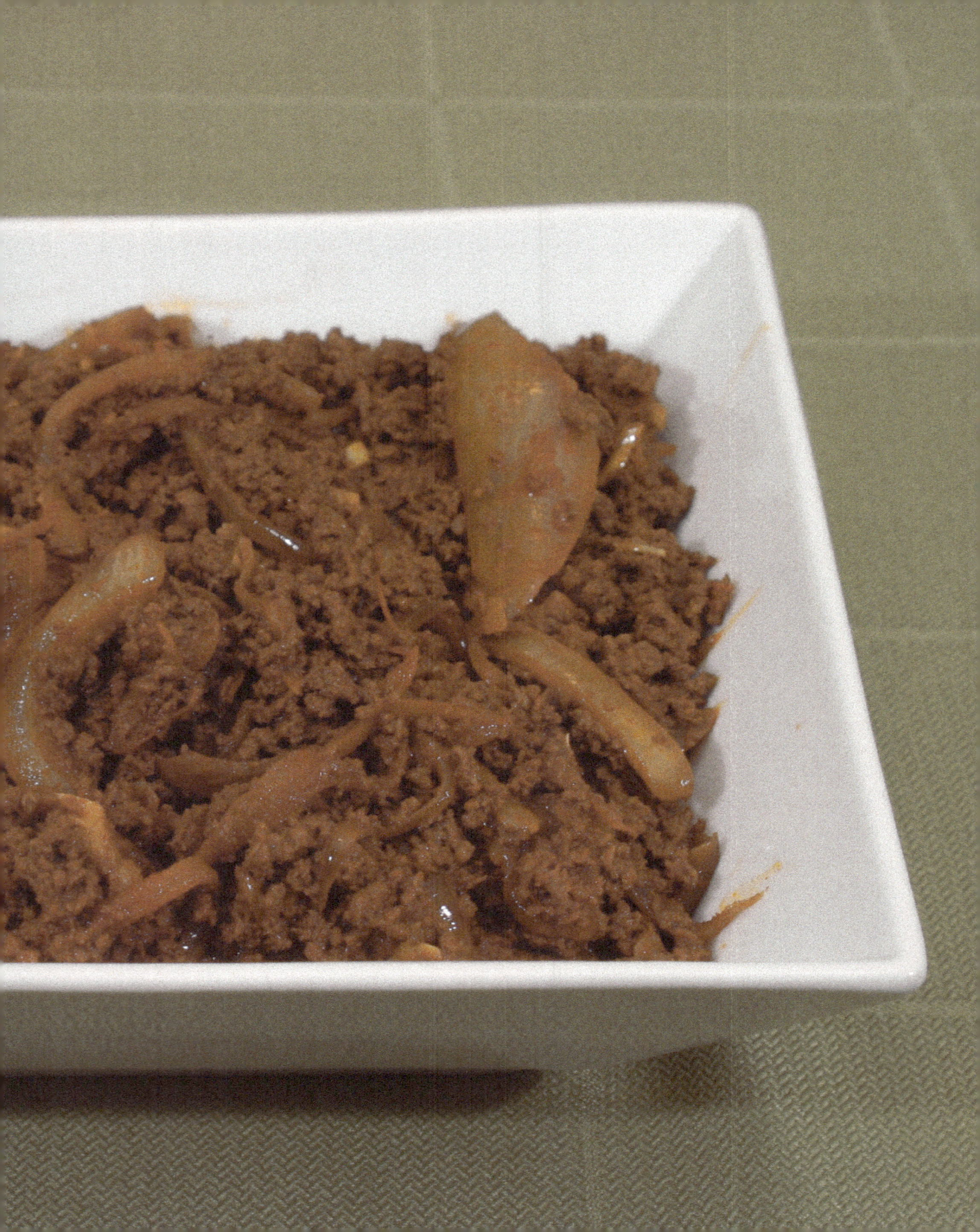

Meat & Seafood

Sautéed Ground Beef
የተፈጨ ስጋ ጥብስ
(Yetefeche Siga Tibbs) GF DF

Time: **20 min**
Serves: **4**
Difficulty:

This hamburger dish is a nice introduction to Ethiopian food for American children.

Ingredients:
Yellow onions, 2 large, cut in half and then in ¼ inch thick wedges
Vegetable oil, ¼ cup
Berberre paste, ½ cup (p. 29)
Salt, 1 tsp
Ground beef, 2 lb
Garlic, 10 cloves, finely minced
Niter Kibe, 1 Tbsp (p. 21)
Q'imam, ½ tsp (p. 25)

Directions:
1. Place onions into medium pot. Cook, uncovered, over medium-high heat for 4 min, stirring occasionally.
2. Add oil, Berberre paste, salt, and stir to mix. Cook 5 min, stirring occasionally.
3. Add beef and stir thoroughly to combine with onion and species. Cook until meat is fully browned, stirring constantly to break up clumps.
4. Add garlic, Niter Kibe and Q'imam and stir to combine. Cover and cook 5 min.

The Crown Jewel of African Cuisine

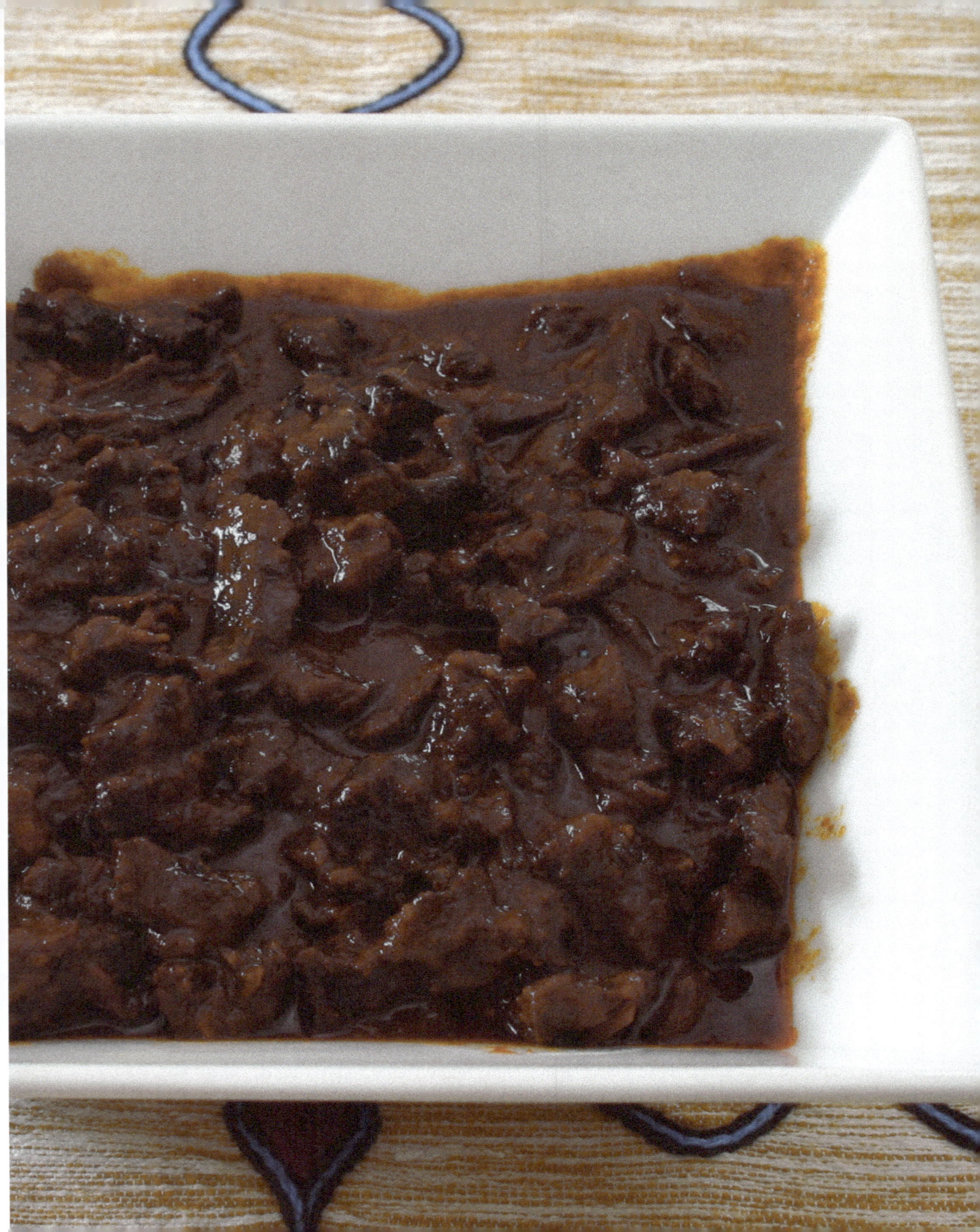

Dried Beef Stew
የቋንጣ ወጥ
(Yequanta Wat) GF DF

Time: 1 hr
Serves: 6
Difficulty: ♦♦♦◊◊

This recipe is a favored tradition because it is made with Beef Jerky (p. 179) and can be enjoyed by anyone, even the many in Ethiopia who are not lucky enough to have a refrigerator.

Ingredients:
Vegetable oil, ⅓ cup
Yellow onion, 1 large, finely diced
Berberre paste, ½ cup (p. 29)
Water, 4 cups total
Ginger-Garlic Paste, 2 Tbsp (p. 23)
Salt, 1 tsp
Beef jerky, ¾ lb, cut into 1½ inch lengths (see beef jerky recipe, p. 179)
Niter Kibe, 2 Tbsp (p. 21)
Q'imam, ¼ tsp (p. 25)

Directions:
1. Heat oil in a large pot over medium-high heat.
2. Add onion to pot and cook, uncovered, for 5 min.
3. Add Berberre paste and cook another 5 min.
4. Add Ginger-Garlic Paste, salt, and ½ cup water, and cook 7 min, stirring occasionally.
5. Add beef jerky pieces and 1½ cups water. Cook 7 min.
6. Reduce heat to medium and cover. Cook 10 min.
7. Add 2 more cups water and increase to medium high. Cook 15 min, partly covered, stirring every 5 min.
8. Add Niter Kibe and Q'imam and stir to mix. Reduce heat to medium and cook 5 min.

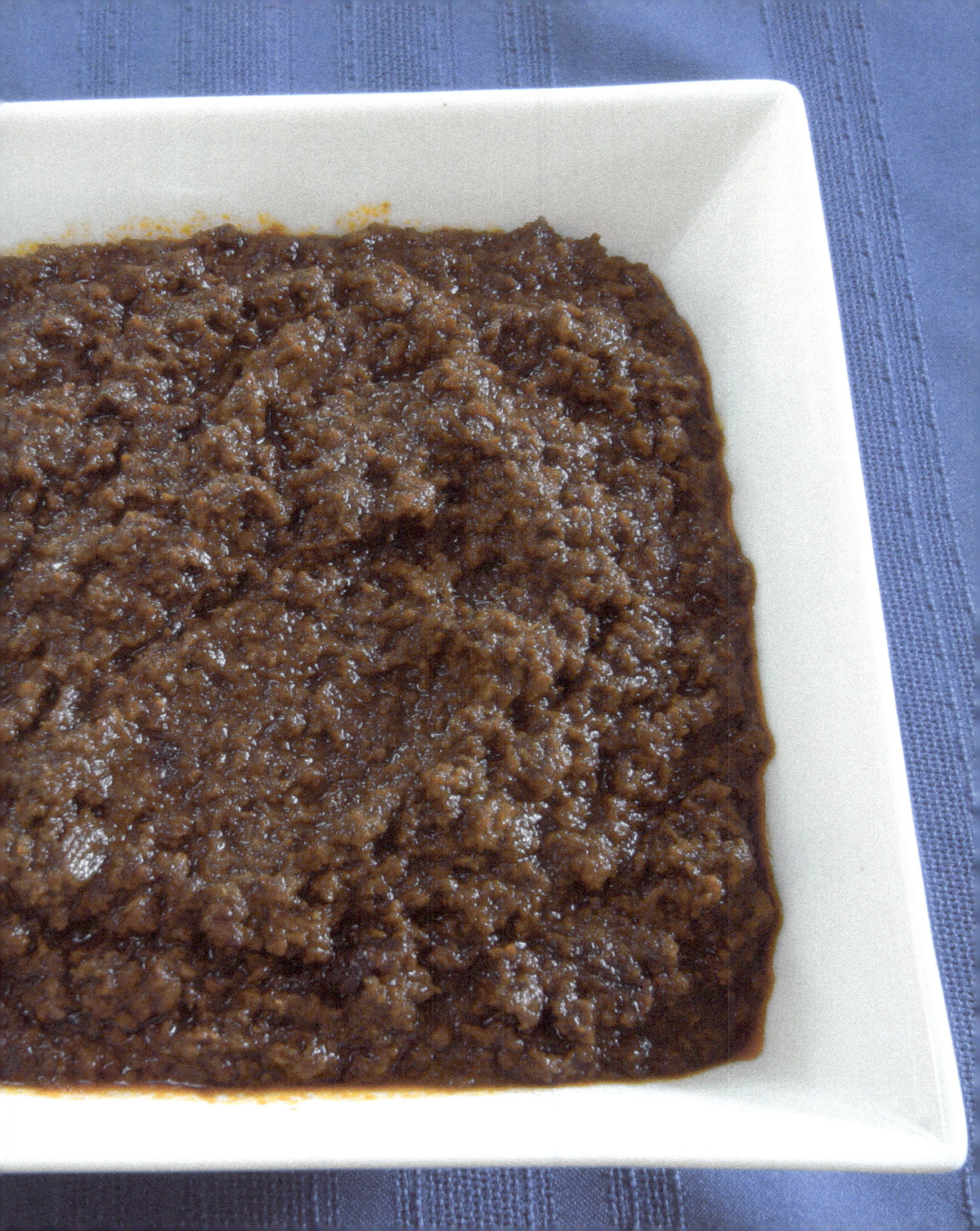

Meat & Seafood

Spicy Ground Beef Stew
ምንቾት አብሽ
(Minchet Abish) GF DF

Time: **1 hr 45 min**
Serves: **5**
Difficulty: ♦♦♦◊◊

Another fiery meat dish that is excellent served on Injera (p. 33) along with non-spicy dishes.

Ingredients:

Top round steak, London broil 2 lb (can substitute ground beef)
Yellow onions, 3 large
Vegetable oil, ½ cup
Niter Kibe, 2 cups total (p. 21)
Water, 3½ cups total
Berberre paste, 3 cups (p. 29)
Ginger-Garlic Paste, 2 Tbsp (p. 23)
Q'imam, 2 tsp (p. 25)
Salt, 3 tsp

Directions:

1. Cut beef into stew-meat sized chunks. In batches, place beef in the bowl of food processor. Process for about 10 seconds, then redistribute meat in bowl. Repeat twice. Remove ground meat and add new batch, continuing until all meat is ground.

   *Note: Ground beef can be substituted but the grind will be somewhat finer and not as fresh. Refrigerate ground beef while preparing other ingredients.

2. Coarsely chop onions and place into bowl of food processor. Process until the onions form a smooth purée with the consistency of mashed potatoes.

3. Place onion purée in a large pot over high heat. Cook 15 min, partially covered. Stir occasionally to prevent sticking.

4. Reduce heat to medium and add oil, 1 cup Niter Kibe, and stir to mix. Cook 8 min.

5. Add Berberre paste, Ginger-Garlic Paste, and ¼ cup water. Increase temperature to high and cook 8 min, uncovered, stirring frequently.

6. Reduce heat to medium-low and continue to cook 10 min, stirring occasionally.

7. Increase heat to high and cook, uncovered, for about 6 min, stirring constantly until the mixture begins to dry a bit.

8. Remove from heat and add ground beef. Stir until thoroughly mixed.

9. Return pot to burner and reduce heat to medium high. Cook 3 min, stirring frequently.

10. Add about ¼ cup water and cook 2 min.

11. Add 1 cup Niter Kibe and 1½ cups water and cook 4 min, stirring frequently.

The Crown Jewel of African Cuisine

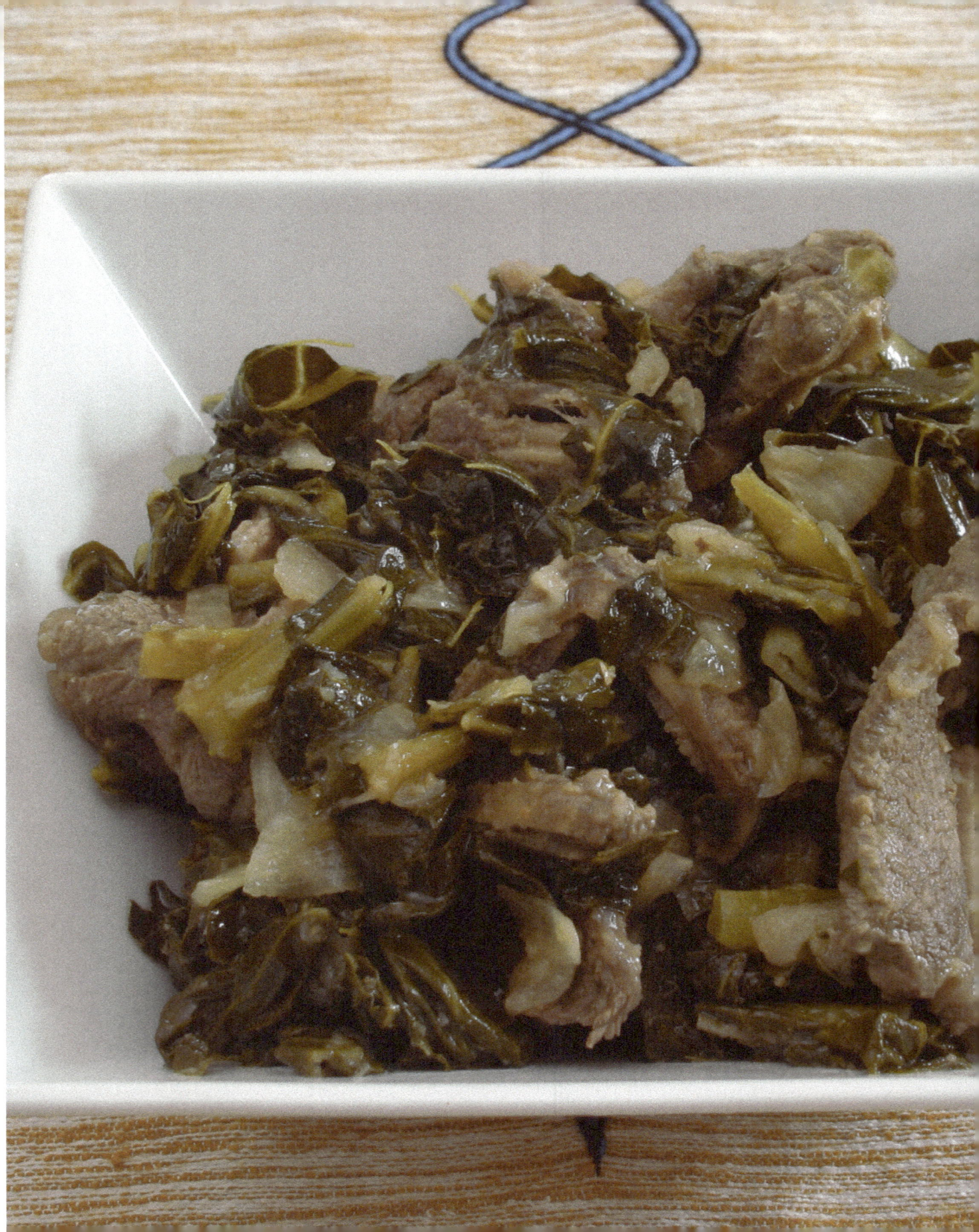

Beef with Collard Greens
ጎድን በ ጎመን
(Godin Be Gomen) GF DF

Time: 1 hr
Serves: 5
Difficulty: ♦♦◇◇◇

This is how we cook short ribs in Ethiopia, complementing the meat with one of our favorite leafy vegetables, collard greens.

Ingredients:

Yellow onion, 1 large, coarsely chopped
Vegetable oil, ½ cup
Collard greens, 3 bunches (about 16 leaves)
Beef short ribs, bone-in, 1 ½ lb
Ginger-Garlic Paste, 2 Tbsp (p. 23)
Water, 2 cups
Salt, 2 tsp
Jalapeño, stemmed and quartered lengthwise

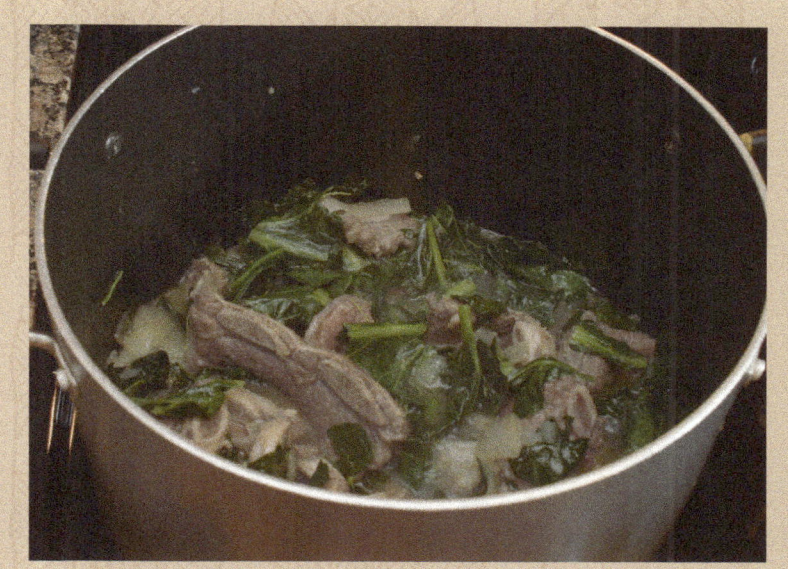

Directions:

1. Cut out midrib (do not discard) of each collard leaf. Tear leaves into large pieces. Peel the tough outer layer off the midribs. Cut peeled midribs into bite sized pieces and set aside with leaves.
2. Place onions in large pot over medium-high heat. Cook 2 min, uncovered.
3. Add vegetable oil. Cook 3 min, stirring once or twice.
4. Add collard leaves and midrib pieces, stir and cook 3 min.
5. Add short ribs, Ginger-Garlic Paste, water and salt and stir to mix. Cover pot, increase heat to high, cook 10 min, then reduce heat to medium high and cook 30 min more.
6. Remove from heat and garnish with jalapeño.

The Crown Jewel of African Cuisine

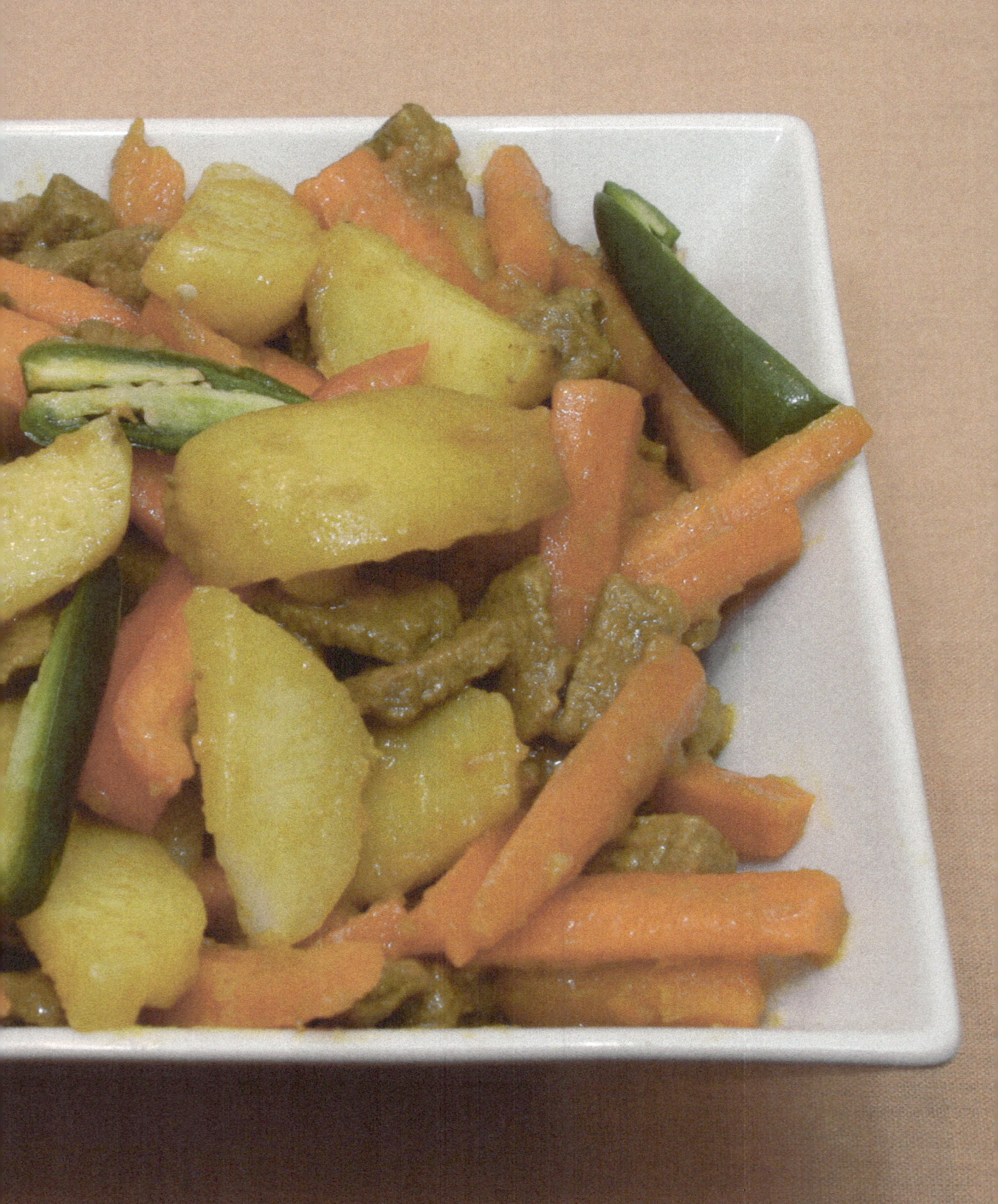

Meat & Seafood

Beef with Carrots and Potatoes
አልጫ ስጋ በ አታክልት
(Alicha Siga Be Atakilt) GF DF

Time: **1 hr**
Serves: **6**
Difficulty:

This dish can practically stand alone on Injera (p. 33). It has everything: meat, vegetables and color.

Ingredients:

Yellow onion, 1 large, cut in half and into ¼ inch wide wedges
Vegetable oil, ½ cup
Turmeric, ½ tsp
Water, 4 cups total
Stew beef, 1 lb, cut into 1 inch by ½ inch by ¼ inch pieces
Ginger-Garlic Paste, 2 tsp (p. 23)
Salt, 2 tsp
Carrots, 1 lb
Red potatoes, 1 lb
Jalapeño, stemmed and cut lengthwise into quarters
Red pepper and yellow pepper, ¼ each, cut into ¼ inch wide strips

Directions:

1. Place onions in large pot over medium-high heat. Cook 2 min, stirring frequently.
2. Add oil, stir and cook 2 min.
3. Add turmeric and ¼ cup water and cook 2 min.
4. Add beef, Ginger-Garlic Paste, salt. Cook 25 min, covered, stirring every few min and adding ~3 Tbsp water each time you stir it to keep it from getting dry. By the end of the 25 min, a total of ~1¾ cup water should have been added.
5. Peel carrots and cut into 3 inch lengths. Slice these lengthwise into 6–8 pieces.
6. Peel potatoes and cut each potato into 8 wedges. Set aside in bowl covered with water.
7. Add carrots and last 2 cups water to beef mixture. Cook 7 min, covered, stirring every few min.
8. Drain potatoes and add to pot. Cook 10–12 min, covered, stirring occasionally.
9. Add jalapeños and red and yellow peppers, stir and immediately remove from heat.

The Crown Jewel of African Cuisine

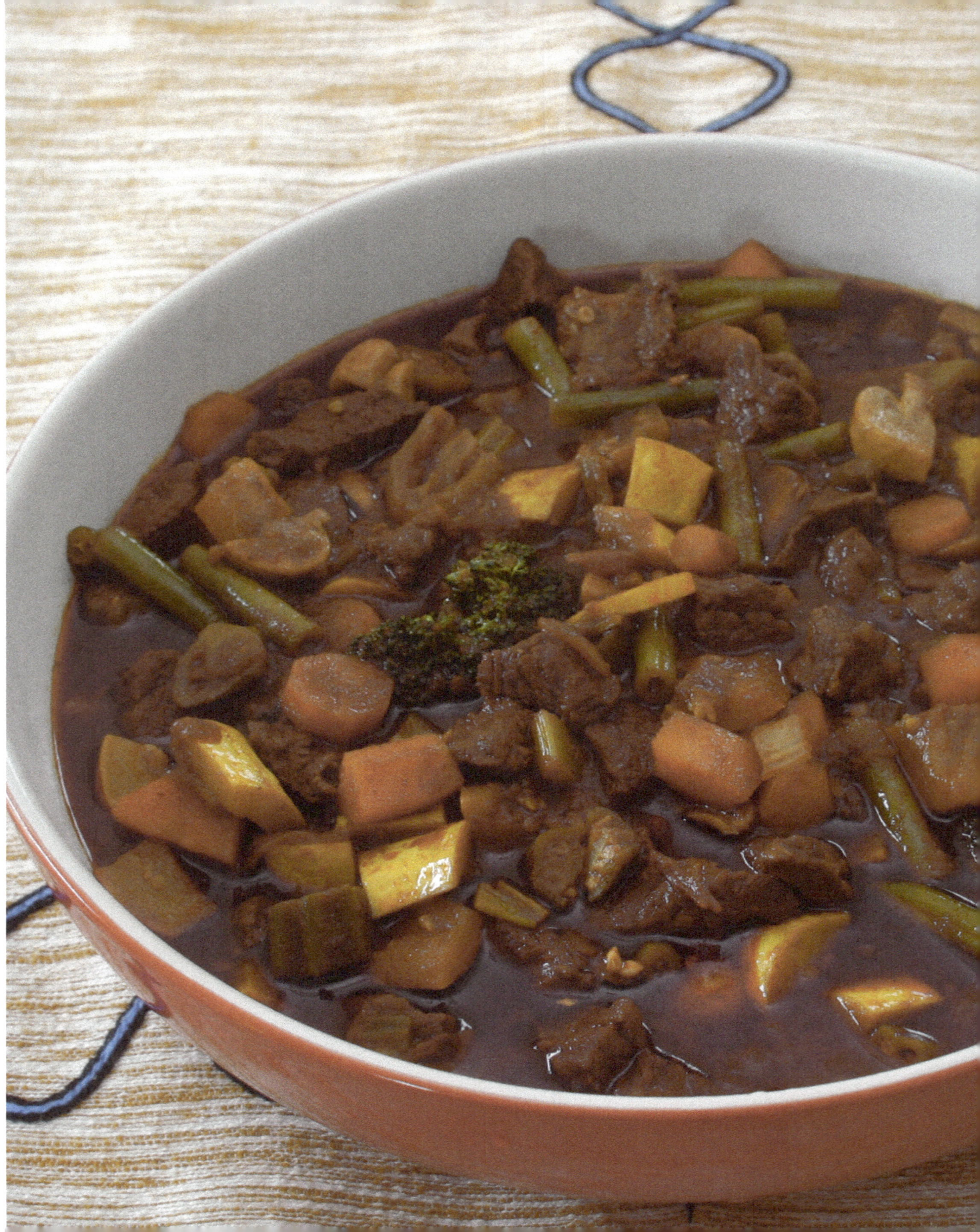

Beef and Vegetable Stew
ቀይ ስጋ በ አታክልት
(Kayeh Siga Be Atakilt) GF DF

A key ingredient in this colorful and flavorful stew is okra, which may have originated in Ethiopia.

Time: 2 hr
Serves: 10
Difficulty: ♦♦♦◊◊

Ingredients:

Yellow onion, 1 large, finely diced
Vegetable oil, ½ cup
Water, 6 cups total
Berberre paste, 1 cup (p. 29)
Ginger-Garlic Paste, ¼ cup (p. 23)
Salt, 2½ tsp
Beef stew meat, 2½ lb, cut into ½ inch dice, rinsed, drained and squeezed dry
Plum tomatoes, 3, coarsely chopped
Carrots, 3, peeled and cut into ½ inch dice
Yellow squash, 2, cut into ½ inch dice
Green beans, ⅓ lb, stemmed and cut into ½ inch lengths
White mushrooms, 8, coarsely chopped
Celery, 2 stalks, each cut lengthwise into 3 strips, then cut into ½ inch lengths
Okra, fresh or frozen, 2 cups, chopped
Niter Kibe, ½ cup (p. 21)
Q'imam, 1 tsp (p. 25)
Broccoli florets, ½ lb, broken into small pieces

Directions:

1. Put onion in very large pot over high heat. Cook 2 min, covered.
2. Add oil, stir and cook 2 min, stirring frequently.
3. Add 1 cup water and stir. Cook 6 min, covered.
4. Add ½ cup water and stir. Cook 5 min, covered.
5. Add Berberre paste, stir to combine and cook 2 min, covered.
6. Add Ginger-Garlic Paste, salt and stir to combine. Cook 8 min, uncovered, stirring continuously.
7. Add ½ cup water and cook 6 min, covered, stirring often.
8. Add beef to pot, stir and cook 5 min, covered.
9. Add tomatoes and cook 15 min, stirring every 5 min.
10. Add 2 cups water, stir and cook 10 min, covered.
11. Add 2 cups water and all of the remaining vegetables, except the broccoli. Stir to combine thoroughly. Cook, covered, for about 25 min or until carrots are tender, stirring a couple times.
12. Add broccoli, reduce heat to medium, and cook 3 min.

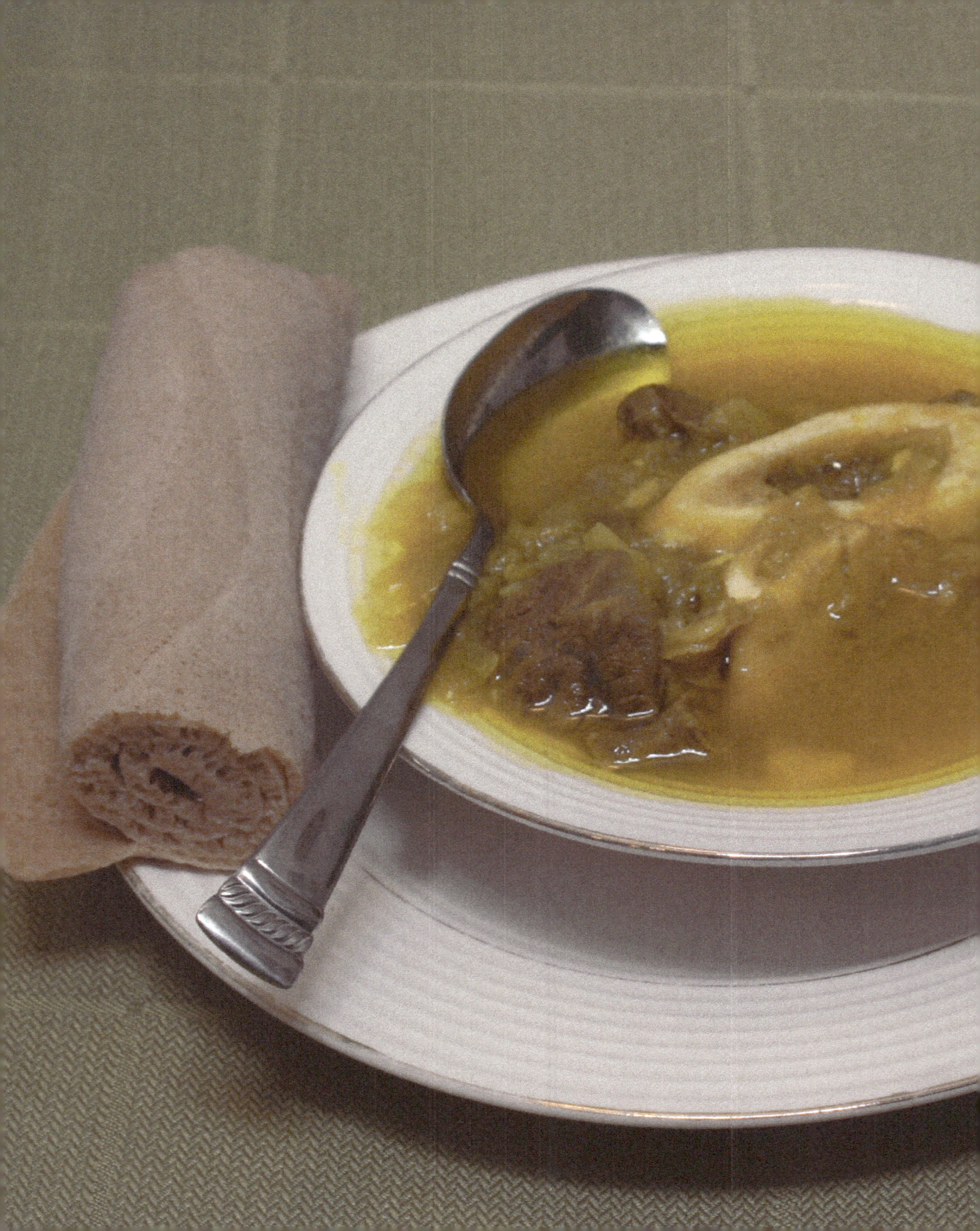

Meat & Seafood

Beef Broth
የስጋ ሾርባ
(Yesiga Shorba) GF DF

Time: 1 hr 45 min
Serves: 8–10
Difficulty: ♦♦♦♦♦

You can serve this broth as a meaty soup or as a beverage consommé. We like to give this to people who have a cold, to help them get better.

Ingredients:

Beef shank, 1½ lb
Beef soup bones, 1½ lb
Beef marrow bones, 1½ lb (these bones are usually available on request from the grocery store butcher.)
Water
Yellow onion, 2 large, chopped into ½ inch dice
Salt, 4 tsp
Turmeric, 1½ tsp
Ginger-Garlic Paste, 1 Tbsp (p. 23)
Garlic cloves, 10, minced
Niter Kibe, ½ cup (p. 21)
Jalapeño, 1, stemmed and quartered lengthwise

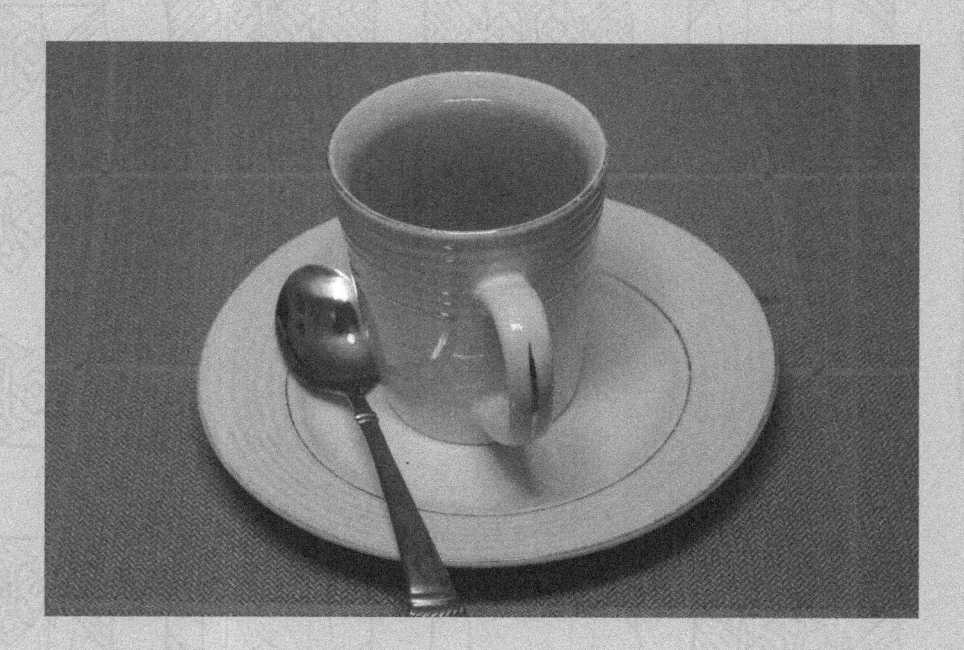

Directions:

1. Remove large pieces of meat from shank and cut into 1 inch cubes. Place these and all bones into a large pot. Rinse with lukewarm water and drain.
2. Add enough water to just cover the meat. Cook 10 min, covered, on high heat, turning the bones periodically.
3. Drain water. Return pot to stove over medium-high heat. Add 12 cups water and all remaining ingredients, except jalapeños. Cook 40 min at a rolling boil, partially covered.
4. Reduce heat to simmer and cook 40 min, covered.
5. Remove from heat and add jalapeños.
6. Serve as a soup with meat and meaty bones or to drink, as a consommé.

The Crown Jewel of African Cuisine

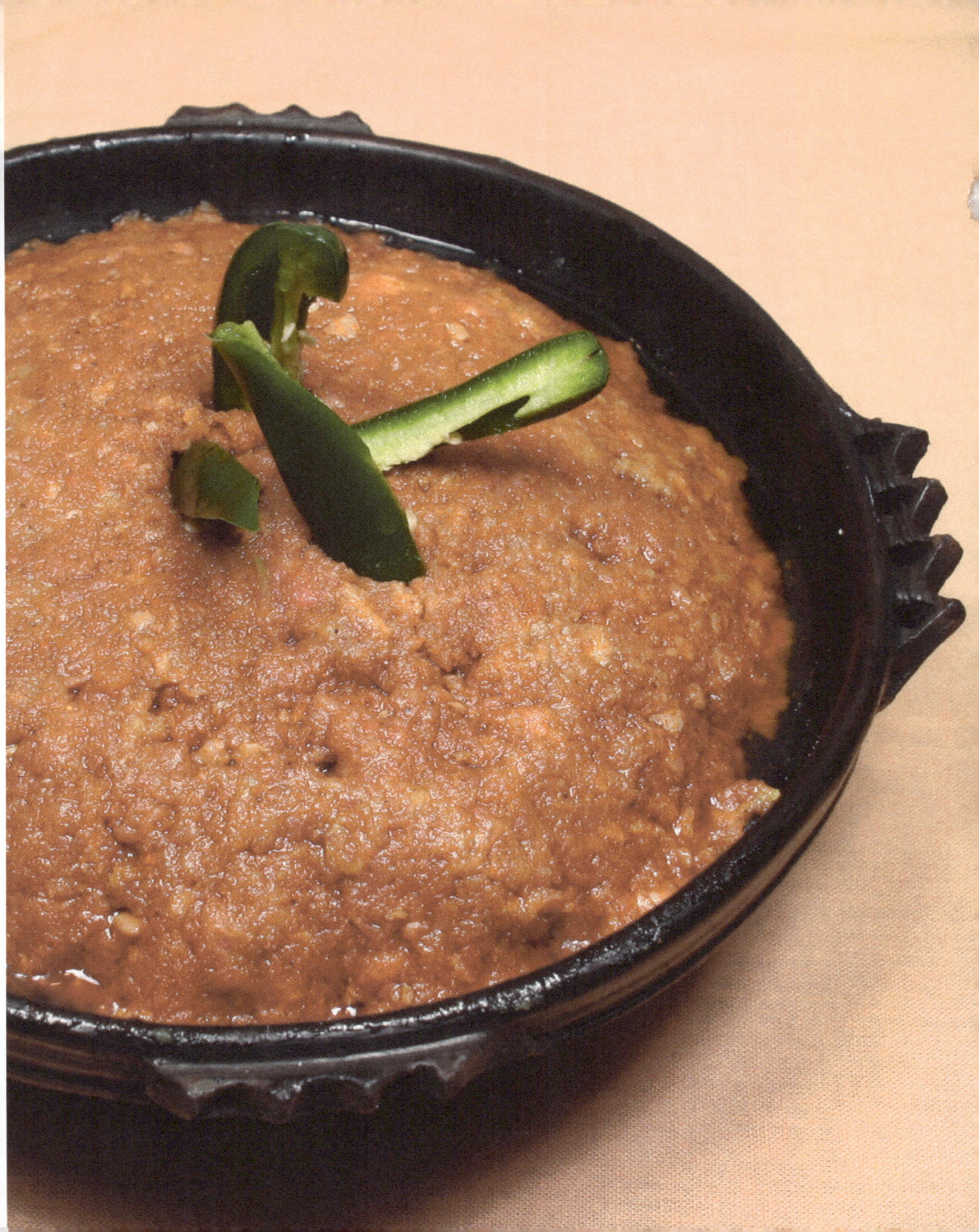

Meat & Seafood

Beef Tartar
ከትፎ
(Kitfo) GF DF

Time: 15 min, plus 2 hr refrigeration
Serves: 8
Difficulty:

In the US, health officials say it is not safe to eat raw beef. This recipe is written to describe our traditional Ethiopian practice of eating raw ground beef. I think the health people would not like it very much, but Beef Tartar is an important Ethiopian tradition, so I wanted to include this recipe.

Ingredients:

Eye of round roast, 2 lb (do NOT substitute store-bought ground beef)
Cardamom, 2 Tbsp
Mitmita*, 3 Tbsp
Niter Kibe, 1 cup (p. 21)
Salt, 1 tsp
Jalapeño, 1, stemmed and quartered lengthwise

*available at specialty stores and online, see p. 17

Directions:

1. Cut meat into 1 inch dice. Place half of the meat into a food processor and process 30 seconds continuously. Transfer to a bowl and repeat with second half.
2. Add cardamom and mitmita. Use disposable kitchen gloves and mix by hand. (Gloves are used for hygiene and to prevent red pepper oils in mitmita from soaking into skin.)
3. Return mixture to food processor and process 10 seconds.
4. Transfer to a bowl and place in refrigerator for 2 hours for the flavors to blend.
5. Once the flavors have been allowed to blend, place Niter Kibe in a large fry pan over medium-high heat.
6. When the Niter Kibe has completely melted, remove pan from heat and add beef and salt. Mix thoroughly by hand, using a new clean pair of gloves and taking care not to burn yourself on the hot pan. Break up any lumps.
7. Return to stove over low heat and cook 3 min.
8. Remove to a serving bowl and garnish with a light glaze of melted Niter Kibe and wedges of jalapeño.

The Crown Jewel of African Cuisine

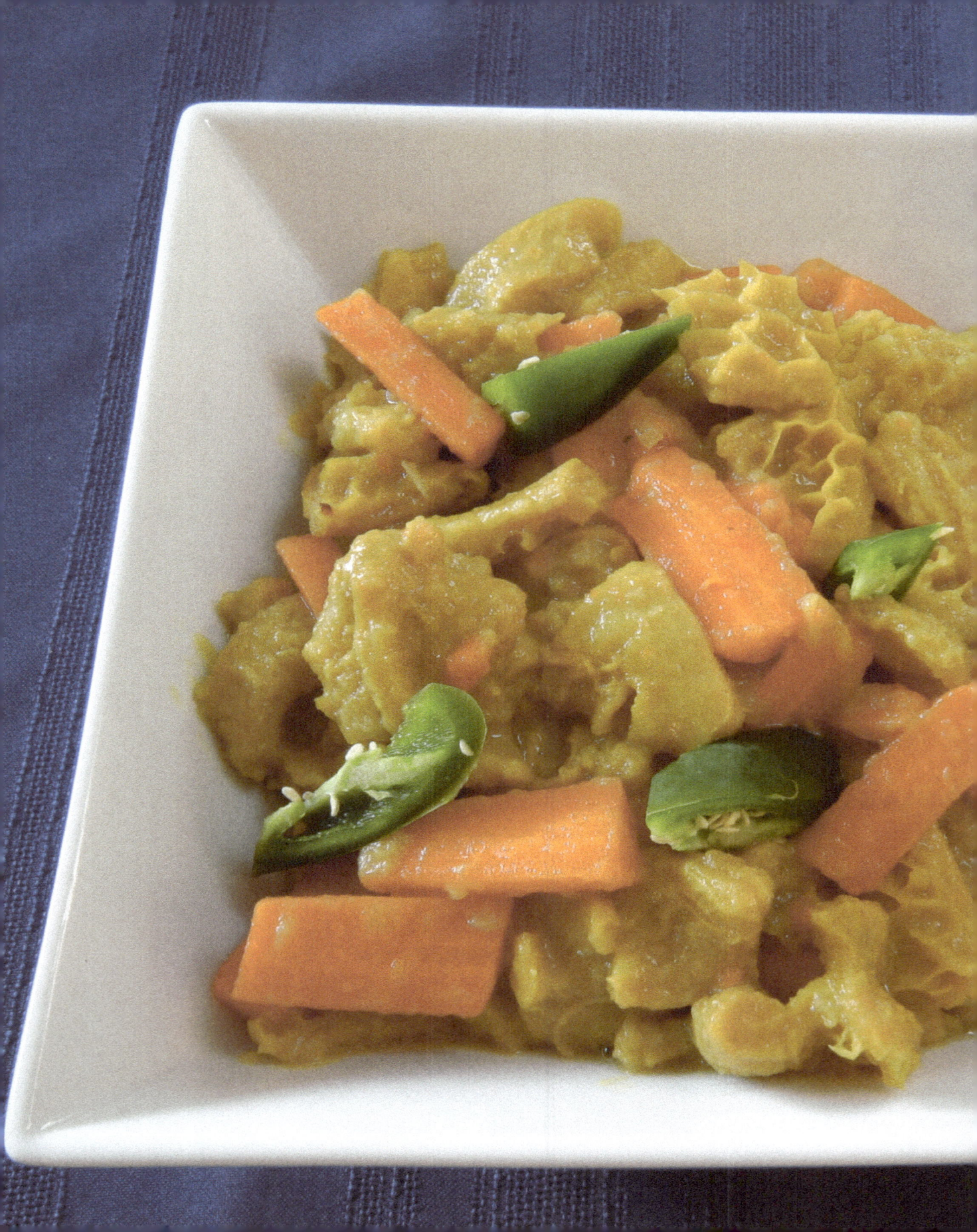

Ethiopian Tripe Stew
የጨጓራ አልጫ
(Yecheguara Alicha) GF DF

Every culture has its version of tripe stew, and this is ours.

Meat & Seafood

Time: 2 hr 15 min
Serves: 8
Difficulty: ♦♦♦◊◊

Ingredients:

Honeycomb tripe, also known as beef stomach, 2 lb
Water, 8 cups total
Yellow onion, 1 large, cut in half and then into ¼ inch thick wedges
Ginger-Garlic Paste, 2 Tbsp (p. 23)
Turmeric, 1 tsp
Salt, 1 tsp
Carrots, 1 lb, peeled, cut in half lengthwise and then cut into 2 inch lengths
Niter Kibe, 2 Tbsp (p. 21)

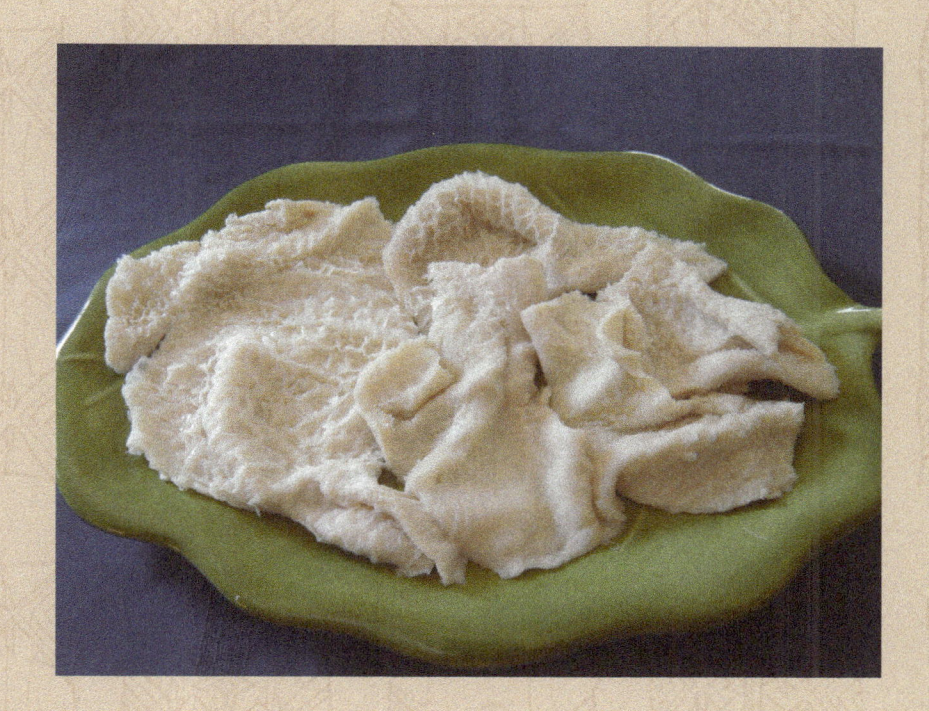

Directions:

1. Thoroughly clean tripe by rinsing under cold water.
2. Cut tripe into bite-sized pieces and place into large pot with enough water to cover.
3. Cover pot, bring it to a boil over high heat, and parboil the tripe for 15 seconds.
4. Drain in colander and rinse thoroughly with water.
5. Rinse pot and return tripe to pot with 4 cups water. Cook 30 min over medium heat, covered.
6. Add 2 cups water and cook 20 min, stirring occasionally.
7. Add onions, Ginger-Garlic Paste, turmeric and salt. Cover and cook 30 min.
8. Add 2 more cups water and cook 20 min, covered.
9. Add carrots and cook 10 min.
10. Add Niter Kibe and cook 3 min.

The Crown Jewel of African Cuisine

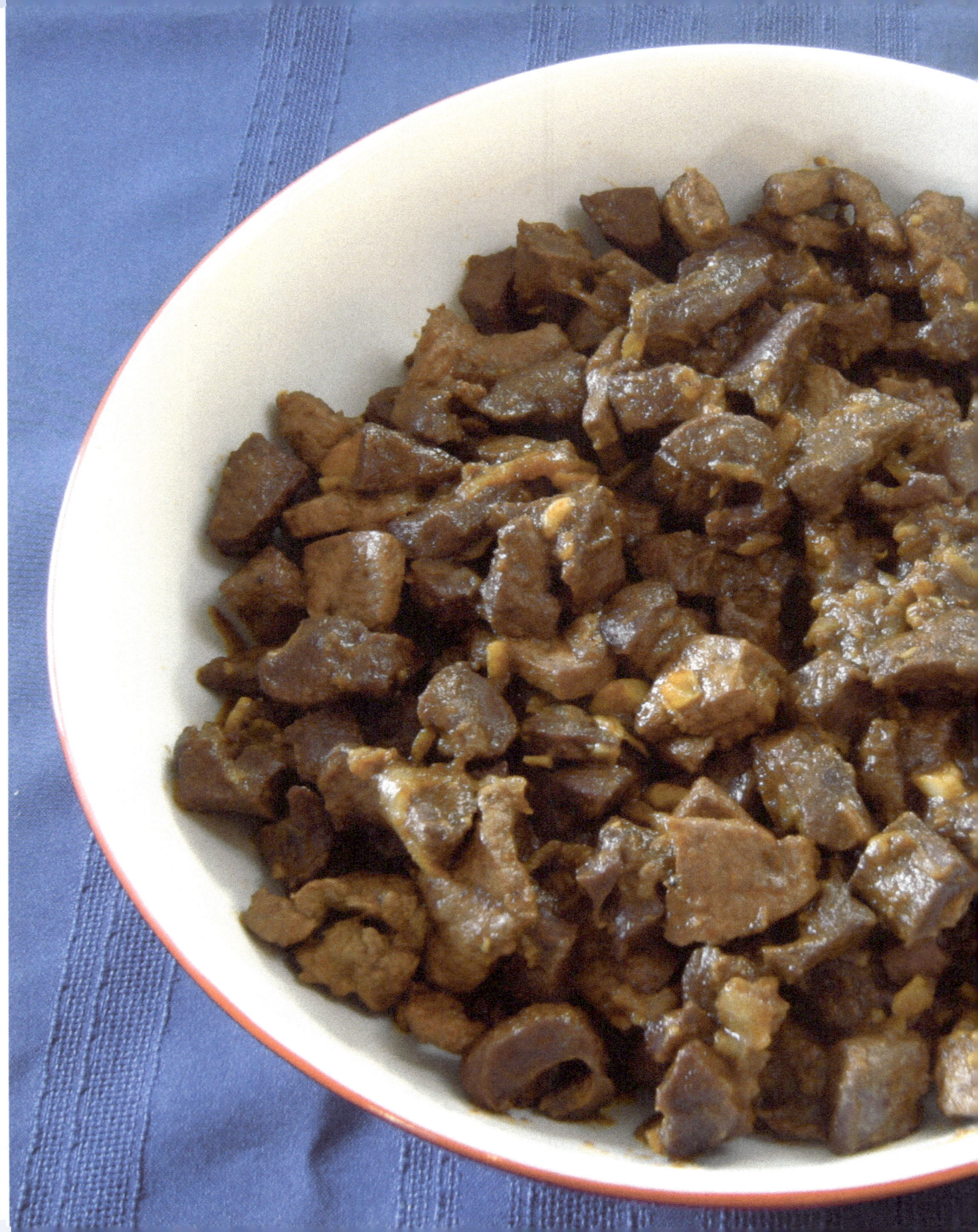

Meat & Seafood

Beef Heart and Liver Stew
ልብ ና ጉበት
(Lib Na Gub'et) GF DF

Time: 45 min
Serves: 8–10
Difficulty:

This is for the liver lovers!

Ingredients:

Vegetable oil, ½ cup
Yellow onion, 1 large, cut in half, sliced into ¼ inch wedges
Garlic, 1 head, cloves peeled and thinly sliced
Berberre paste, 1 Tbsp (p. 29)
Beef heart, 2 lb, rinsed and cut to 1 inch dice
Salt, 1 tsp
Beef liver, 1 lb, rinsed and cut to 1 inch dice
Niter Kibe, ¼ cup (p. 21)

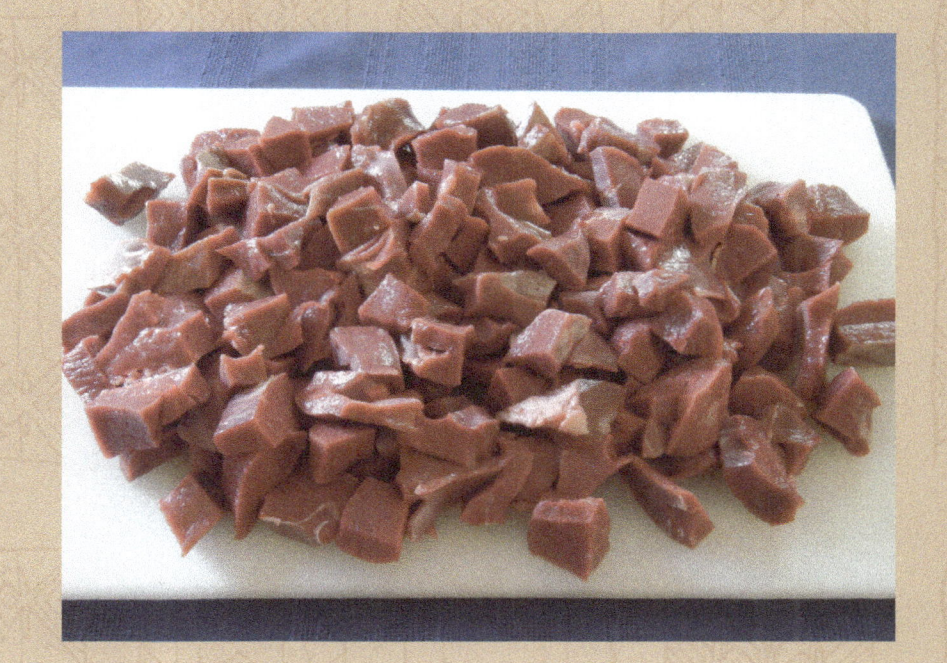

Directions:

1. Heat oil in large frypan over high heat. Add onions and garlic. Cook 4 min, stirring occasionally.
2. Add Berberre paste and cook 5 min, stirring frequently.
3. Add heart pieces, salt and stir to mix. Cook 6 min, partially covered, stirring occasionally.
4. Remove lid, cook 7 min, stirring occasionally and making sure that all pieces are cooked through.
5. Add liver and Niter Kibe and stir to mix. Cook 10 min, uncovered, stirring occasionally.

The Crown Jewel of African Cuisine

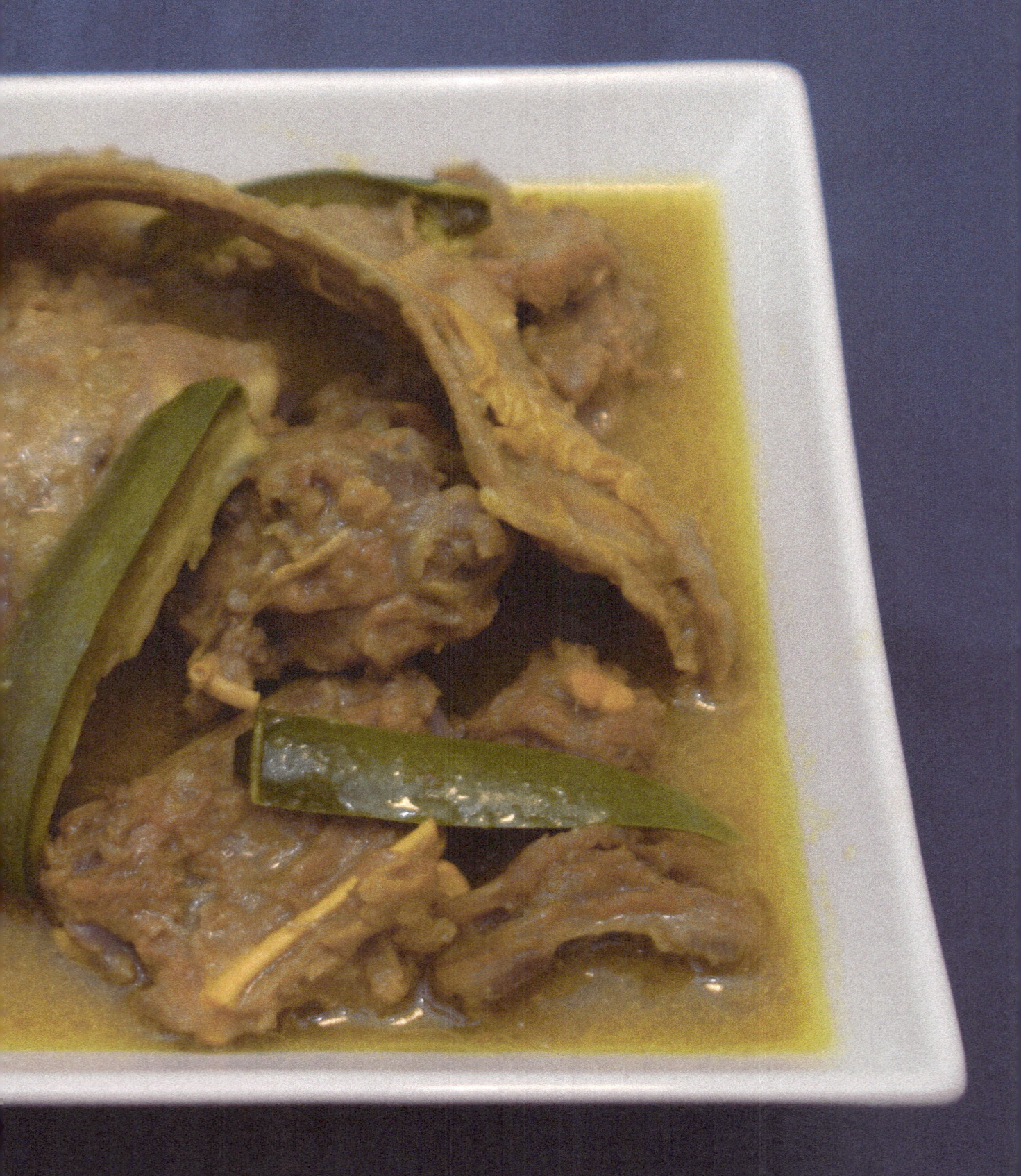

Lamb Stew
የበግ አልጫ ወጥ
(Yebeg Alicha Wat) GF DF

Time: 2 hr 30 min
Serves: 5–6
Difficulty: ▲▲△△△

This rich stew is a perennial favorite at my restaurant.

Ingredients:
- Lamb, bone-in, 3 lb, any cut including ribs, leg, shank, chops, shoulder
- Water, 7 cups total, plus enough to cover lamb
- Yellow onion, 2 large, coarsely chopped
- Vegetable oil, ⅓ cup
- Ginger-Garlic Paste, 2 Tbsp (p. 23)
- Turmeric, 1 tsp
- Salt, 2 tsp
- Niter Kibe, ½ cup (p. 21)
- Jalapeño, 1, stemmed and quartered lengthwise

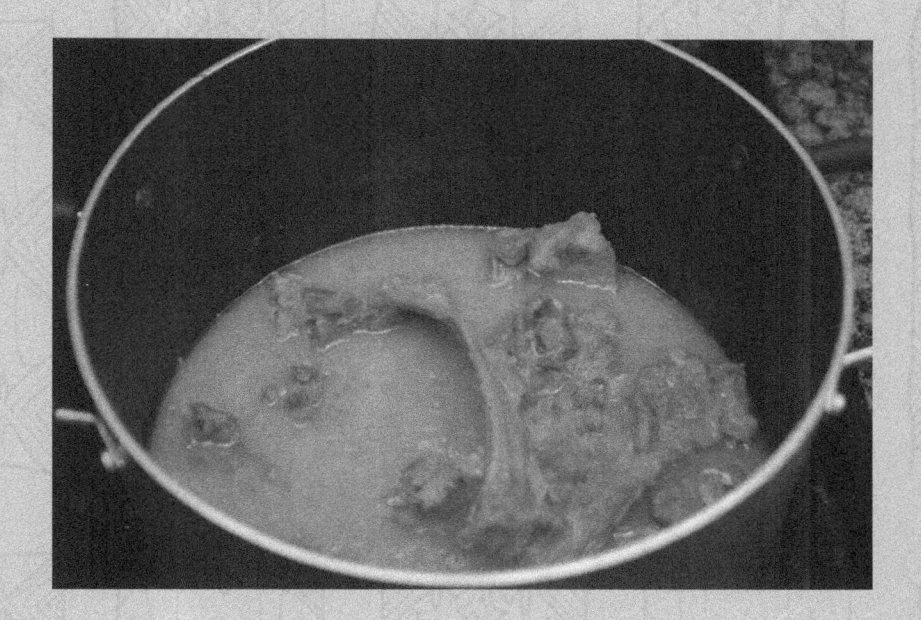

Directions:
1. Cut meat (with bone still in) into manageable 3–4 inch long sections. Cut wherever easiest, such as at joints or between ribs. If bones are small enough, carefully use heavy knife to cut crosswise and expose marrow.
2. Place lamb in large pot and add enough water to cover. Cook 10 min over high heat, covered. Drain in large colander and rinse thoroughly.
3. Place onions in another large pot and cook 7 min over medium-high heat until the onions become translucent, stirring occasionally to prevent burning.
4. Add oil, stir, and cook 5 min.
5. Add Ginger-Garlic Paste, turmeric, salt, 2 cups water, stir, and cook 5 min.
6. Add lamb to pot with onions and 2 additional cups water and stir to mix. Cook 30 min over medium-high heat, covered, stirring every few min.
7. Add 3 cups water and Niter Kibe and bring to a simmer. Simmer covered for an hour or until the meat is tender, stirring occasionally.
8. Remove from heat and garnish with jalapeño.

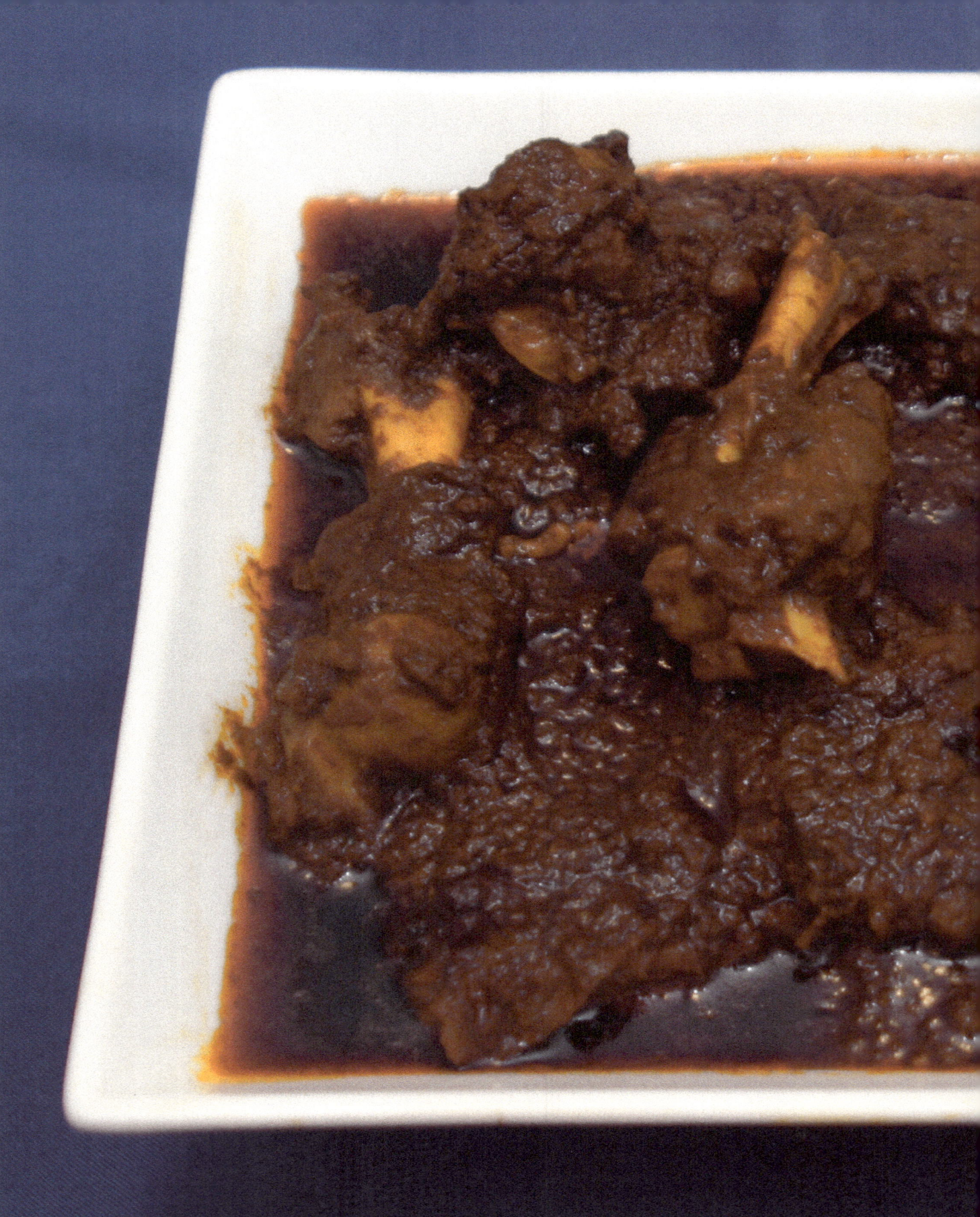

Meat & Seafood

Spicy Lamb Stew
የበግ ቀይ ወጥ
(Yebeg Key Wat) GF DF

Time: 2 hr 45 min
Serves: 5–6
Difficulty: ▲▲▲▲△

A spicy and heartier version of Lamb Stew (p. 95).

Ingredients:

Lamb, bone-in, 3 lb, any cut including ribs, leg, shank, chops, or shoulder
Water, 3½ cups, plus enough to cover lamb
Yellow onions, 4 large, coarsely chopped
Vegetable oil, ½ cup
Berberre paste 1½ cups (p. 29)
Ginger-Garlic Paste, 2 Tbsp, (p. 23)
Niter Kibe, 1 cup (p. 21)
Q'imam, 1 tsp (p. 25)
Salt, 1½ tsp

Directions:

1. Cut meat (with bone still in) into managable 3–4 inch long sections. Cut wherever easiest, such as at joints or between ribs. If bones are small enough, carefully use heavy knife to cut crosswise and expose marrow.
2. Place lamb into large pot and add water to cover. Cook 10 min over high heat, covered.
3. Place onions in bowl of food processor and process until the onions form a smooth purée.
4. Remove the lamb to a colander and rinse well. Once the lamb is cool enough to handle, trim the meat from the bone. Cut the meat into ¾ inch dice and score each piece with a deep cut.
5. Place onion purée into another large pot. Cook, uncovered, over high heat, stirring occasionally for 20 min.
6. Add oil to onion purée, stir to mix. Cook 4 min, stirring frequently.
7. Add Berberre paste and Ginger-Garlic Paste and stir to mix. Remove cover and cook 8 min, stirring frequently.
8. Reduce heat to medium, add Niter Kibe and stir to mix. Cook 15 min, stirring occasionally.
9. Add ¼ cup water, stir, and cook 5 min, covered, stirring occasionally.
10. Add ½ cup water, stir, and cook 5 min.
11. Add lamb to pot along with 1¼ cups water. Bring it to a simmer and cook 30 min, partly covered, stirring occasionally.
12. Add 1½ cups water, Q'imam and salt and stir to mix. Cook 45 min, uncovered, or until the lamb is very tender, stirring every few min.

The Crown Jewel of African Cuisine

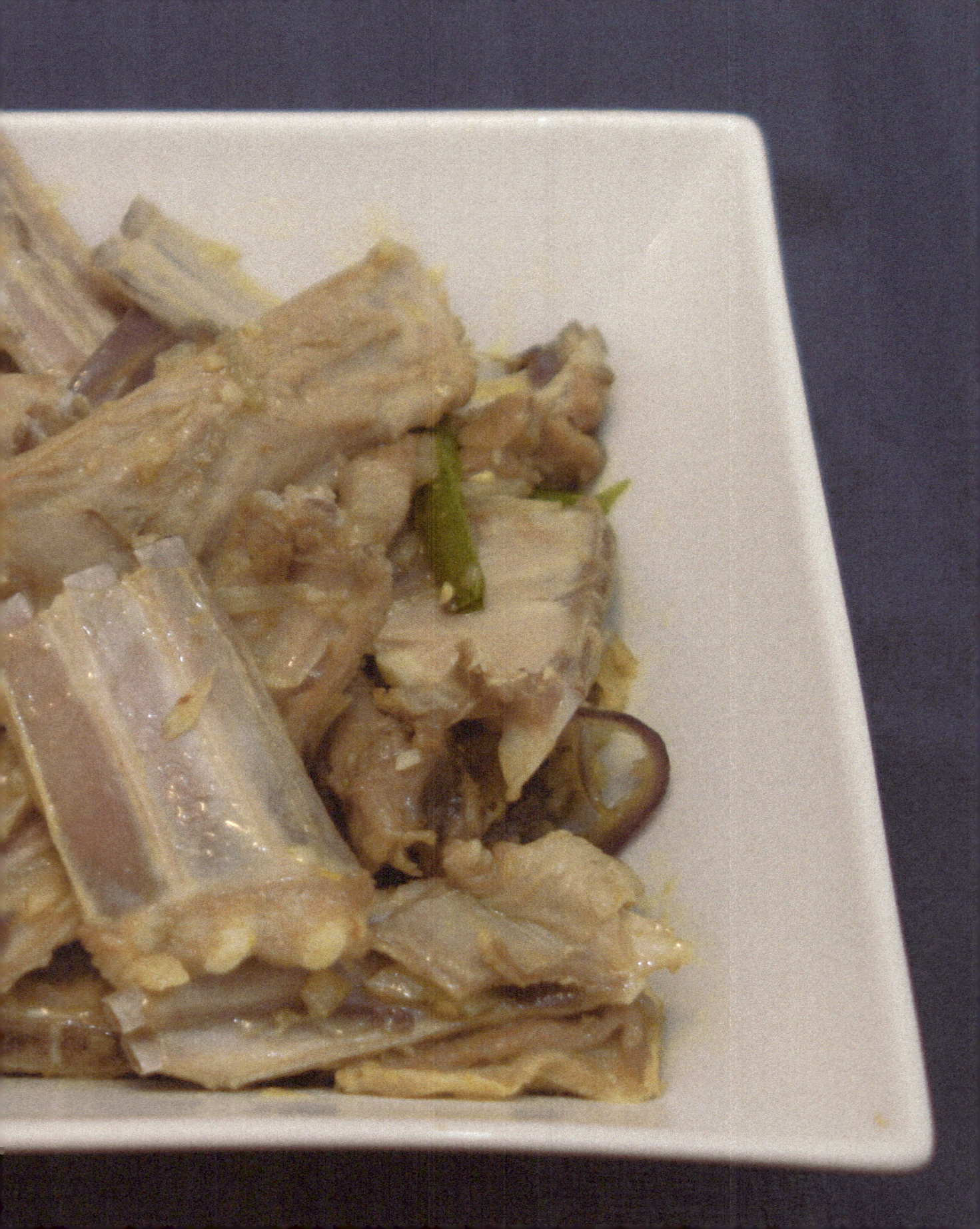

Meat & Seafood

Sautéed Lamb
የበግ ትብስ
(Yebeg Tibbs) GF DF

Time: **20 min**
Serves: **5**
Difficulty:

One of the most popular dishes at my restaurant. If you don't get there early on the day I cook this, you might just be out of luck!

Ingredients:

Lamb, bone-in, 2 lb, ribs or chops
Vegetable oil, 2 Tbsp
Red onion, ½ medium, sliced thinly
Garlic, 4-5 cloves, thinly sliced
Jalapeño, 1, stemmed and quartered lengthwise
Niter Kibe, ½ cup (p. 21)
Salt, ½ tsp

Directions:

1. If using ribs, separate into groups of 3 ribs each and using a heavy knife carefully cut ribs crosswise to expose marrow.
2. Heat oil into a large fry pan over medium-high heat.
3. Add lamb, cook 4–5 min or until meat is seared on all sides.
4. Add onions, garlic, jalapeño, Niter Kibe and salt and stir to mix. Cook 8 min, or until the meat is cooked through.

The Crown Jewel of African Cuisine

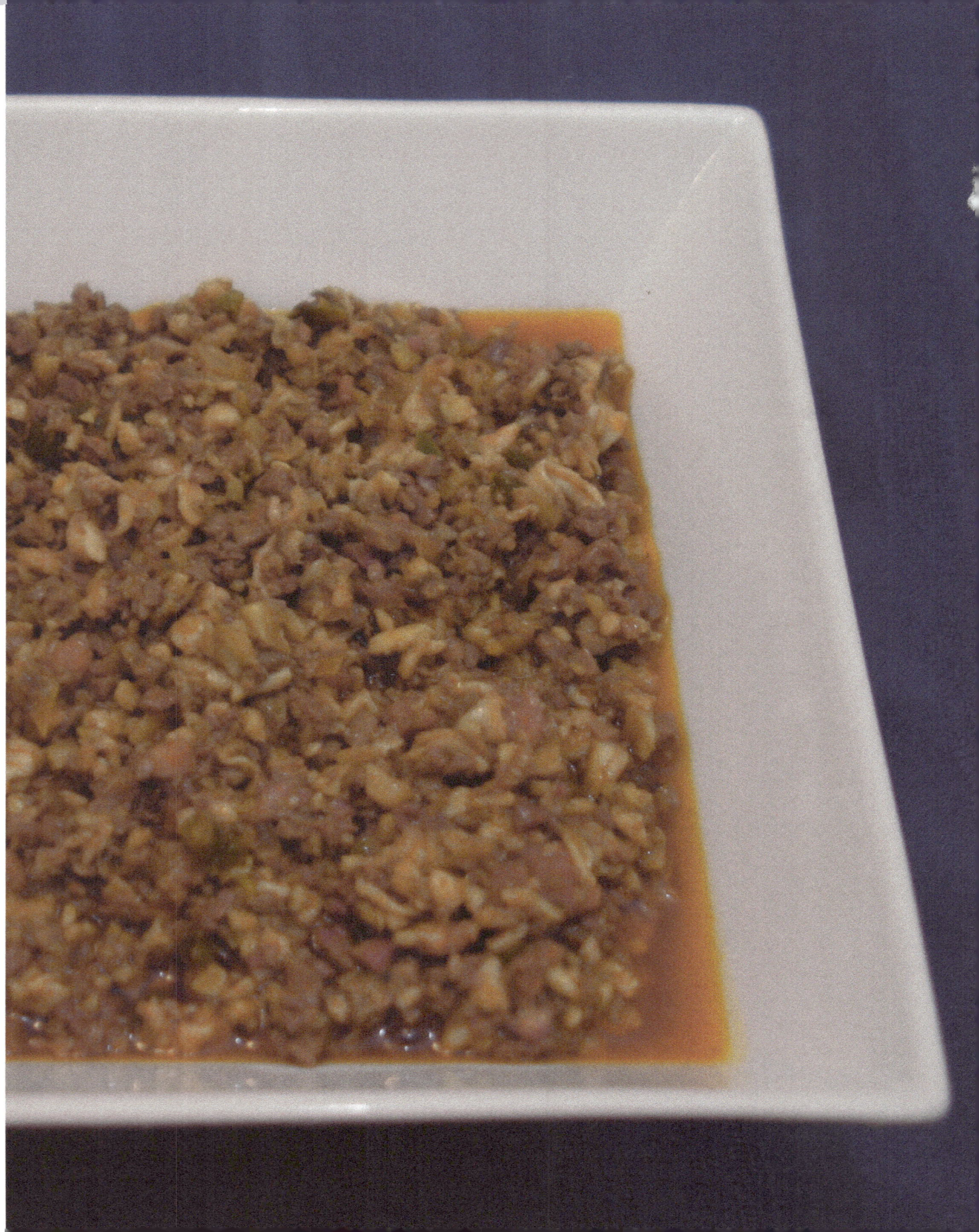

Meat & Seafood

Lamb Dullet
የበግ ዱለት
(Yebeg Dullet) GF DF

Time: 2 hr 30 min
Serves: 6–8
Difficulty: ◆◆◆◆◇

This popular Ethiopian dish features what Americans would describe as undercooked meat along with well cooked meat. As I say in my restaurant, please know that undercooked meat can pose health risks.

Ingredients:

Lamb tripe, 1–1½ lb
Water, ~½ cup total, plus enough to parboil the tripe
Lime, 1
Lamb kidneys, 2
Lamb liver, 1
Lamb tenderloin, 2
Leeks, white part only, ¼ lb, finely minced
Garlic, 1 head, peeled and finely minced
Red onion, ½ medium, finely minced
Jalapeño, 1, stemmed and seeded, finely minced
Vegetable oil, ⅓ cup
Salt, 1 tsp
Niter Kibe, 1 cup (p. 21)
Mitmita*, 2 Tbsp

*available at specialty stores and online, see p. 17

Directions:

1. Bring a large pot of water to a boil, and parboil the tripe for 15 seconds. Remove tripe to cutting board. Use a knife to scrape away the fuzzy lining. If some of the lining remains difficult to remove, parboil a second time and scrape again.

2. Rinse the cleaned tripe thoroughly. Place in bowl and squeeze the juice of one lime over it. Add ½ cup water, mix thoroughly, and marinate 10 min.

3. Trim off any discolored parts and rinse again.

4. Mince tripe finely and place in fine meshed strainer and rinse with cold water. Remove to bowl and set aside in refrigerator.

5. Rinse the liver and kidneys under cold water, and peel away their membranous coverings.

6. Coarsely chop liver and kidneys. Place in food processor and process until finely minced. Set aside in bowl and refrigerate.

7. Peel away the membranous covering of tenderloin. Coarsely chop tenderloin and process in a food processor until finely minced. Place processed tenderloin in bowl and refrigerate.

8. Heat a medium sized pot over medium high. Add leek, garlic, onions and jalapeños. Cook 5 min, stirring to prevent sticking.

9. Add vegetable oil and salt, stir, and cook 10 min, stirring often (if needed, add 2–3 Tbsp water at a time to prevent sticking).

10. Add Niter Kibe, reduce to low heat and simmer about 5 min, until onions are tender and translucent.

11. Remove from heat, add processed meats and mitmita, and stir to mix. Return the pan to medium-low heat. Cook 2 min, which is just long enough to warm it for serving.

The Crown Jewel of African Cuisine

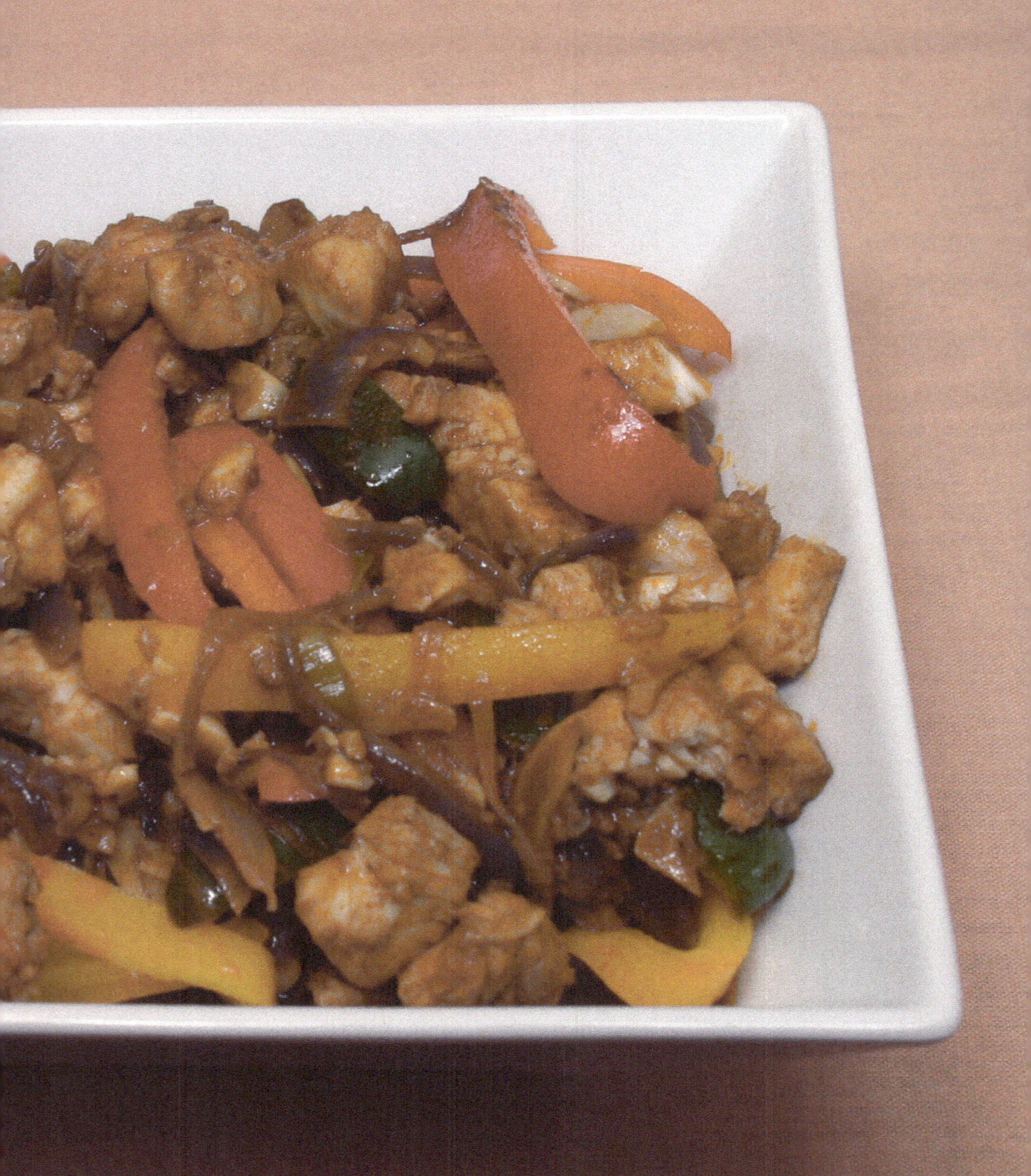

Meat & Seafood

Sautéed Tilapia
የዓሣ ትብስ

(Yeasa Tibbs) GF DF

Time: 20 min
Serves: 5
Difficulty:

Ethiopians traditionally do not eat a lot of fish, but when fish is served, it is almost always the freshwater fish tilapia.

Ingredients:

Tilapia fillets, 2 lb
Lime, 1
Salt, 1 tsp
Vegetable oil, ½ cup
Garlic, 6 cloves, sliced thin
Leek, 1, white and tender green parts, cut crosswise into ¼ inch thick slices
Red onion, ½ large, sliced into ¼ inch thick wedges
Niter Kibe, 2 Tbsp (p. 21)
Berberre paste, 2 Tbsp (p. 29)
Salt, 1 tsp
Cardamom, ½ tsp
Water, ⅓ cup
Red bell pepper, ⅓, julienned to ¼ inch thick pieces
Yellow bell pepper, ⅓, julienned to ¼ inch thick pieces
Jalapeño, 1, stemmed and quartered lengthwise

Directions:

1. Place tilapia fillets in large bowl and squeeze the juice of the lime over them. Mix well with hands to distribute lime juice and then rinse fish.

2. Place fish in a clean bowl and add salt and enough water to cover the fish. Mix with hands. Pour off water. Add enough water again to cover, mix with hands and pour off water. Pat tilapia dry with paper towels.

3. Cut fish into 1 inch dice and set aside.

4. Heat oil in large pot over medium-high heat. Add garlic, leek and onion. Cook 4 min, uncovered, stirring occasionally.

5. Add Niter Kibe, Berberre paste and salt. Cook 2 min, stirring occasionally.

6. Add cardamom, ⅓ cup water, and the fish, and stir gently to mix. Cook 2 min, covered. Gently turn fish and cook 2 min more, covered.

7. Add bell peppers and jalapeños, stir gently to mix, and remove from heat.

The Crown Jewel of African Cuisine

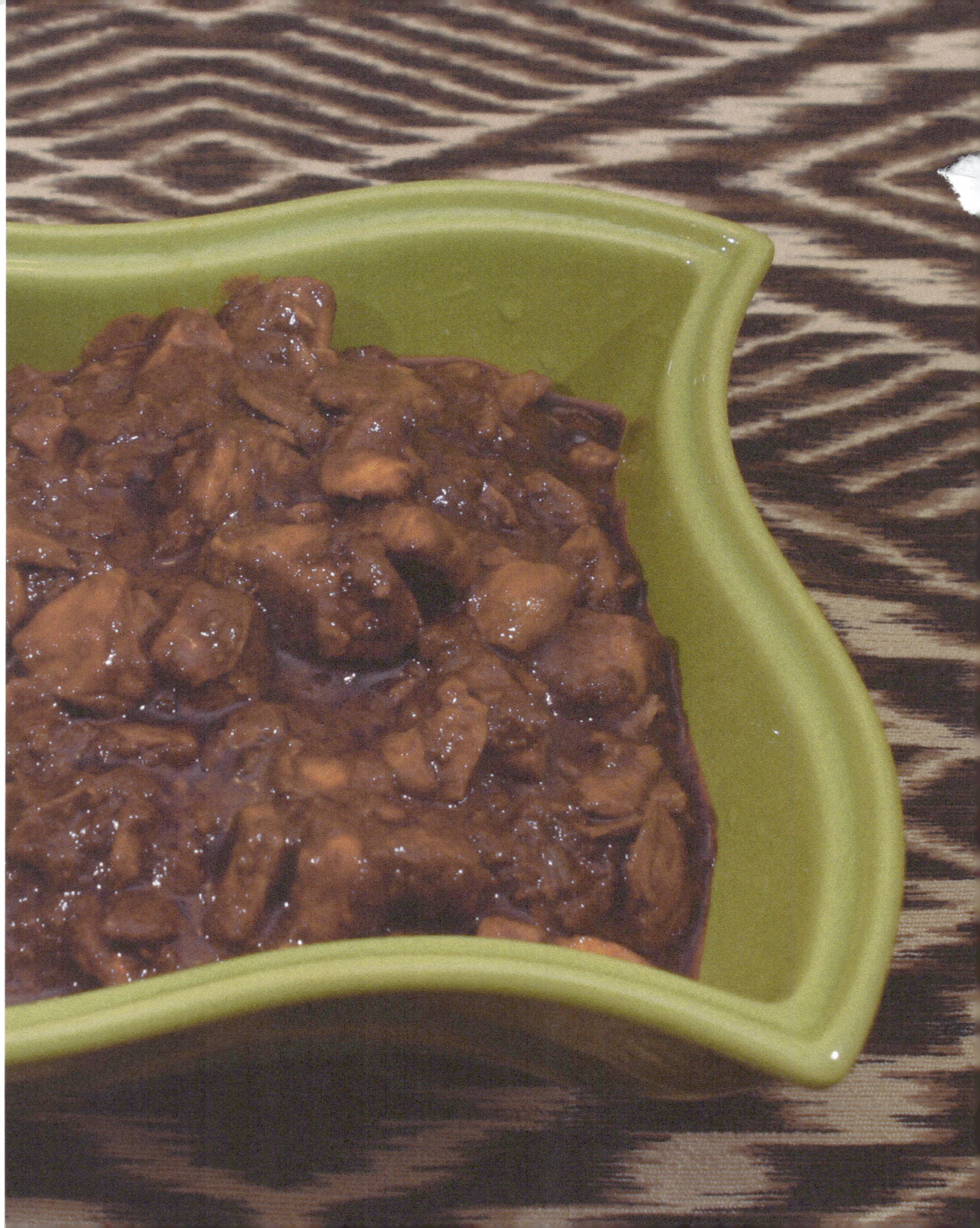

Salmon Stew
የዓሳ ወጥ
(Yeasa Wat) GF DF

Meat & Seafood

Time: **1 hr 30 min**
Serves: **6**
Difficulty:

In Ethiopia, we usually make this fish stew, which requires a firm fish, with tuna. I have lived for many years in the Pacific Northwest and now use salmon to create this striking version of Asa Wat.

Ingredients:
Salmon fillets, 2½–3 lb
Lime, 1
Yellow onion, 2 large, finely chopped
Vegetable oil, ½ cup
Water, 10 cups total
Berberre paste, 1 cup (p. 29)
Ginger-Garlic Paste, 1 tsp (p. 23)
Salt, 1½ tsp
Niter Kibe, 2 Tbsp (p. 21)
Q'imam, ½ tsp (p. 25)

Directions:
1. Rinse salmon in cold water. Squeeze juice of lime over the salmon. Rinse salmon again and pat dry with paper towels.
2. Remove the salmon skin and cut the meat into 1 inch dice.
3. Place onions and 6 cups water in large pot over medium-high heat. Cook 25 min, partially covered, or until onions are translucent but not browned. During this time, stir frequently and add water, ½ cup at a time, to prevent sticking.
4. Add oil, stir to mix, and cook 7 min, uncovered, stirring occasionally.
5. Add Berberre paste and cook 8 min, stirring occasionally, adding ½ cup water twice during this time.
6. Add Ginger-Garlic Paste and reduce heat to medium low. Cook 25 min, stirring occasionally. During this time, add 3 cups water, ½ cup at a time, to prevent sticking.
7. Add salmon, salt, Niter Kibe and Q'imam and stir to mix. Cook another 5 min, stirring occasionally.

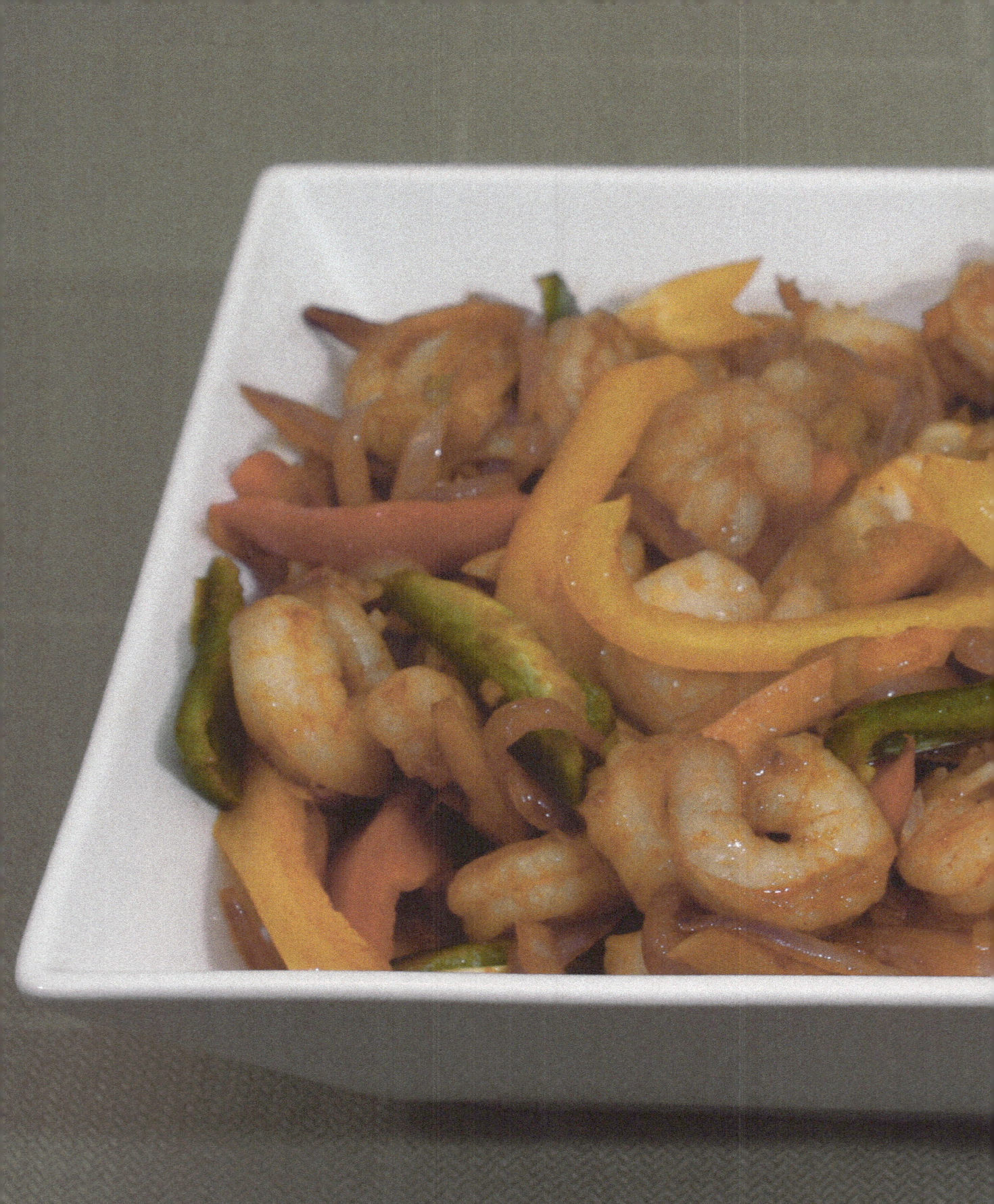

Meat & Seafood

Ethiopian Style Shrimp Scampi
እንቁርካር ትብስ
(Ankurkar Tibbs) GF DF

Time: 30 min
Serves: 3–4
Difficulty: ♨♨♧♧♧

Where I live now, seafood is abundant, so I created this scampi in Ethiopian style (shrimp is not traditionally eaten in Ethiopia). Enjoy this Tibbs with the freshest available shrimp.

Ingredients:

- Shrimp, ½ lb (~50–60 medium)
- Lime, ½
- Vegetable oil, ⅓ cup
- Leek, 1, removing all but bottom 4 inches
- Red onion, 1, cut in half and then into ¼ inch wedges
- Garlic, 10 cloves, thinly sliced
- Niter Kibe, 1 Tbsp (p. 21)
- Berberre paste, 1 Tbsp (p. 29)
- Salt, 1 tsp
- Jalapeño, stemmed and seeded, cut into 2 inch by ¼ inch strips
- Red, yellow, orange bell pepper, ⅕ of each, cut into 2 inch by ¼ inch strips

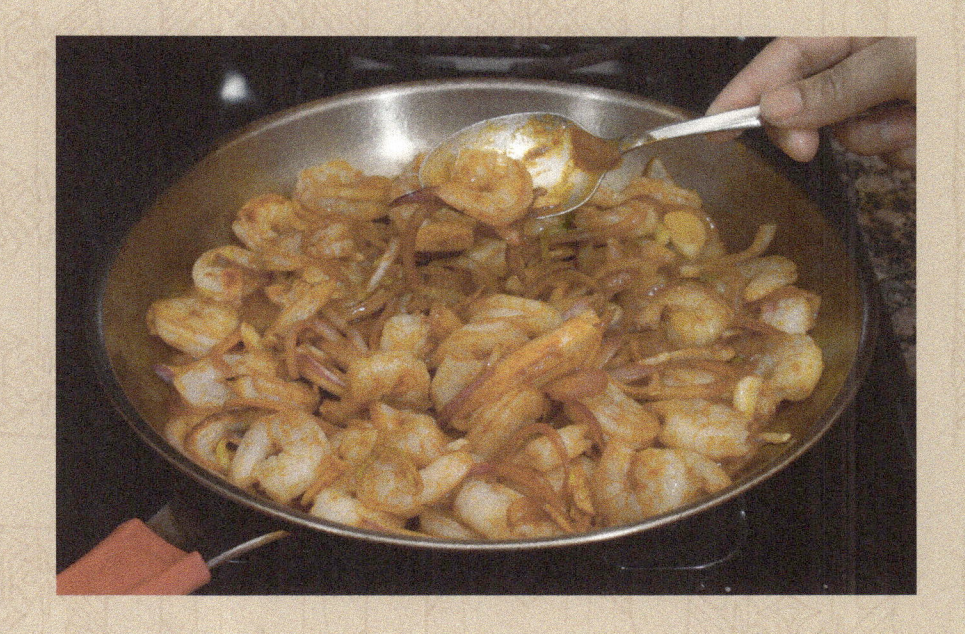

Directions:

1. Peel and devein shrimp and place into bowl. Squeeze juice of lime over it. Mix thoroughly with hands. Rinse under cold water and drain in a colander.
2. Cut leek in half lengthwise, then slice crosswise into ⅛ inch wide slices.
3. Heat oil in large frying pan over high heat. Add leek, onion and garlic and cook 5 min, stirring frequently.
4. Add Niter Kibe, Berberre paste and salt and stir well. Add shrimp and stir to combine, and cook 5 min, stirring constantly.
5. Add jalapeño and bell peppers and remove from heat. Let stand a few min before serving.

The Crown Jewel of African Cuisine

Buttermilk Cheese with Kale (p. 119).

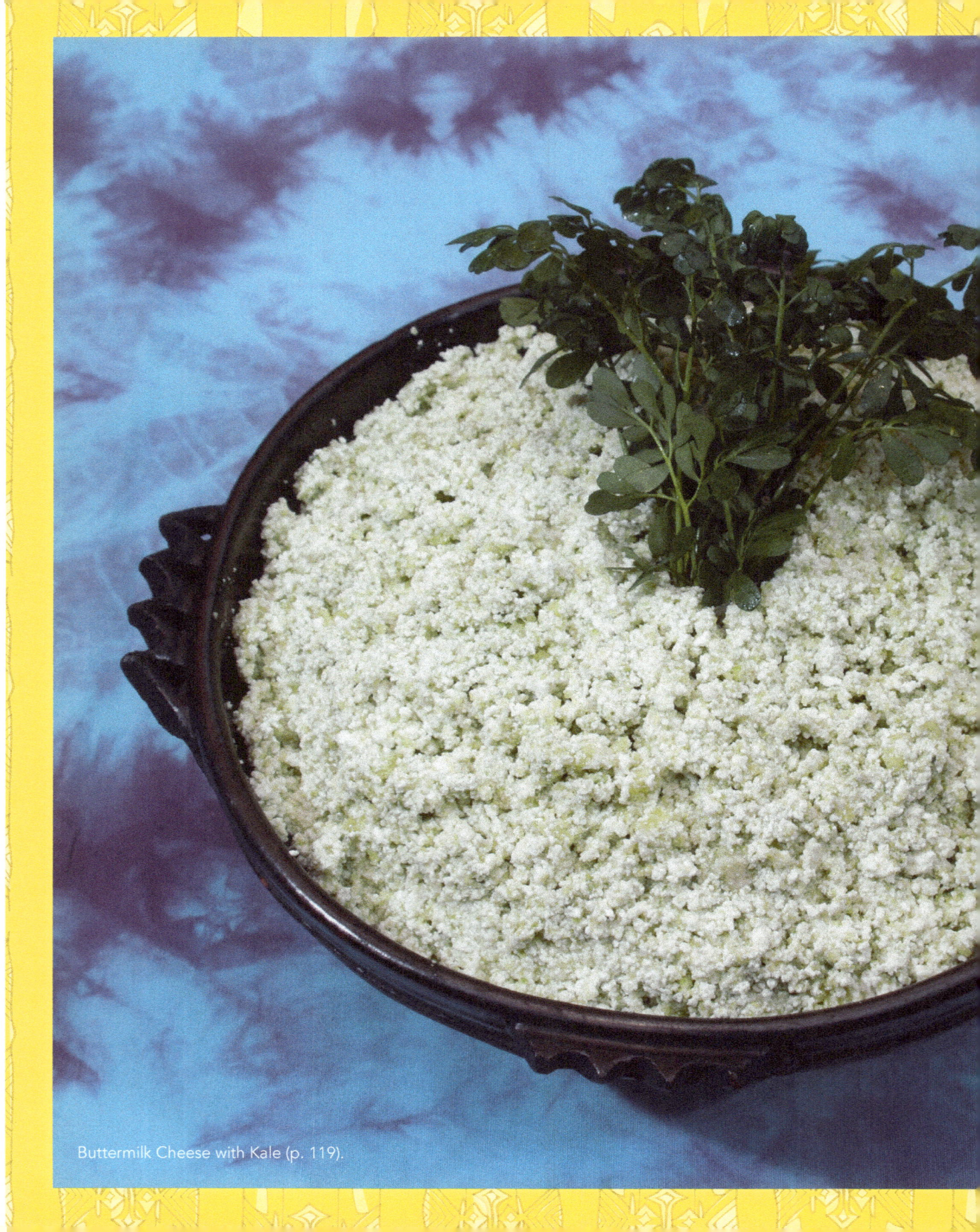

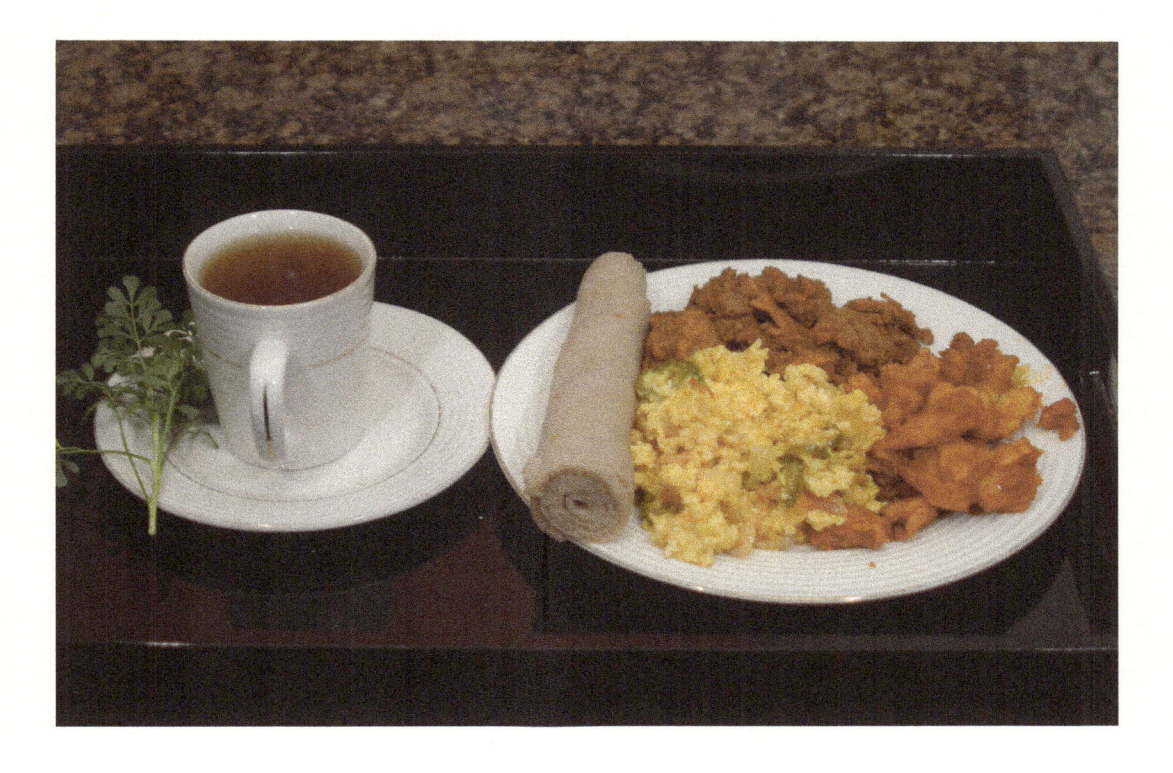

Farm Fresh:
Cheese and Eggs

When I was a girl, we always had chickens running in the yard. I love using eggs and fresh made cheeses to liven up a meal. Like Americans, we enjoy eggs for breakfast in Ethiopia. Here are some spicy egg stews and homemade cottage cheese recipes to add to your breakfast or brunch routine. They also make excellent side dishes for lunch or dinner.

Above: Traditional Ethiopian breakfast, clockwise from front: Ethiopian Style Scrambled Eggs (p. 115), Spicy Eggs Fitfit (p. 113) and Spicy Torn Bread (p. 47).

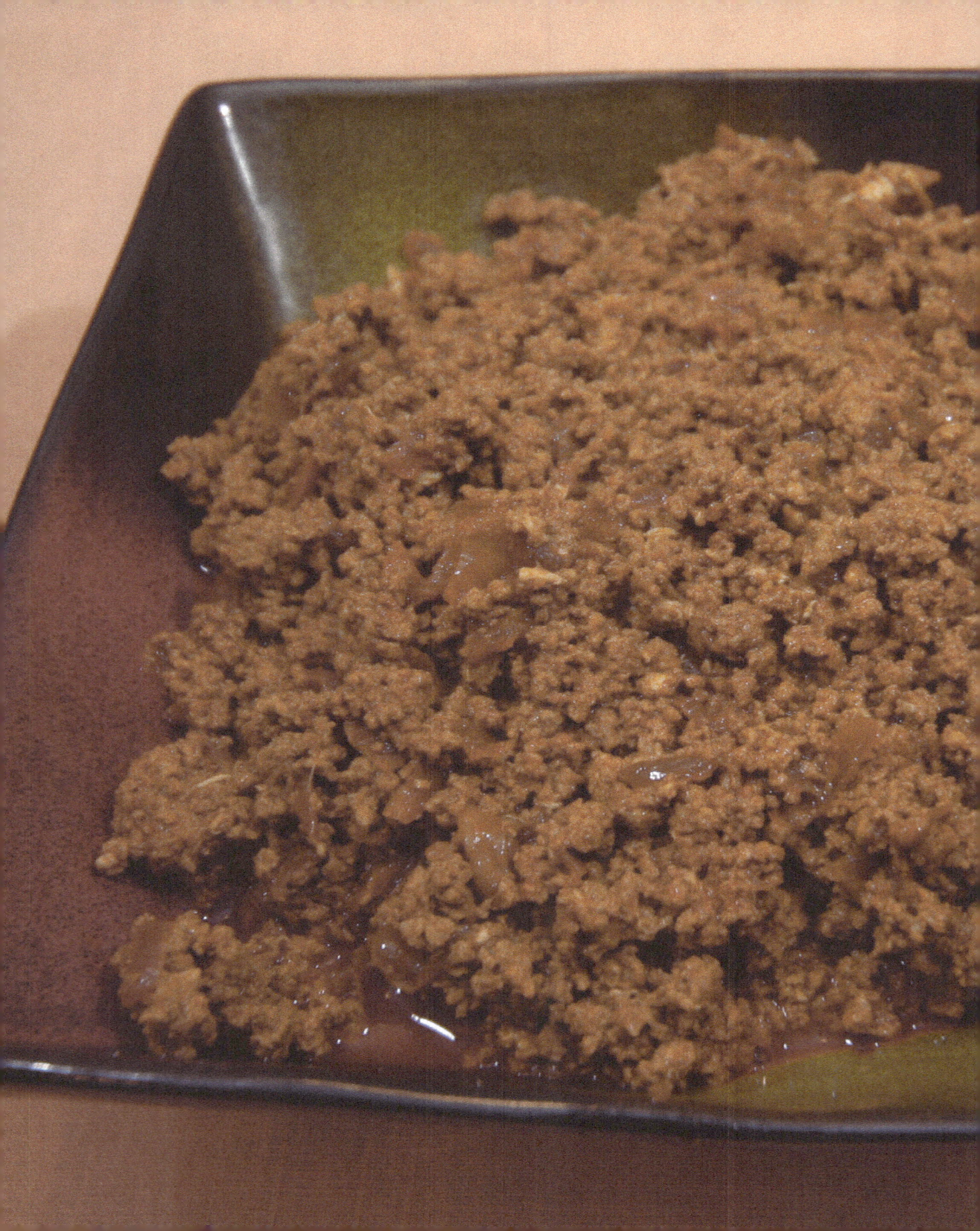

Spicy Egg Stew
የእንቁላል ወጥ
(Yeenqulal Wat) (V) (GF) (DF)

Traditional Ethiopian egg dish that makes a tasty weekend brunch on Injera (p. 33).

Cheese & Eggs

Time: 40 min
Serves: 5
Difficulty: ♦♦♦◇◇

Ingredients:

Yellow onion, 1 large, finely diced
Vegetable oil, ½ cup
Berberre paste, ½ cup (p. 29)
Ginger-Garlic Paste, 1 tsp (p. 23)
Water, ~2 cups total
Salt, 1½ tsp
Eggs, 8
Niter Kibe, ¼ cup (p. 21)
Q'imam, ½ cup (p. 25)

Directions:

1. Heat a large pot over high heat.
2. Add onions and cook 4 min, stirring occasionally.
3. Add oil and cook 4 min, stirring occasionally.
4. Add Berberre paste and 2 Tbsp water and stir to mix. Immediately add Ginger-Garlic Paste, salt and ½ cup water and stir to mix.
5. Reduce heat to medium and cook 15 min, stirring occasionally to prevent sticking. When the mixture gets dry and begins to stick, add 2 Tbsp water at a time, as necessary. You will likely end up adding around ½ cup water.
6. Whisk 8 eggs in a medium sized bowl. Add eggs and ½ cup water to the pot. Cook 3 min, stirring frequently until mixture thickens.
7. Add Niter Kibe, stir, and cook 4 min, stirring frequently.
8. Add Q'imam, stir, and cook 5 min, covered, stirring occasionally.

The Crown Jewel of African Cuisine

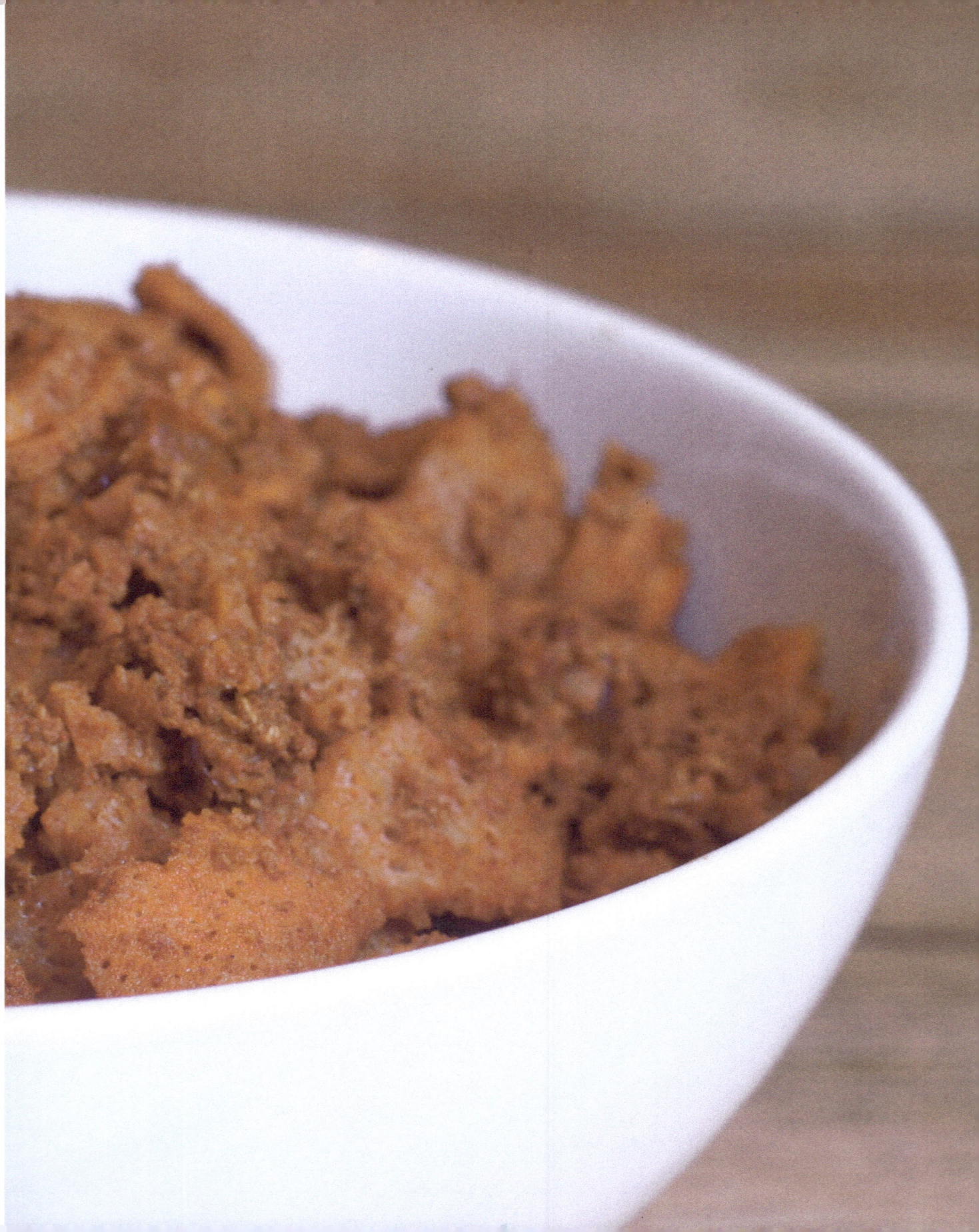

Cheese & Eggs

Spicy Eggs Fitfit
የእንቁላል ፍትፍት
(Yeenqulal Fitfit) (V) (GF) (DF)

Time: 20 min
Serves: 5–6
Difficulty:

A variation on Spicy Egg Stew (p. 111) to take advantage of leftover Injera (p. 33).

Ingredients:

Vegetable oil, ½ cup
Yellow onion, 1 large, diced
Water, 2½ cups, divided
Berberre paste, ¾ cup (p. 29)
Niter Kibe, ½ cup (p. 21)
Salt, 2 Tbsp
Eggs, 5
Injera, 3 rounds

Directions:

1. Heat oil in pot over medium-high heat. Add onion and cook 5 min, stirring to prevent sticking.
2. Add Berberre paste, Niter Kibe, salt, and ¼ water. Simmer 4 min, stirring occasionally.
3. Add another 1¾ cup water, stir to mix, and cook 3 min, covered.
4. Whisk eggs in small bowl.
5. Add eggs to pot and stir quickly with rapid strokes. Add ½ cup water, mix. Cook 5 min, covered.
6. Remove from heat.
7. Break up Injera into bite-sized pieces. Add to egg mixture and gently stir to combine thoroughly.

The Crown Jewel of African Cuisine

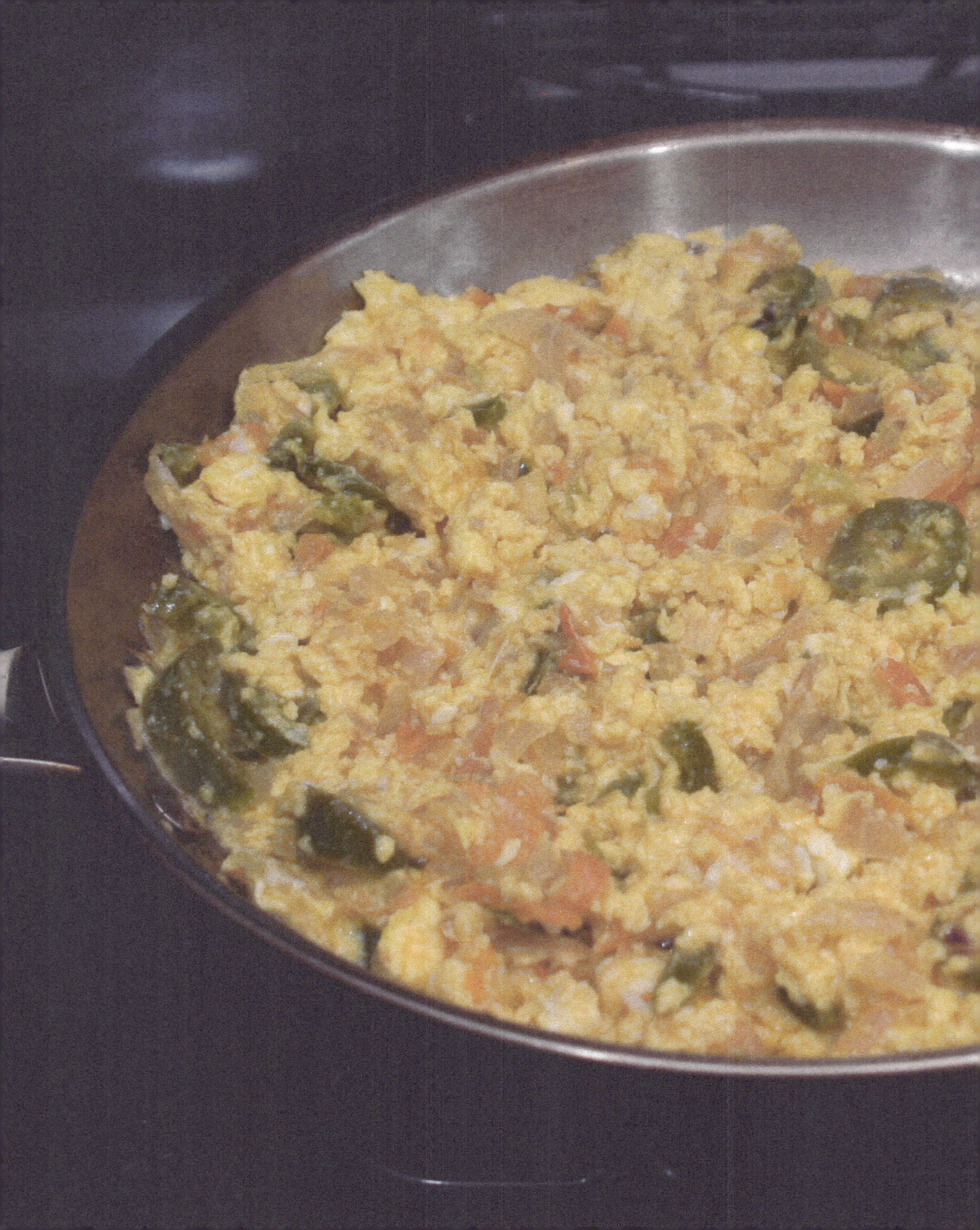

Ethiopian Style Scrambled Eggs
የእንቁላል ትብስ
(Yeenqulal Tibbs) (V) (GF) (DF)

Time: 15 min
Serves: 5
Difficulty:

For the ultimate Ethiopian brunch, serve these eggs with Spicy Egg Stew (p. 111), Spicy Eggs Fitfit (p. 113), Spicy Torn Bread (p. 47), and Spicy Breakfast Bread (p. 45).

Ingredients:
Vegetable oil, ¼ cup
Red onion, 1 medium, finely diced
Plum tomatoes, 3, diced
Jalapeños, 2, cut into ¼ inch thick rings
Niter Kibe, ½ cup (p. 21)
Salt, pinch
Eggs, 10

Directions:
1. Heat oil in a nonstick frying pan over medium-high heat.
2. Add onion, tomatoes, jalapeños, Niter Kibe, and salt, stir to mix, and simmer 10 min, stirring occasionally.
3. While the vegetables are simmering, crack 10 eggs into a bowl and set aside.
4. After 10 min of simmering, add eggs to pan, stir quickly to combine. Stir eggs until they are fully cooked and scrambled, about 2 min.

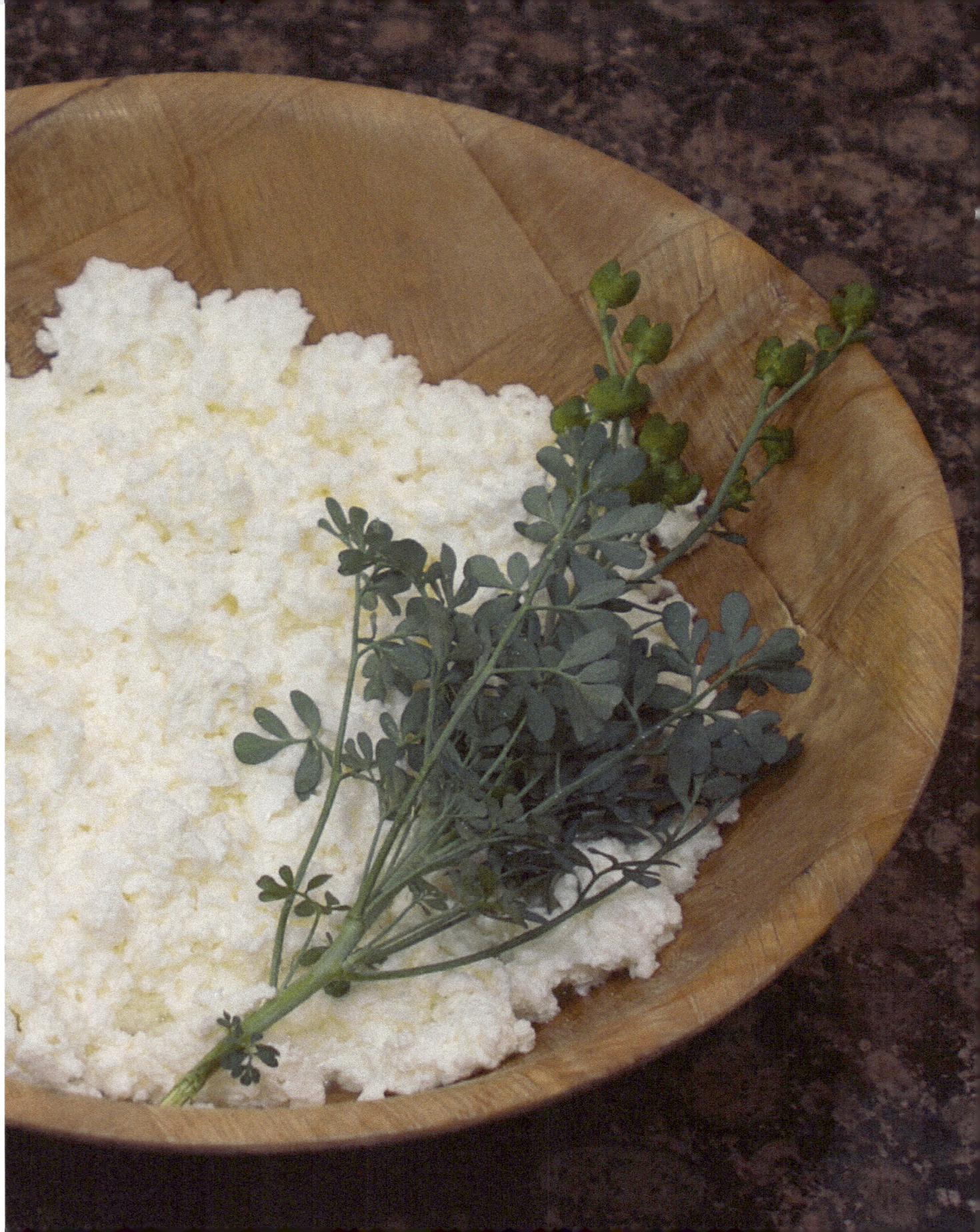

Cheese & Eggs

Basic & Spicy Cottage Cheese
አይብ, አይብ በ ቅቤ ና ምትምጣ
(Ayib, Ayib Be Qibe Na Mitmita) (V) (GF)

Time: 15 min, plus 1 hr to cool
Serves: 6–8
Difficulty: ♦◊◊◊◊

You can add this refreshing side dish to cool the palate in any spicy Ethiopian meal.

Ingredients:

Buttermilk, ½ gallon (can substitute 1 gallon 2% or whole milk, but if you do this, add 1¾ cup white vinegar)

Directions:

1. Pour buttermilk into a large pot. Cook over high heat, uncovered, for 6 min without stirring.
2. Reduce heat to medium low. Cook 7 min without stirring.
3. Remove from heat. Cover and refrigerate at least 1 hour until cooled.
4. Pour the cheese and the watery whey into a fine strainer (or colander lined with cheese cloth) and let it drain thoroughly.
5. Place the cheese in a serving bowl and refrigerate.

For a Spicy Variation (pictured as side dish for "Traditional Spicy Breakfast Cake" on page 51:

Melt ¼ cup Niter Kibe (p. 21). Add 2 tsp Berberre powder*, or if you want it even spicier, use mitmita* and thoroughly mix. Pour over top of cheese and mix. For a very different spicy variation, add Jalapeño Relish (p. 27) to taste, instead of Berberre powder or mitmita.

*available at specialty stores and online, see p. 15

The Crown Jewel of African Cuisine

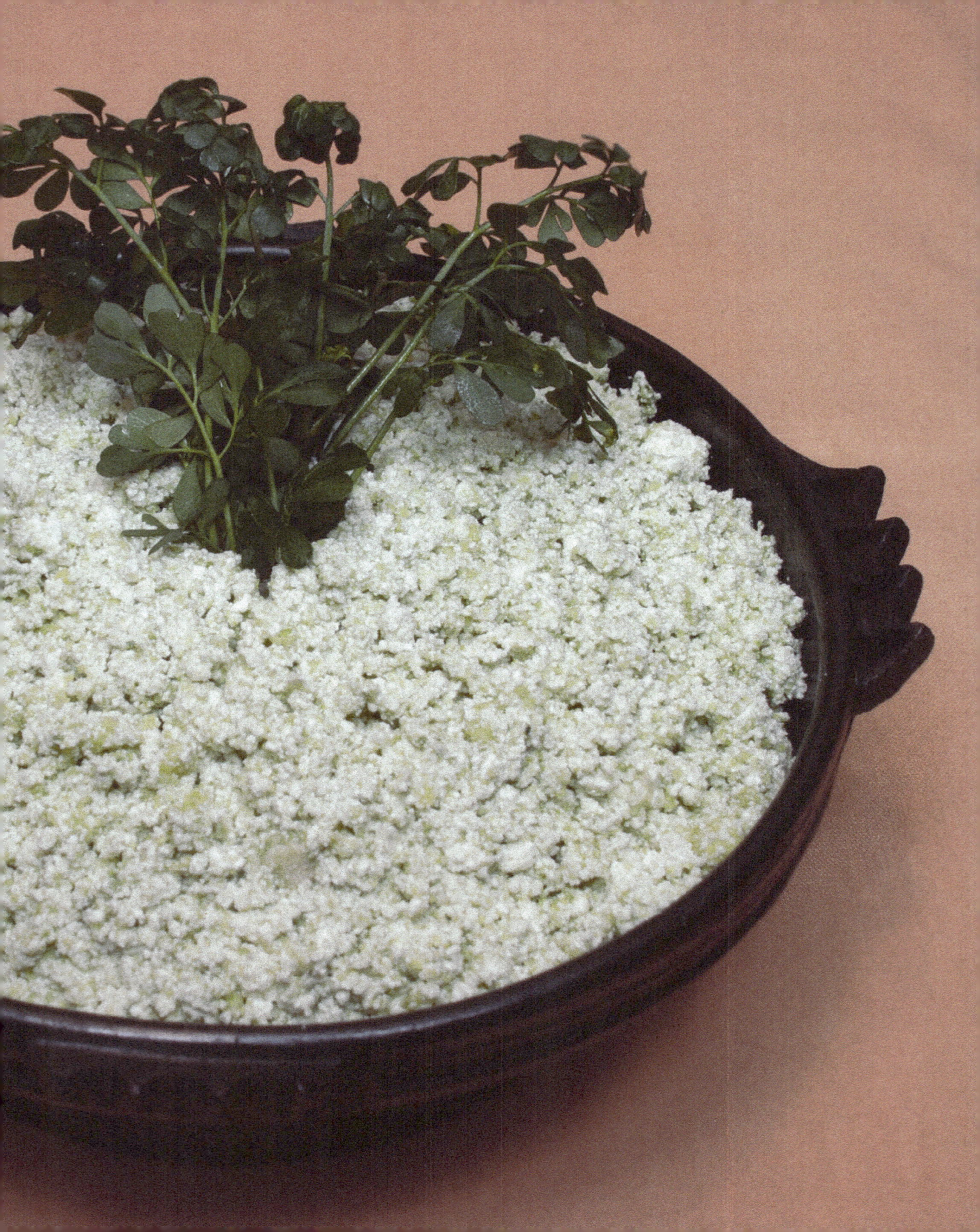

Cheese & Eggs

Buttermilk Cheese with Kale
ዓይብ በጎመን
(Ayib Be Gomen) (V) (GF)

Time: 1 hr 15 min
Serves: 6–8
Difficulty:

I love this splash of brightness on a platter of Injera (p. 33). This variation of buttermilk cheese is particularly popular in the Gurage region of Southwestern Ethiopia.

Ingredients:

Buttermilk, ½ gallon (can substitute 1 gallon 2% or whole milk, but if you do this, add 1¾ cup white vinegar)
Kale, 1 large leaf
Garlic, 2 large cloves, peeled
Jalapeño, 1, cut into large chunks, without removing seeds
Salt, ½ tsp
Water, ¼ cup
Niter Kibe, ¼ cup (p. 21)

Directions:

Make the cheese

1. Pour buttermilk into large pot over high heat, uncovered, and cook 6 min, without stirring.
2. Reduce heat to medium-low, and cook 7 more min, without stirring.
3. Turn off heat, cover the pot, and put it in the refrigerator to cool for 1 hour (while cooling, prepare the kale mix, following the directions below).
4. Pour the cheese and the watery whey into a fine strainer (or colander lined with cheese cloth) and let it drain thoroughly.
5. Place the cheese in a serving bowl and refrigerate.

Prepare the kale mix

1. Put kale in a small pot, add enough water to cover it, and cook over high heat, uncovered, for 25 min.
2. After the kale is cooked, chop it into large pieces and place it in a blender, along with the garlic, jalapeño chunks, salt, and water. Blend 1 min, until smooth.
3. Add spiced clarified butter (Niter Kibe) to a small pot and cook over medium-high heat. Once the Niter Kibe is melted, add the blended kale mixture, stir to combine, and cover. Cook 4 min, then remove the pot from the heat and allow it to cool for several min.

Combine the kale mixture with the cheese

1. Once the strained cheese and kale/butter mixture are both cool, pour the kale/butter mixture over the cheese and stir with a spoon until thoroughly combined.
2. Serve over Injera.

The Crown Jewel of African Cuisine

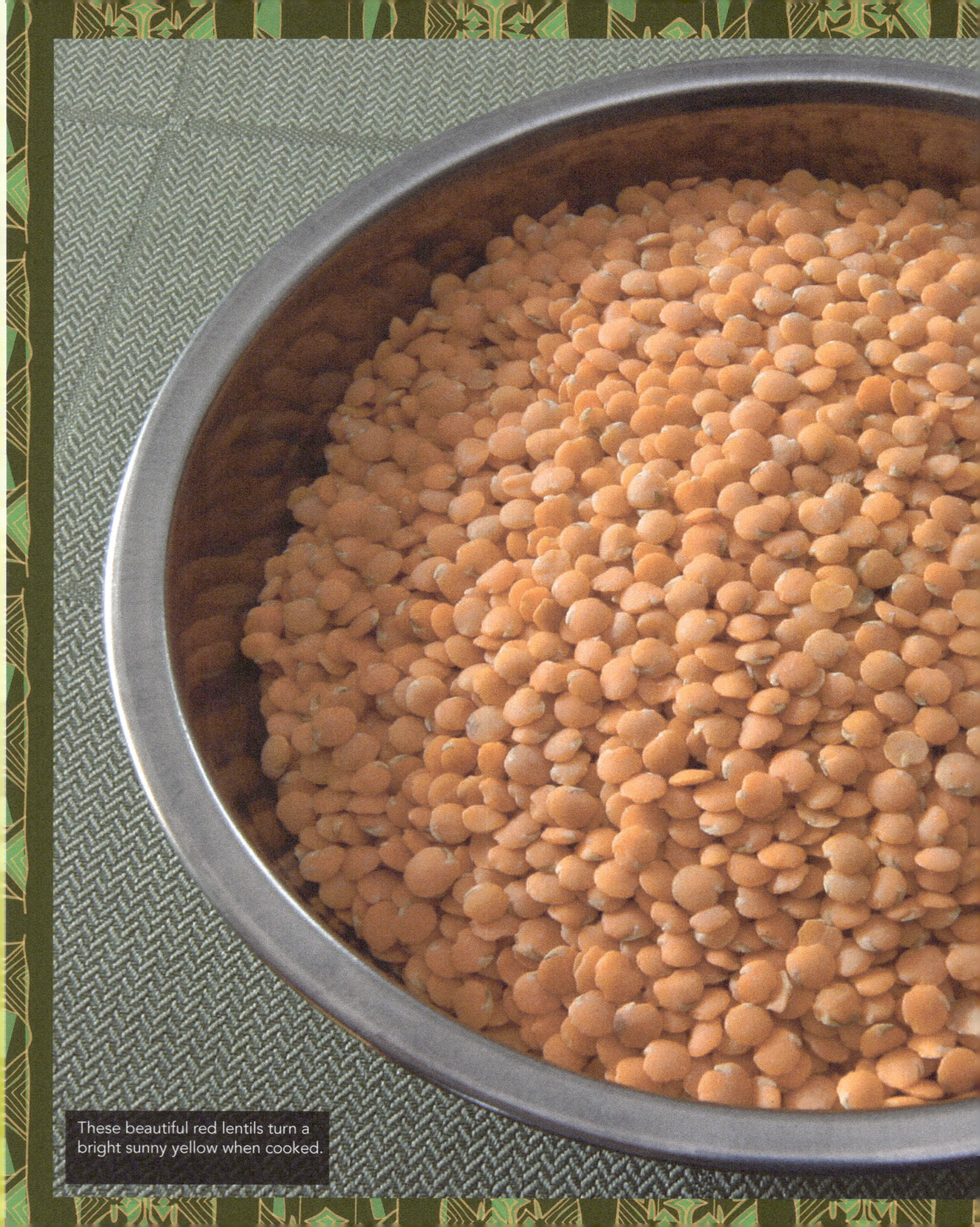

These beautiful red lentils turn a bright sunny yellow when cooked.

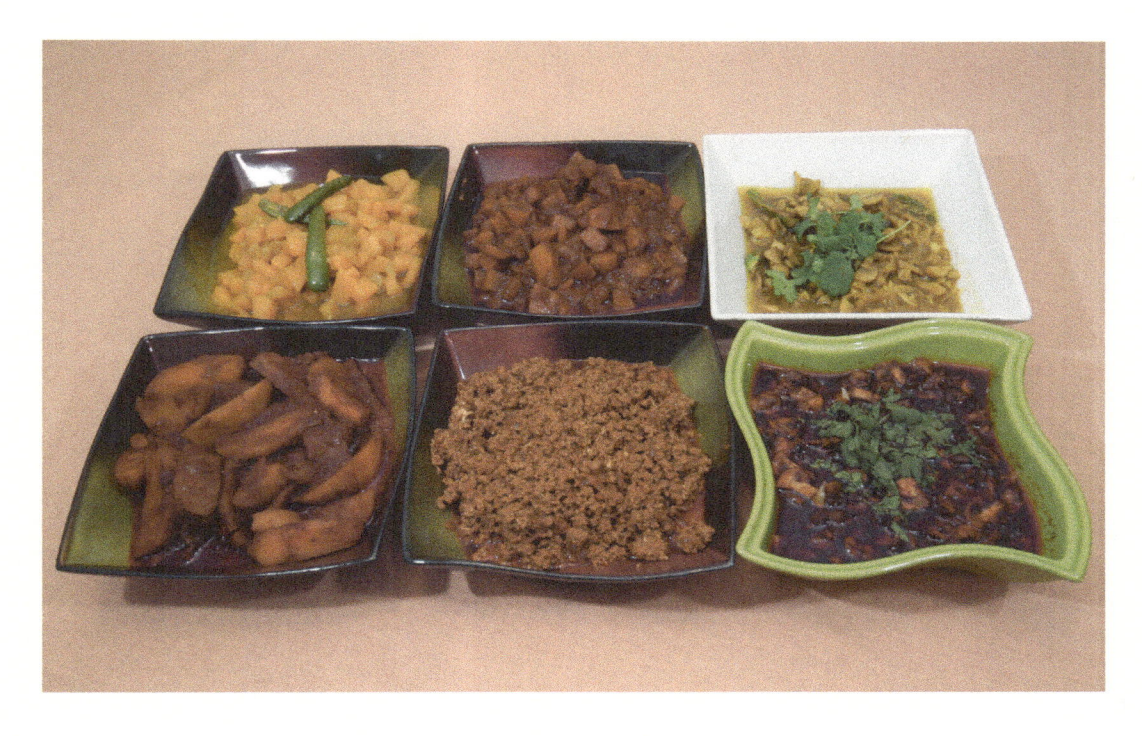

Hearty Vegetables: Lentil Stews

In Ethiopia, meat is considered the very best. If a woman serves lentils to guests, they say, oh she did a very bad job. If she serves chicken, they say, oh what a good job she did! Even though I grew up this way, these days my favorite foods are vegetables, especially lentils. They are healthier for all of us and there are so many different kinds of vegetables. In Ethiopia, we do our best cooking with what is common and not so expensive. So we have many wonderful vegetable dishes.

Lentils and split peas are very popular staples. Here are recipes for traditional lentil stews and split pea stews. We also enjoy squash in Ethiopia. Here are my recipes for cooking turban squash, acorn squash and butternut squash. They are very filling and have very beautiful colors, red, yellow, and gold.

I now live in the Pacific Northwest where there are so many kinds of mushrooms. I love eating them in Ethiopian-style, and have shared a couple of my recipes here.

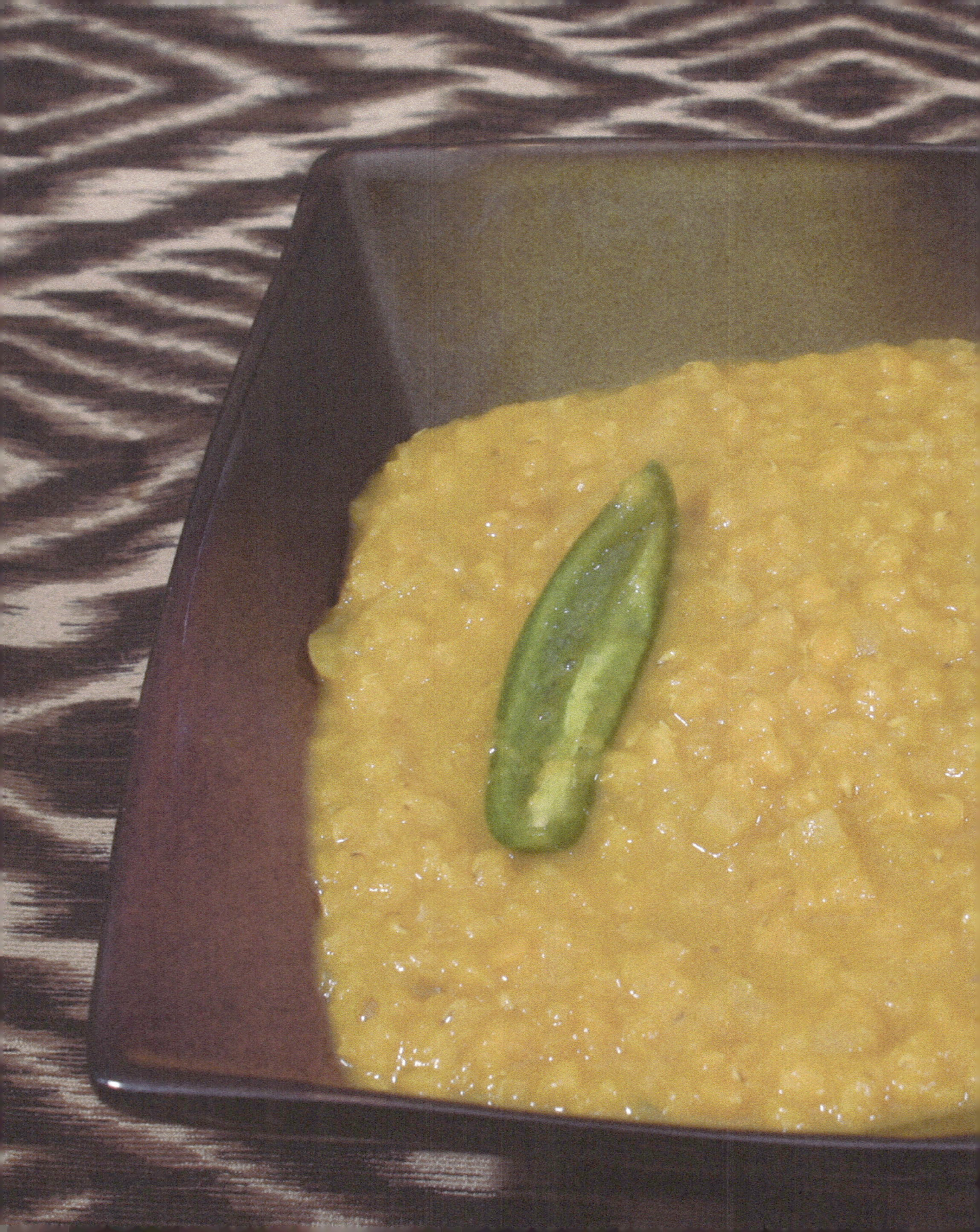

Vegetarian Stews

Red Lentil Stew
የምስር አልጫ
(Yemiser Alicha) V VG GF DF

Time: 50 min
Serves: 5–6
Difficulty:

The lentil dishes (red, green) describe the color of the before cooked.

Ingredients:

Yellow onion, 1 large, finely diced
Water, 6 cups total
Vegetable oil, ½ cup
Turmeric, ½ tsp
Ginger-Garlic Paste, 1 tsp (p. 23)
Salt, 1 tsp
Dried red lentils, 2 cups, rinsed (be sure to remove any stones)
Jalapeño, 1, stemmed and seeded, quartered lengthwise

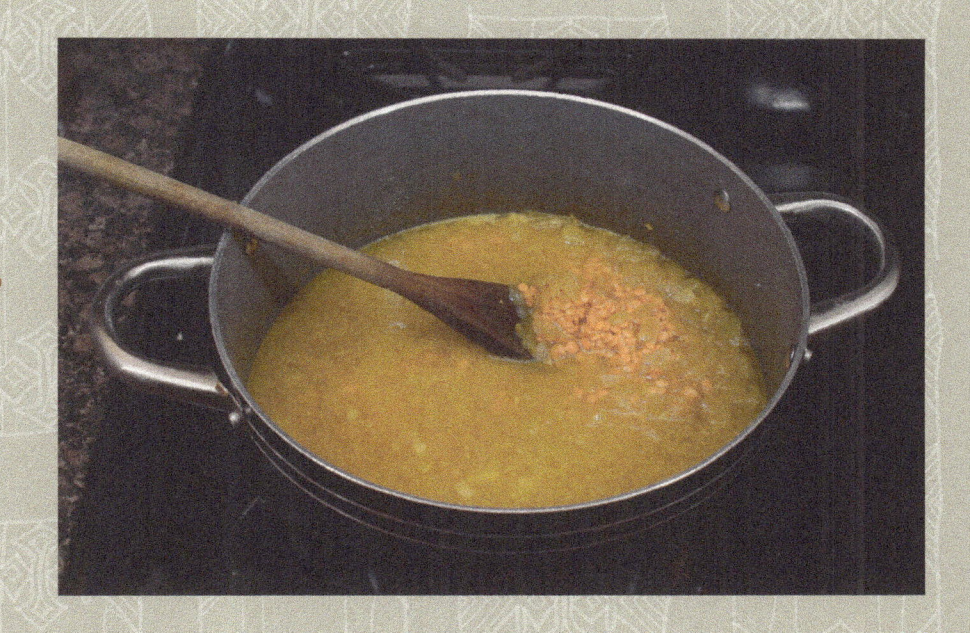

Directions:

1. Heat a medium saucepan over medium-high heat.
2. Place onions in saucepan and cook 8 min, uncovered, stirring occasionally to prevent sticking.
3. Add 1 cup water and cook 5 min.
4. Add oil, stir to mix and cook 4 min, stirring occasionally.
5. Add ½ cup water and stir to mix. Cook 4 min.
6. Add turmeric, Ginger-Garlic Paste, salt, ½ cup water, stir, and cook 7 min.
7. Add lentils and remaining 4 cups water. Cook 20 min, stirring occasionally to prevent sticking.
8. Remove from heat to a serving bowl. Garnish with jalapeño.

The Crown Jewel of African Cuisine

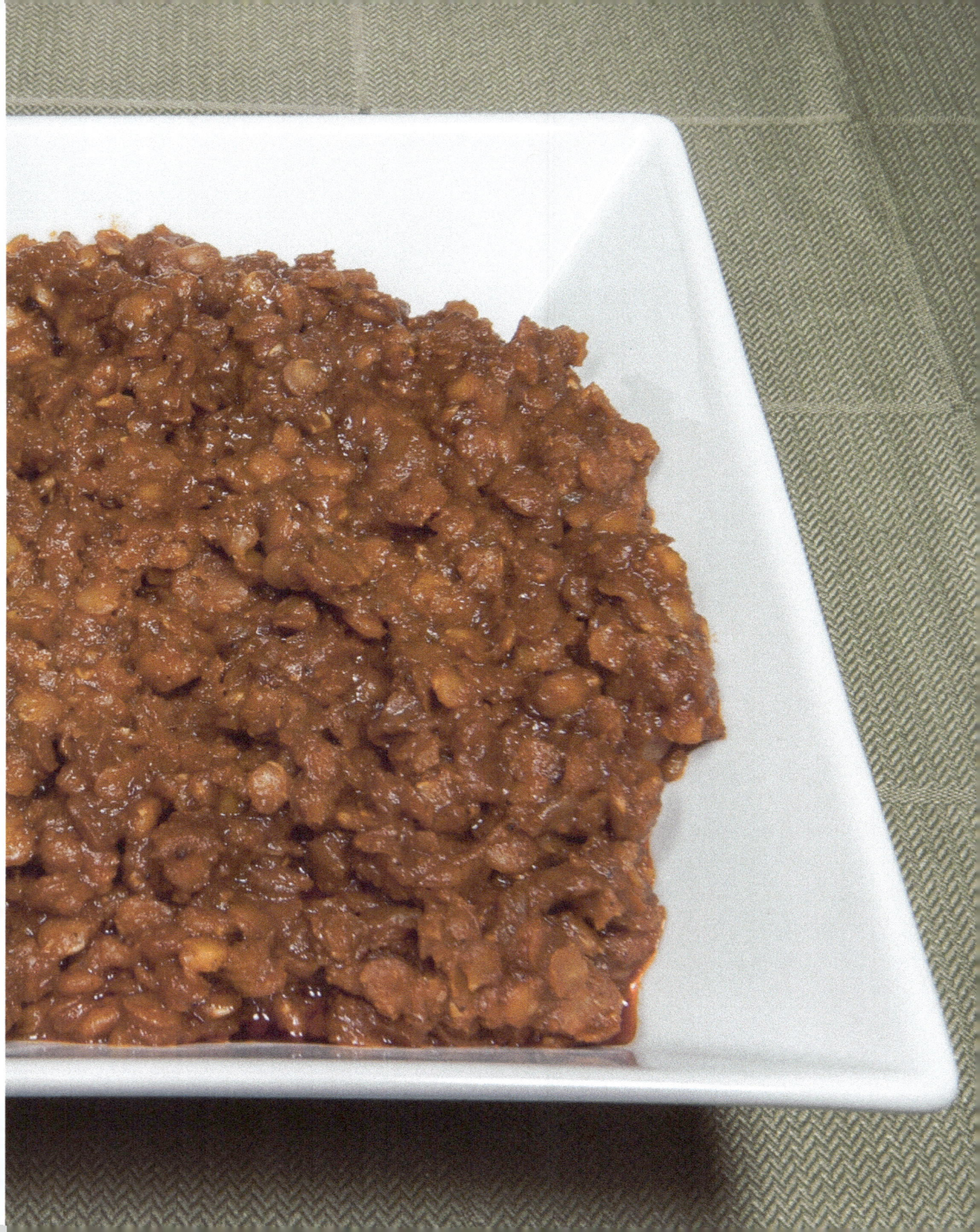

Vegetarian Stews

Spicy Red Lentil Stew
የምስር ወጥ
(Yemiser Wat) (V) (VG) (GF) (DF)

Time: 1 hr
Serves: 6-8
Difficulty: ♦♦♦◊◊

When we cannot eat meat, either during Lent or if meat is unavailable, Ethiopians prefer lentils. We eat these along with greens and other vegetables to make a complete meal.

Ingredients:
- Yellow onions, 2 large, finely diced
- Vegetable oil, 1 cup
- Water, 6 cups total
- Berberre paste, 1 cup (p. 29)
- Ginger-Garlic Paste, 1½ Tbsp (p. 23)
- Salt, 3 tsp
- Red lentils, 3 cups, rinsed (be sure to remove any stones)
- Q'imam, 1 tsp (p. 25)

Directions:
1. Set aside 6 cups water.
2. Put diced onions and ¼ cup of the water in a large pot over medium-high heat, and cook, covered, for 15 min, or until the onions are translucent, stirring after 5–7 min, and then every 2–3 min after that, to prevent sticking. Each time you stir the onions, add ¼ cup water or less, as needed to prevent sticking.
3. Add oil, scrape pan bottom, stir to mix, reduce heat to medium, and cook, covered, for 8 min, stirring every few min and adding ¼ cup of the water with each stirring, if necessary, to prevent sticking.
4. Add Berberre paste, stir, and cook 3 min, covered.
5. Add Ginger-Garlic Paste, salt, and ¼ cup water, scrape the bottom and cook 12 min, uncovered. During this time, stir and scrape the bottom every couple min and add a small amount of the water (no more than ¼ cup at at time), to prevent sticking.
6. Add lentils and all but 1 cup of the remaining water, stir to mix thoroughly, and increase heat to high. Cover, bring to a boil, reduce heat to medium, scrape the bottom, and simmer 6 min.
7. Stir, scrape the bottom again, add the finishing spice mix (Q'imam) the last 1 cup of water, and simmer until lentils are tender (~8 min), stirring and scraping the bottom frequently to prevent sticking. If the lentils are still not tender after 8 min, stir in an additional ½ cup water and cook a few more min. Repeat if necessary.
8. Serve over Injera.

The Crown Jewel of African Cuisine

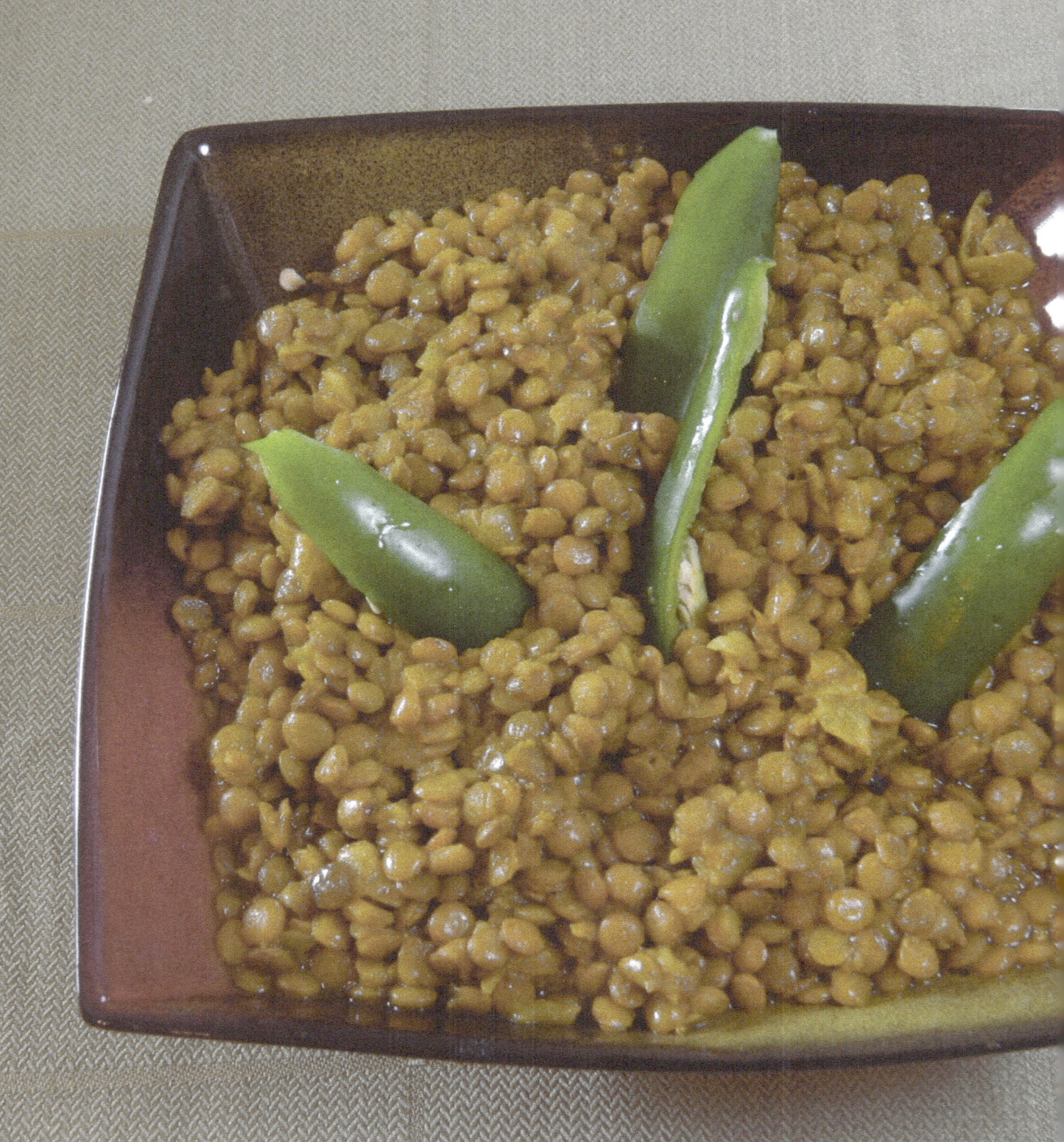

Green Lentil Stew
የድፍን ምሰር አልጫ
(Yediffin Miser Alicha) (V) (VG) (GF) (DF)

A mild lentil dish that is a lunch and dinner staple on Injera (p. 33).

Time: 1 hr
Serves: 5–6
Difficulty: ♦♦◇◇◇

Ingredients:

Dried green lentils, 2 cups, rinsed (be sure to remove any stones)
Water, 5 cups total, plus enough to cover lentils in pot
Yellow onion, 1 medium, finely diced
Vegetable oil, 1 cup
Turmeric, 1 tsp
Ginger-Garlic Paste, 1 Tbsp (p. 23)
Salt, 1 tsp
Jalapeños, 2, stemmed but not seeded, quartered lengthwise

Directions:

1. Place lentils in large pot and add enough cold water to cover by an inch.
2. Place over high heat and cook 25 min, stirring occasionally.
3. While lentils are cooking, put the onions in a medium pot and cook 2 min over medium-high heat, stirring once or twice. Add ¼ cup water. Cook another 10 min, covered.
4. Add oil, turmeric and ginger-garlic to the onions. Cook 3 min, stirring frequently.
5. Add ½ cup water to the onion mixture. Cook 4 min, covered. Remove from heat and set aside.
6. When the lentils are done cooking, remove from heat and drain in a colander.
7. Add drained lentils to pot with onion mixture. Add the salt and 4¼ cups water, and stir to mix. Cook 15 min, covered, stirring occasionally.
8. Add jalapeños, stir and remove from heat.

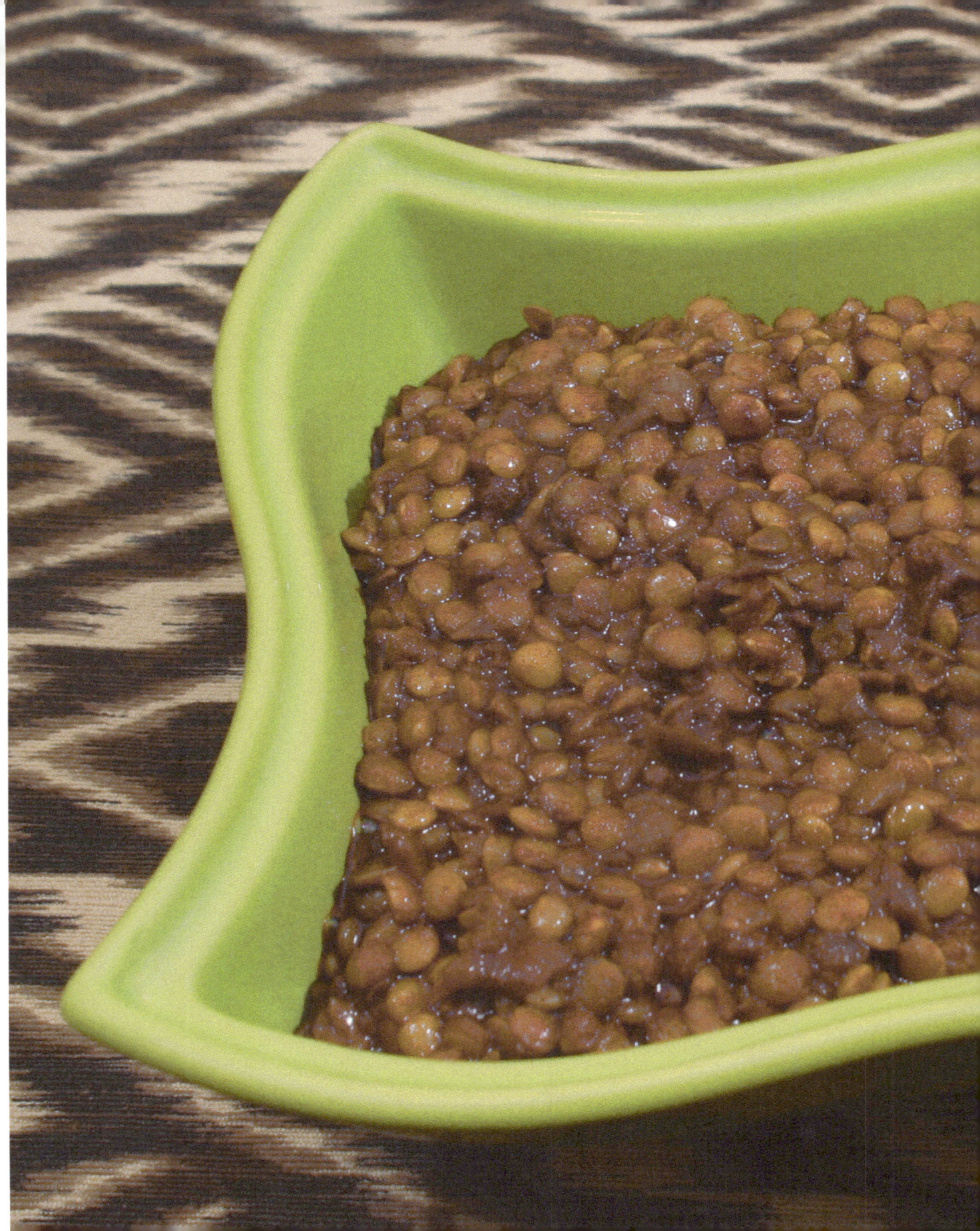

Vegetarian Stews

Spicy Green Lentil Stew
የደፍን ምስር ወጥ
(Yediffin Miser Wat) (V) (VG) (GF) (DF)

Time: 1 hr 15 min
Serves: 5–6
Difficulty: ♨♨♨

A spicy variation of the previous recipe.

Ingredients:
Dried green lentils, 2 cups, rinsed (be sure to remove any stones)
Water, 5 cups total, plus enough to cover the lentils
Yellow onion, 1 large, finely diced
Vegetable oil, ½ cup
Berberre paste, ½ cup (p. 29)
Ginger-Garlic Paste, 1 tsp (p. 23)
Salt, 1 tsp
Q'imam, ½ tsp (p. 25)

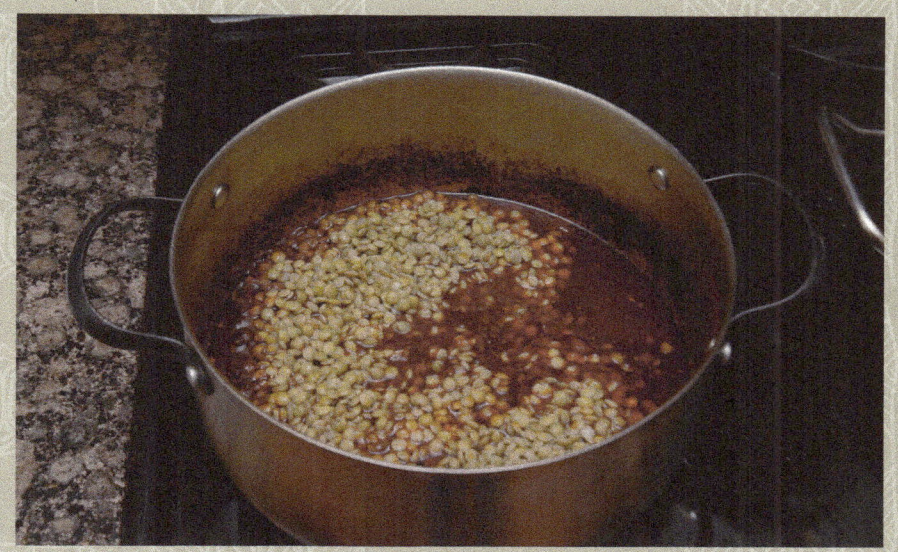

Directions:
1. Place lentils in medium saucepan and add enough cold water to cover by an inch.
2. Cook over high heat for 12 min, stirring to prevent sticking.
3. While lentils are cooking, place onions in large pot with ½ cup water. Cook 15 min, partially covered, over high heat, until onions are translucent but not browned, stirring occasionally. During this time, if onions begin to stick, add a second ½ cup water and continue cooking.
4. Drain lentils in a colander. They will not be completely cooked at this time.
5. Add oil to onions. Cook, uncovered, for 7 min, stirring occasionally.
6. Add Berberre paste to onions and stir to mix. Add ½ cup water. Cook 8 min, stirring occasionally. If the mixture starts to dry, add ¼ cup water and continue cooking.
7. Add Ginger-Garlic Paste and ¼ cup water to onion mixture and reduce heat to medium low. Cook 15 min, stirring occasionally to prevent sticking.
8. Add 2 cups water, stir, and cook 15 min.
9. Add cooked lentils and salt. Increase heat to medium high, and cook 2 min.
10. Add Q'imam and 1 cup water and cook 5 min, partly covered, stirring occasionally.

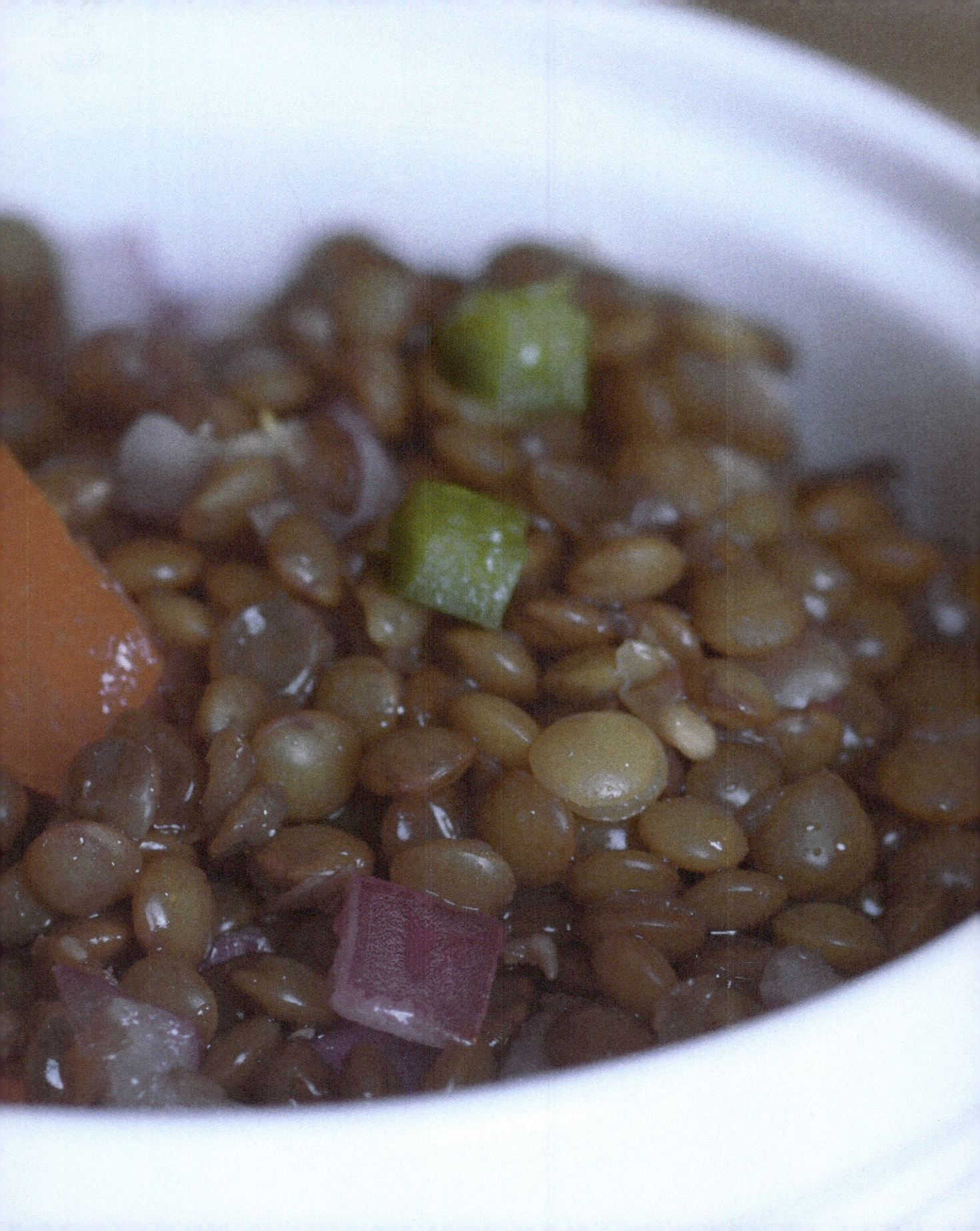

Vegetarian Stews

Green Lentil Salad
የምስር ሳላጣ
(Yemiser Salata) Ⓥ ⓋⒼ ⒼⒻ ⒹⒻ

Time: 30 min, plus 1 hr to cool
Serves: 5
Difficulty: ♦♦◊◊◊

A perfect cold lentil salad to have as a summer side dish.

Ingredients:
- Dried green lentils, 2 cups, rinsed (be sure to remove stones)
- Red onion, ½ medium, minced
- Plum tomato, 1, diced
- Jalapeño, 1, stemmed and seeded, diced
- Lemon, 1, juiced
- Vegetable oil, ½ cup
- Salt, 2 tsp

Directions:
1. Place lentils in a medium-sized saucepan. Add enough water to cover by 1 inch. Bring to a boil and cook 25 min, or until lentils are slightly al dente.
2. Drain lentils in a colander.
3. Remove to a serving bowl.
4. Add onions, tomato, jalapeño, lemon, oil and salt. Mix and refrigerate at least 1 hour.

The Crown Jewel of African Cuisine

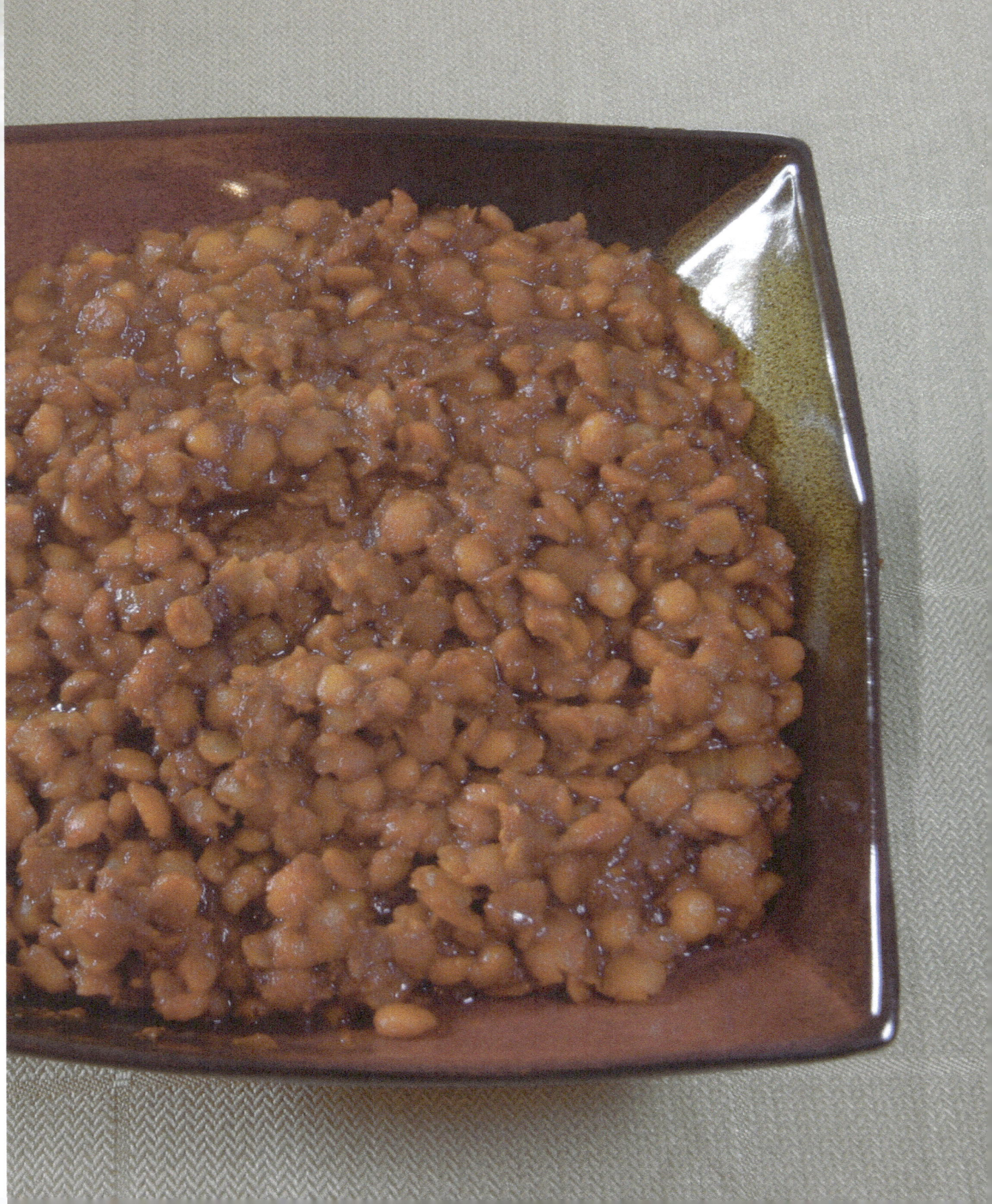

Vegetarian Stews

Spicy Yellow Split Pea Stew
የአተርክክ ወጥ
(Yeaterkik Wat) (V) (VG) (GF) (DF)

Time: 1 hr 30 min
Serves: 6–8
Difficulty: ♦♦♦◊◊

In Ethiopia, we make this dish with yellow peas still in their skin (not split), but it is just as delicious using the easier-to-obtain split peas.

Ingredients:

Dried yellow split peas, 3 cups
Yellow onion, 2 medium, finely diced
Water, 8¼ cups, total, plus enough to cover split peas
Vegetable oil, ½ cup
Berberre paste, 1 cup (p. 29)
Ginger-Garlic Paste, 2 Tbsp (p. 23)
Salt, 2 tsp
Q'imam, 1 tsp (p. 25)
Niter Kibe, ⅓ cup, optional (p. 21)

Directions:

1. Heat medium-sized fry pan over medium-high heat.
2. Add yellow split peas and dry roast, stirring constantly for 3 min or until fragrant.
3. Pour into bowl to cool.
4. Heat a large pot over medium-high heat. Add onions and cook 2 min. Add ¾ cup water, stir and cover. Cook 6 min.
5. Add oil and cook 4 more min, stirring constantly.
6. Add ½ cup water, Berberre paste, Ginger-Garlic Paste and stir to mix. Reduce heat to medium. Cook 5 min.
7. Add 1 cup water and cook another 15 min, stirring occasionally to prevent sticking.
8. In a second large pot, rinse split peas with cold water. Add enough water to cover peas by 1 inch. Cook 8 min over high heat, uncovered.
9. Remove from heat and drain.
10. When onion mix is complete, add peas to onion mix, along with 6 cups water and salt. Cook 25 min over medium heat, stirring occasionally.
11. Increase heat to medium high and cook 10 min, stirring frequently.
12. Add Q'imam and, if you like, the Niter Kibe, and stir. Cook 4 min.

The Crown Jewel of African Cuisine

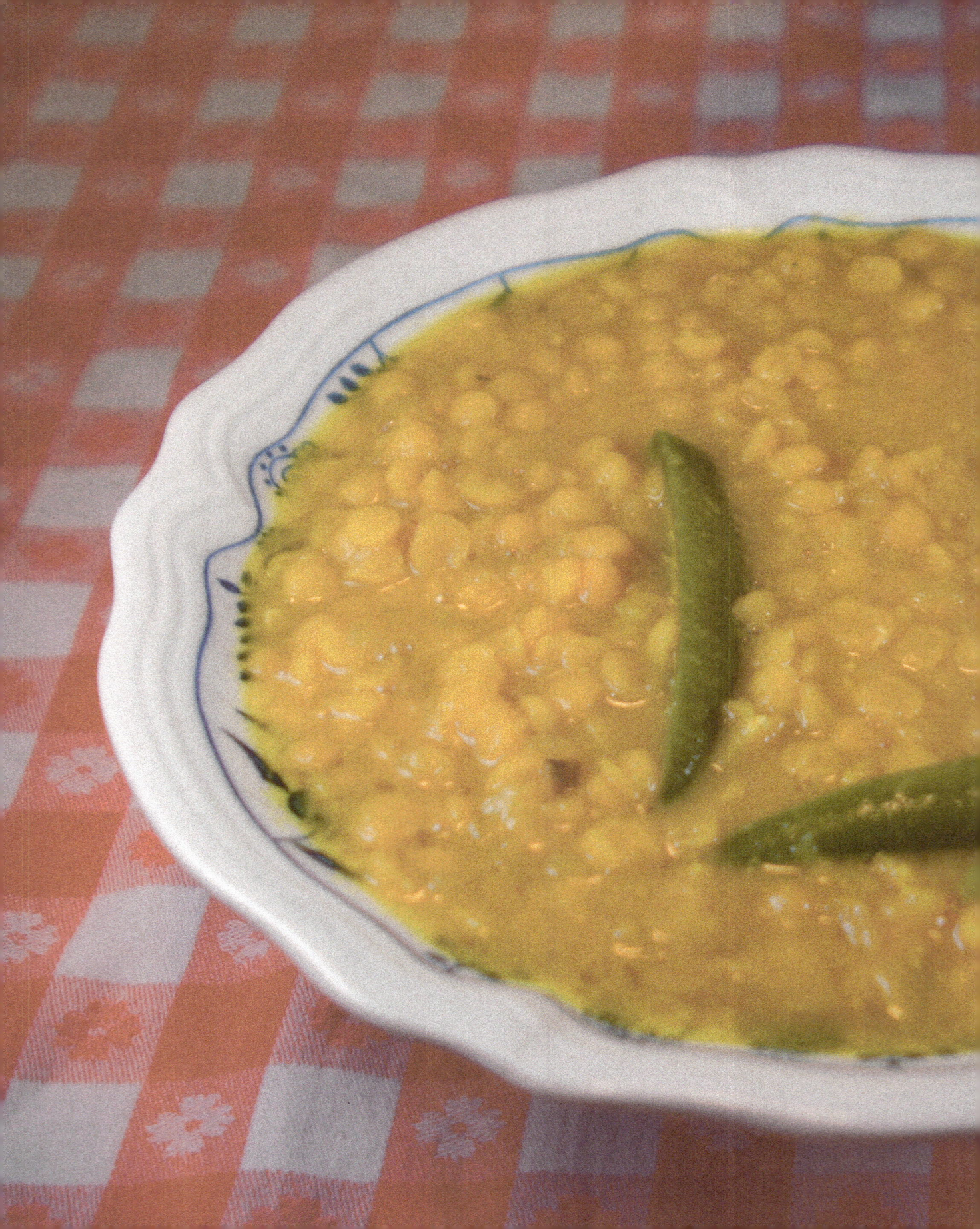

Vegetarian Stews

Yellow Split Pea Stew
የአተርክክ አልጫ
(Yeaterkik Alicha) (V) (VG) (GF) (DF)

Time: 50 min
Serves: 6–8
Difficulty: ♦♦♢♢♢

People who want something hearty but not spicy like to order this sunny yellow dish. The jalapeño is just a garnish.

Ingredients:

Yellow split peas, 2 cups
Yellow onion, 1 large, finely diced
Water, 6 cups total, plus enough to cover split peas
Vegetable oil, ½ cup
Ginger-Garlic Paste, 2 tsp (p. 23)
Turmeric, ½ tsp
Salt, 1½ tsp
Jalapeño, ½, stemmed but not seeded, cut lengthwise

Directions:

1. Heat medium-sized fry pan over medium-high heat.
2. Add yellow split peas and dry roast, stirring constantly for 3 min or until fragrant.
3. Pour into medium saucepan. Add 2 cups water. Stir and cook 6 min over high heat, uncovered. Reduce heat to medium high. Cook 10 min. Remove from heat and set aside.
4. Place onions into a large pot with ¼ cup water. Cover and cook 8 min over medium-high heat, stirring occasionally.
5. Add oil, Ginger-Garlic Paste, turmeric and salt. Cook 4 min. Add ¼ cup water and cook 8 min, covered, stirring occasionally.
6. Add 3½ cups water, stir in split peas. Cook 20 min, covered, stirring occasionally.
7. Remove to serving bowl and garnish with jalapeño.

The Crown Jewel of African Cuisine

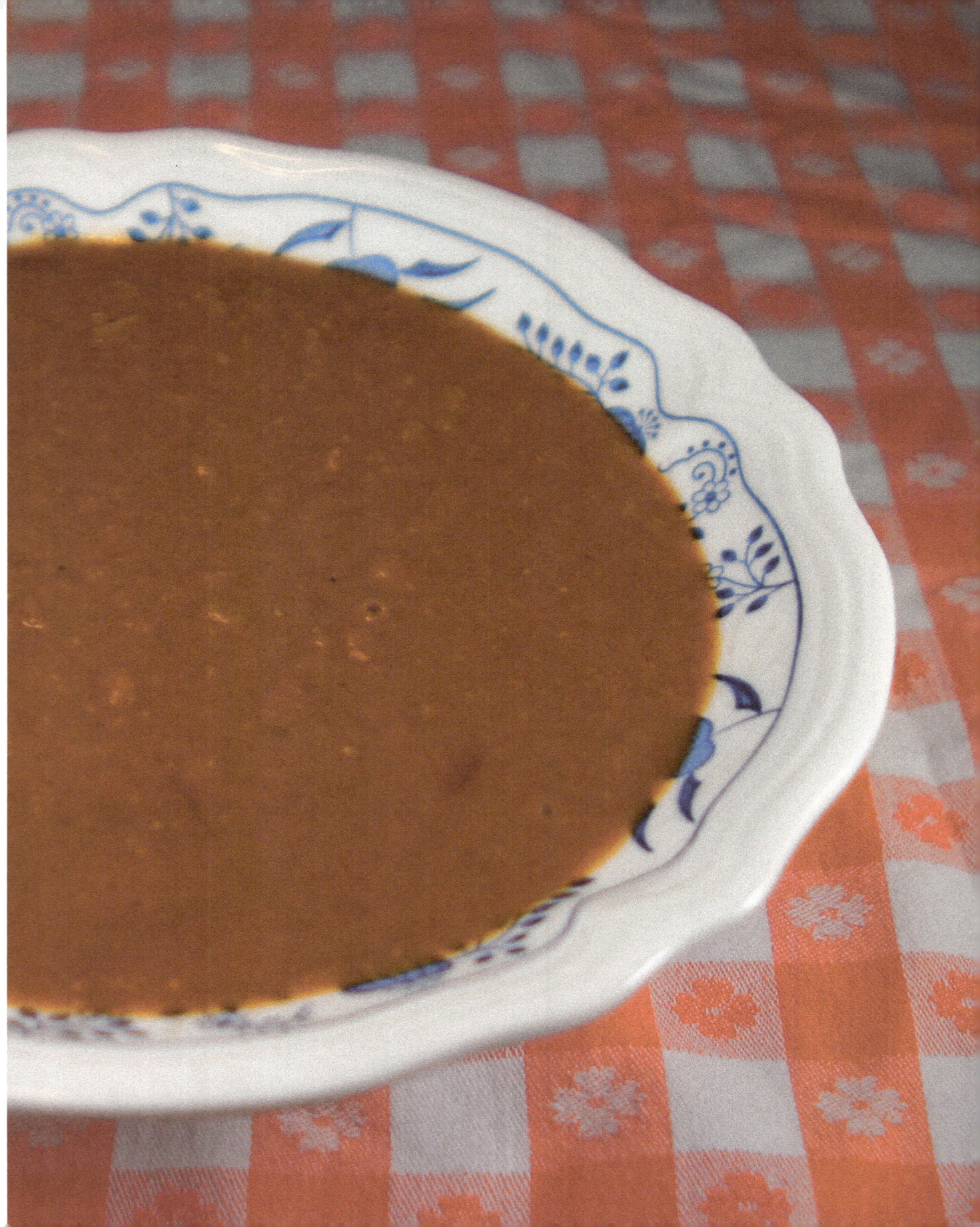

Vegetarian Stews

Ground Roasted Yellow Split Pea Stew
ሽሮ

(Shiro) V VG GF DF

Time: 1 hr
Serves: 6–8
Difficulty:

To many people this dish looks like just a sauce. But it is a hearty entrée and an Ethiopian favorite. Serve this with Ethiopian Kale (p. 161) on Injera (p. 33).

Ingredients:

Yellow onion, 1 large, finely diced
Olive oil, ¾ cup
Berberre paste, ½ cup (p. 29)
Ginger-Garlic Paste, 2 tsp (p. 23)
Water, 6 cups total
Shiro powder*, 1 cup
Salt, 1 tsp
Q'imam, ½ tsp (p. 25)

*available at specialty stores and online, see p. 17

Directions:

1. Place onions and olive oil in large pot over medium-high heat. Cook 10 min, uncovered, stirring occasionally to prevent sticking.

2. Add Berberre paste, Ginger-Garlic Paste, ½ cup water and stir. Cook 5 min. Add 3½ cups water. Cook 10 min, stirring occasionally.

3. Add shiro powder, salt, Q'imam and 2 cups water and stir. Reduce heat to medium and simmer 30 min, stirring frequently to prevent sticking and to mix to a smooth consistenty.

The Crown Jewel of African Cuisine

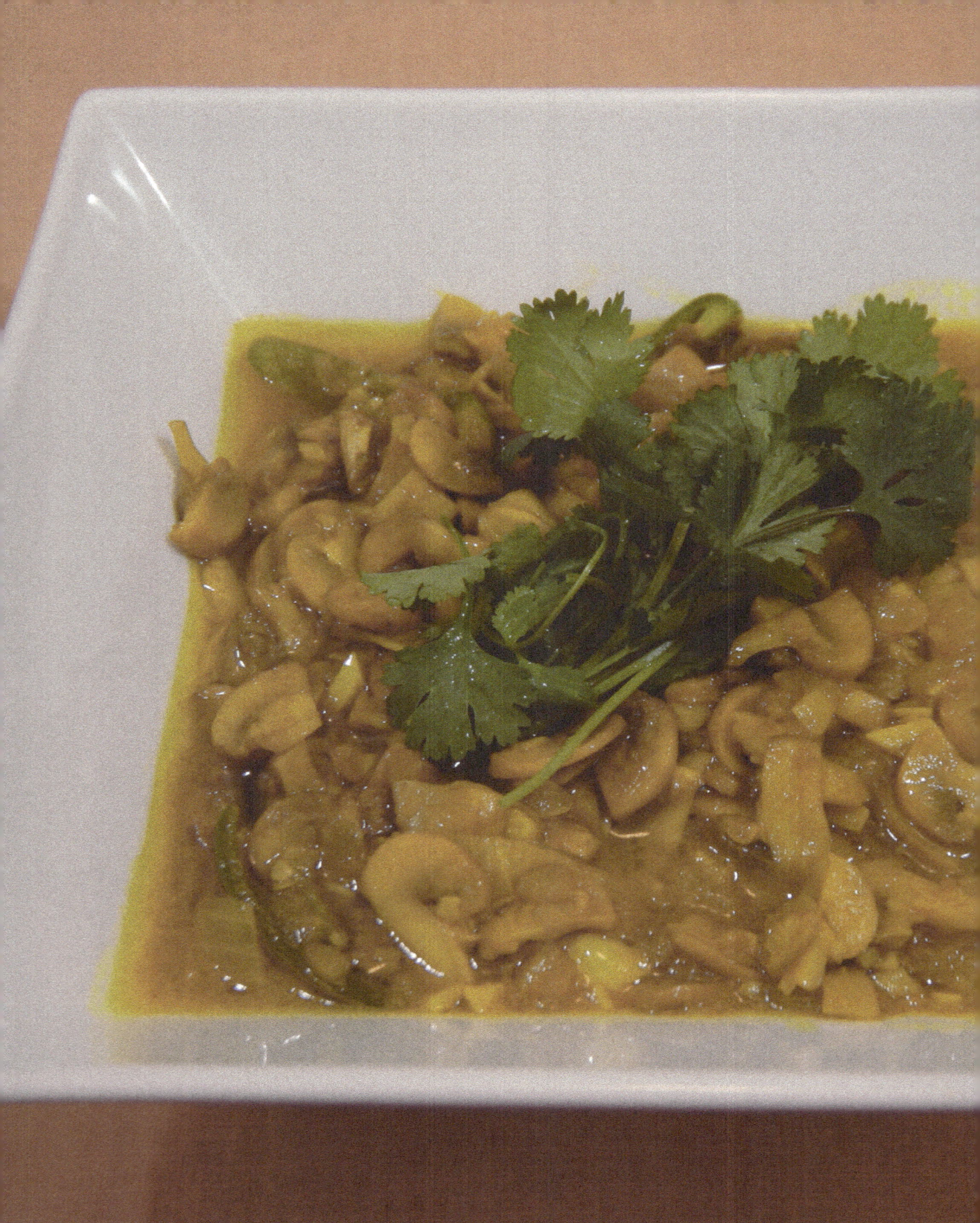

Mushroom Stew
የእንጉዳይ አልጫ ወጥ
(Yeengudai Alicha Wat) V VG GF DF

This mild mushroom stew is a hearty dish for vegetarians.

Time: 25 min
Serves: 4
Difficulty: ♦♦◊◊◊

Ingredients:

Yellow onion, 1 large, finely diced
Vegetable oil, ⅓ cup
Garlic, 4 large cloves, minced
Niter Kibe, ¼ cup (p. 21)
Turmeric, 1½ tsp
Salt, 1 tsp
Mushrooms, 1 lb, cleaned and sliced to ¼ inch thickness
Jalapeño, cut lengthwise into quarters
Cilantro, a few sprigs, coarsely chopped

Directions:

1. Place onions in large pot over high heat. Cook 3 min, uncovered, stirring frequently to prevent sticking.
2. Add oil, stir. Reduce heat to medium. Cook 7 min, stirring occasionally.
3. Add garlic, Niter Kibe, turmeric and salt. Cook 2 min, then add mushrooms. Mix thoroughly to combine. Increase heat to medium high. Cook 10 min, stirring occasionally.
4. Remove to bowl. Garnish with jalapeño and cilantro.

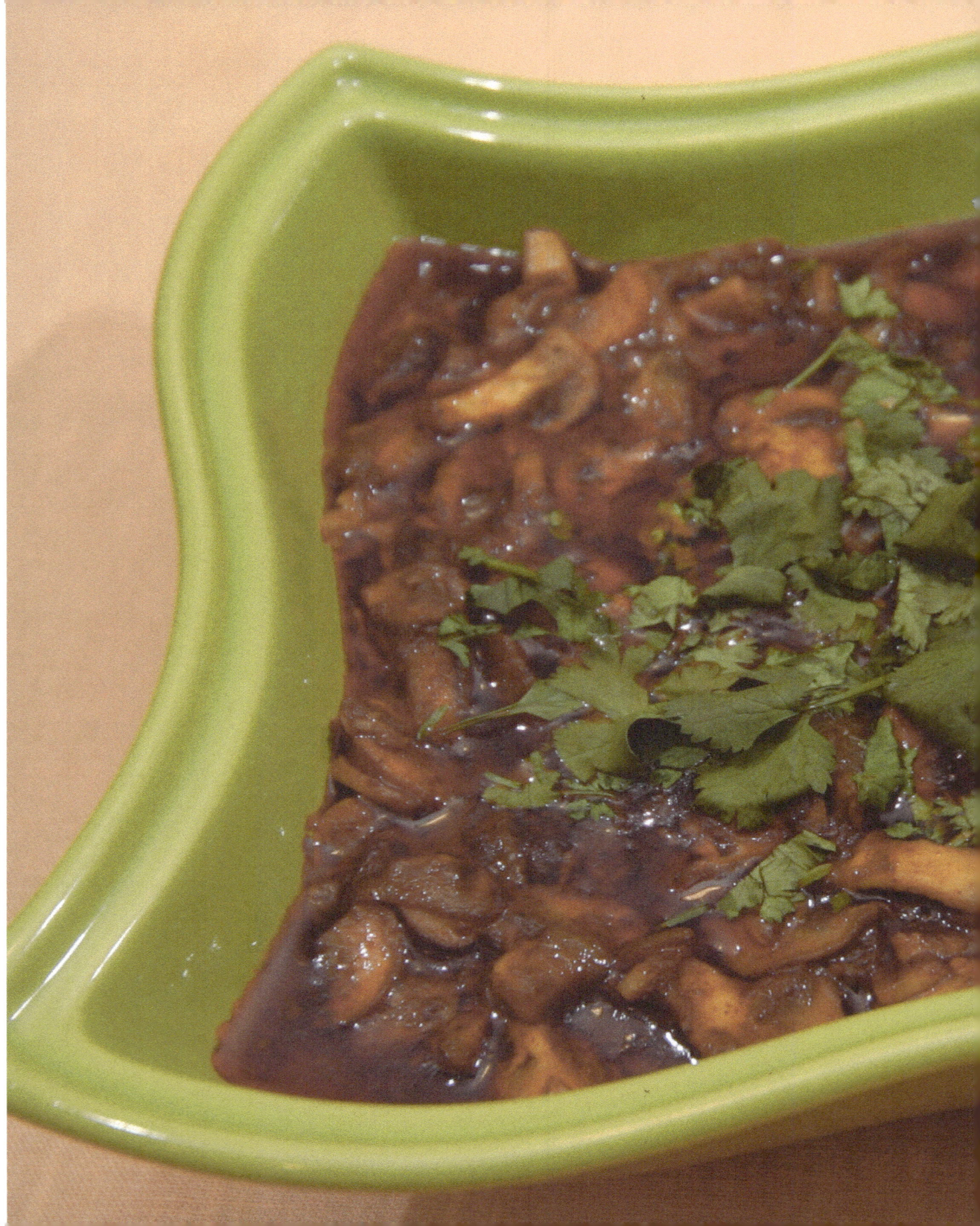

Vegetarian Stews

Spicy Mushroom Stew
የእንጉዳይ ቀይ ወጥ
(Yeengudai Key Wat) (V) (VG) (GF) (DF)

Time: 15 min
Serves: 4
Difficulty:

Try this version of mushroom stew if you like a spicy kick.

Ingredients:
- Yellow onion, 1 large, finely diced
- Vegetable oil, ⅓ cup
- Garlic cloves, 4 large, minced
- Berberre paste, ⅓ cup (p. 29)
- Niter Kibe, ¼ cup (p. 21)
- Salt, 1 tsp
- Mushrooms, 1 lb, cleaned and sliced to ¼ inch thickness
- Cilantro, a few sprigs, coarsely chopped

Directions:
1. Place onions in large pot over high heat. Cook 3 min, uncovered, stirring frequently to prevent sticking.
2. Add oil, stir. Reduce heat to medium. Cook 7 min, stirring occasionally.
3. Add Berberre paste and garlic. Cook 2 min.
4. Add Niter Kibe and salt. Cook 2 min.
5. Add mushrooms. Mix thoroughly to combine. Increase heat to medium high. Cook 10 min, stirring occasionally.
6. Remove to bowl. Garnish with cilantro.

The Crown Jewel of African Cuisine

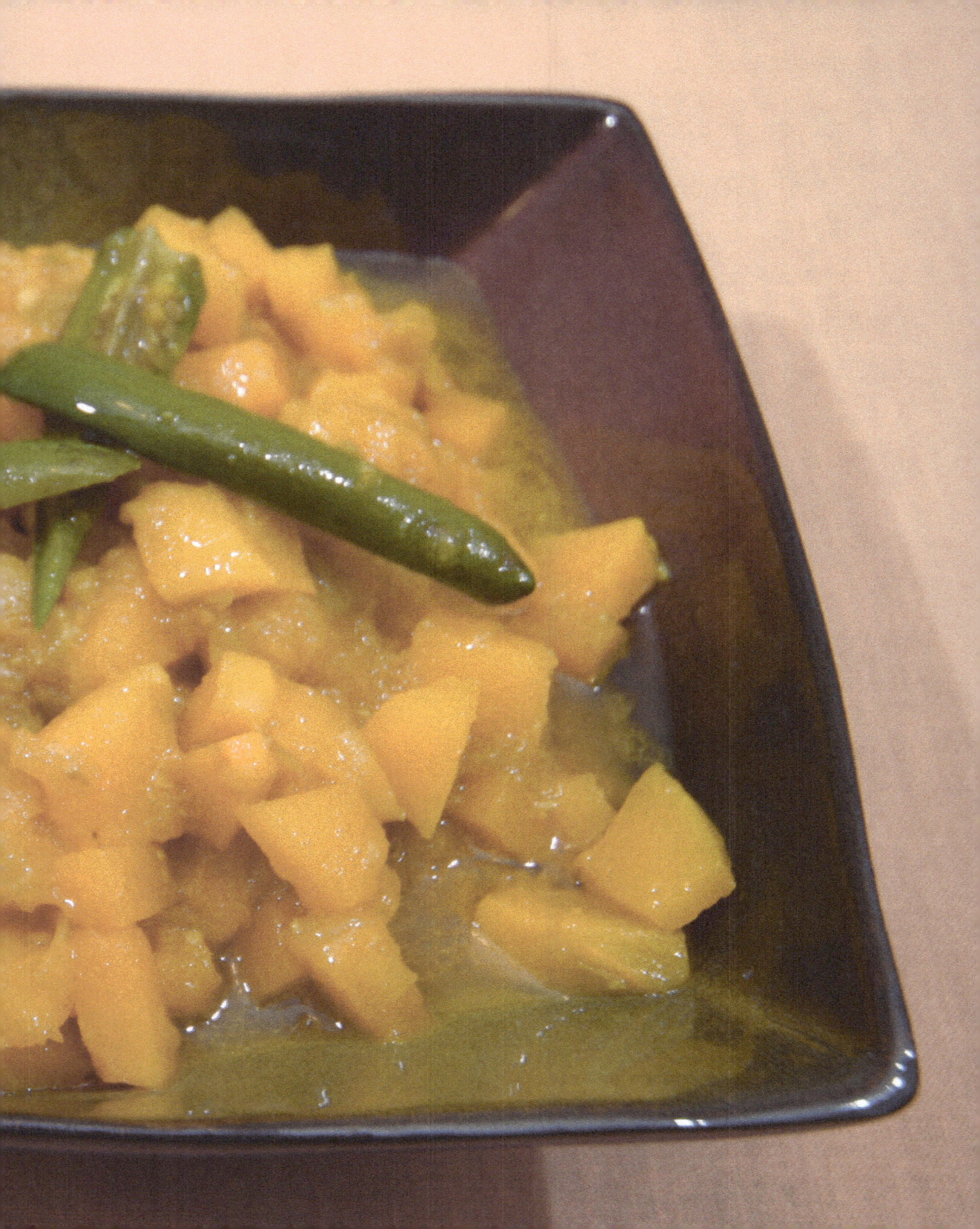

Vegetarian Stews

Squash Stew
የዱባ አልጫ ወጥ
(Yedubba Alicha Wat) (V) (VG) (GF) (DF)

Time: 1 hr 15 min
Serves: 6–8
Difficulty: ●●●○○

In Ethiopia, we dry the diced squash in the sun for a couple hours before cooking, but you can skip this step and still have a delicious stew.

Ingredients:

Yellow onion, 1½ large, finely diced
Water, 4 cups total
Turban, butternut or acorn squash, 2 lb, peeled, seeded, and cut to ¾ inch dice
Vegetable oil, ½ cup
Turmeric, 1 tsp
Salt, 2½ tsp
Ginger-Garlic Paste, 1 Tbsp (p. 23)
Niter Kibe, ¼ cup (p. 21)
Jalapeño, sliced into quarters lengthwise, seeds intact

Directions:

1. Place onions and ½ cup water in large pot over medium-high heat. Cook 7 min, covered, stirring occasionally. Reduce heat to low and cook 13 min, covered.
2. While onion is cooking, peel, seed and dice the squash.
3. Add 1½ cup water to onion and increase heat to medium high. Cook 15 min, stirring occasionally.
4. Add oil to onions and cook 10 min, stirring occasionally. Onions should be soft and translucent. Add ¼ cup water if mixture starts to dry out.
5. Add turmeric, salt, Ginger-Garlic Paste and stir to mix. Cook 7 min.
6. While onion mixture is cooking, rinse the squash and drain it in a colander.
7. Add squash and 2 cups water to onion mixture. Cover and cook (12 min for acorn squash, 18 min for turban squash and 30 min for butternut squash). Stir occasionally to prevent sticking.
8. Add Niter Kibe and jalapeño. Stir to mix and serve.

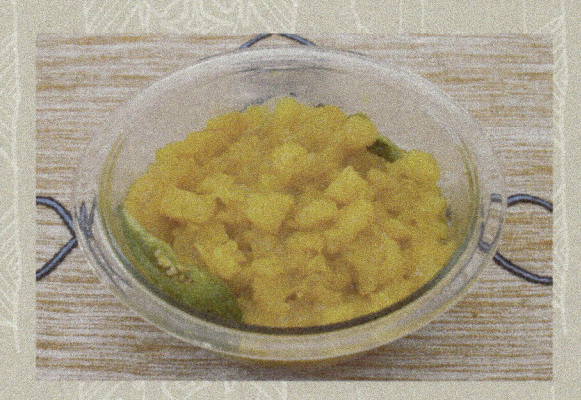

Left: Turban squash. Right: Acorn squash.

The Crown Jewel of African Cuisine

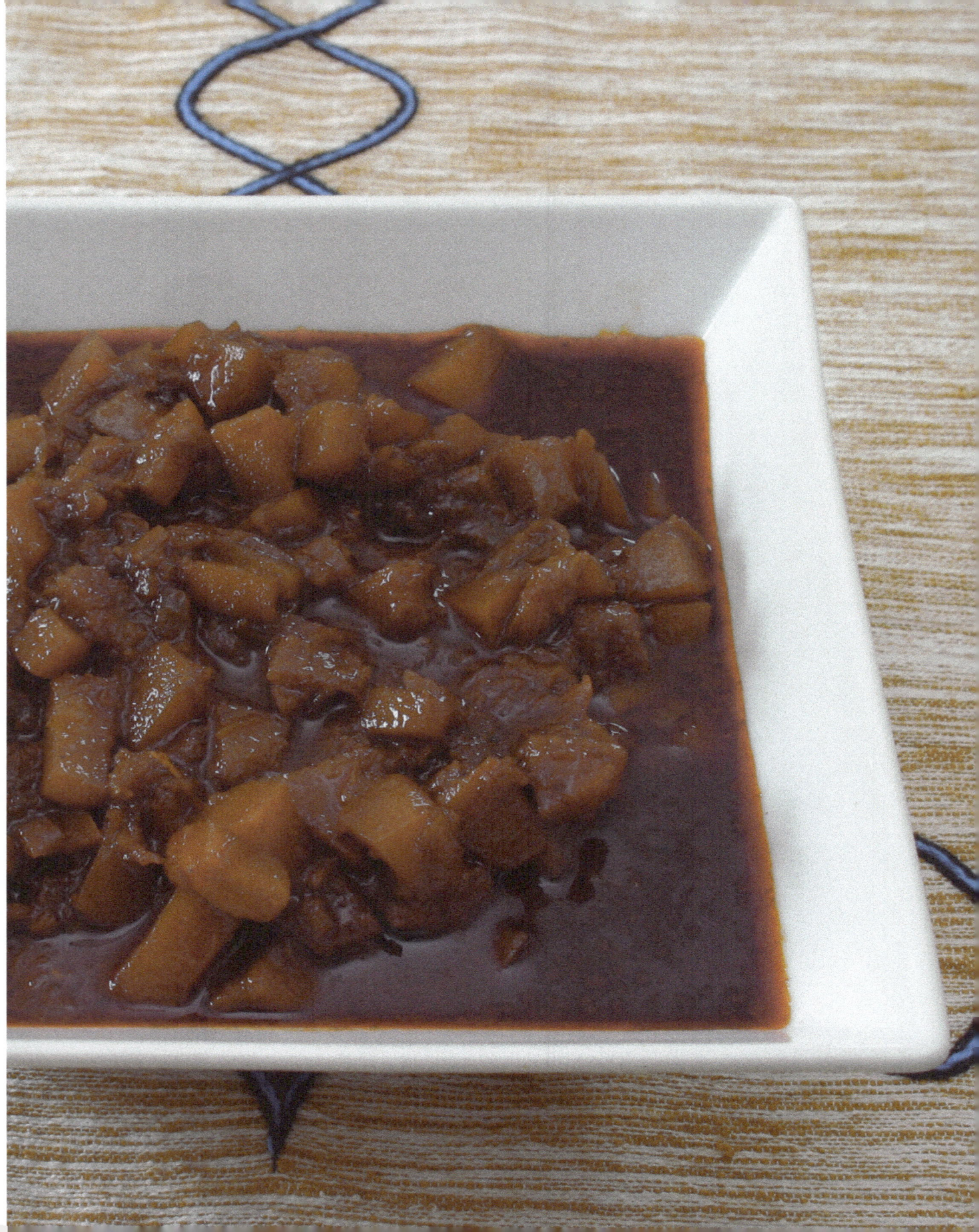

Vegetarian Stews

Spicy Squash Stew
የዱባ ቀይ ወጥ
(Yedubba Key Wat) (V) (VG) (GF) (DF)

Time: **1 hr 15 min**
Serves: **6–8**
Difficulty: ♦♦♦◊◊

Here is a spicy version of squash stew to use to round out your Ethiopian feast!

Ingredients:

- Yellow onion, 1½ large, finely diced
- Water, 4 cups total
- Turban, butternut or acorn squash, 2 lb, peeled, seeded, and cut to ¾ inch dice
- Vegetable oil, ½ cup
- Berberre paste, ½ cup (p. 29)
- Salt, 2½ tsp
- Ginger-Garlic Paste, 1 Tbsp (p. 23)
- Niter Kibe, ¼ cup (p. 21)
- Q'imam, ½ tsp (p. 25)

Directions:

1. Place onions and ½ cup water in large pot over medium-high heat. Cook 7 min, covered, stirring occasionally. Reduce heat to low and cook 13 min, covered.
2. While onion is cooking, peel, seed and dice the squash.
3. Add 1½ cup water to onions and increase heat to medium high. Cook 15 min, uncovered, stirring occasionally.
4. Add oil to onions and cook 10 min, stirring occasionally. Onions should become soft and translucent. Add ¼ cup water if mixture starts to dry out.
5. Add salt, Ginger-Garlic Paste and Berberre paste and stir to mix. Cook 7 min.
6. While onion mixture is cooking, rinse the squash and drain it in a colander.
7. Add squash and 2 cups water to onion mixture. Cover and cook (12 min for acorn squash, 18 min for turban squash and 30 min for butternut squash). Stir occasionally to prevent sticking.
8. Add Niter Kibe and Q'imam. Stir to mix and serve.

Pictured: Butternut squash.

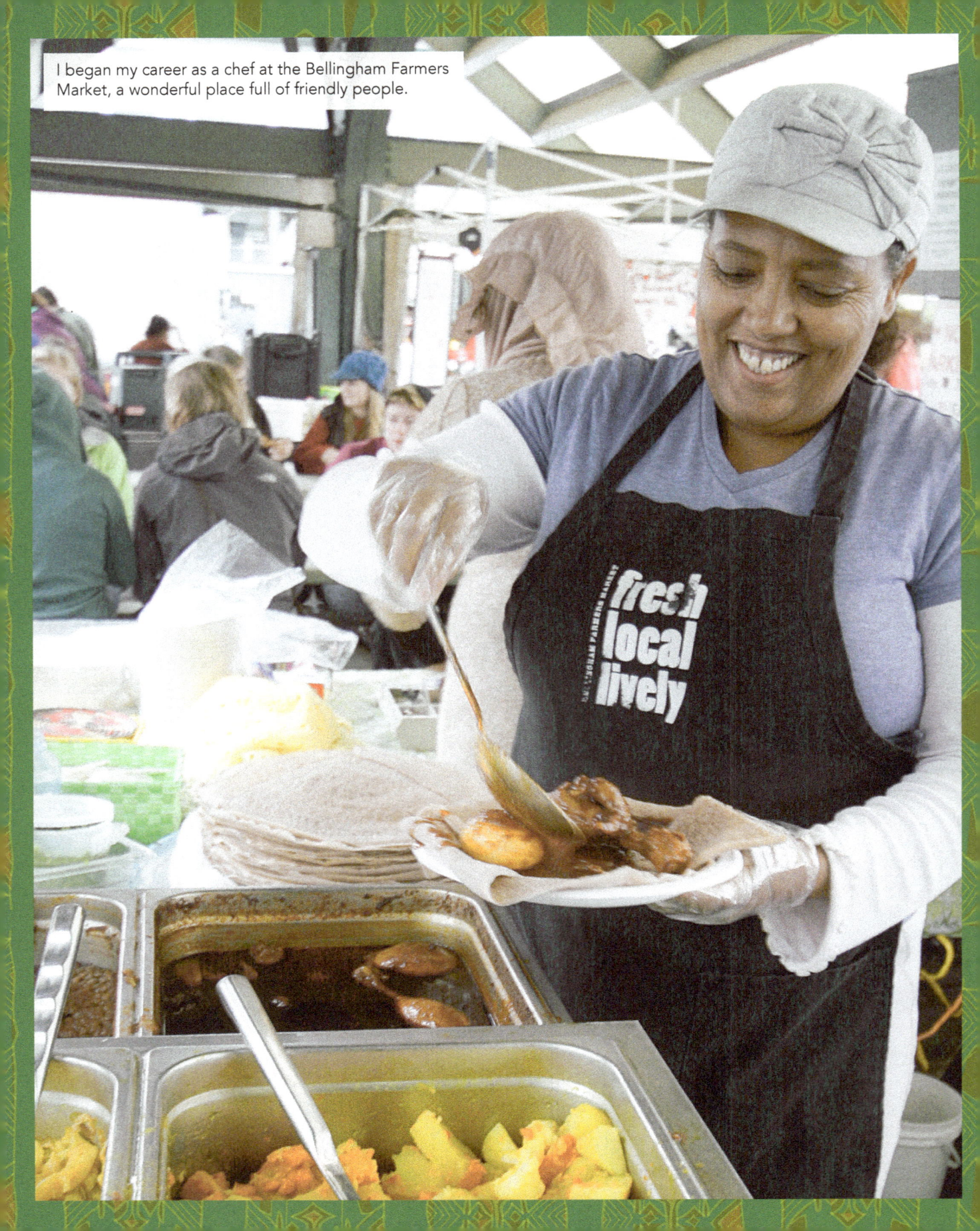

I began my career as a chef at the Bellingham Farmers Market, a wonderful place full of friendly people.

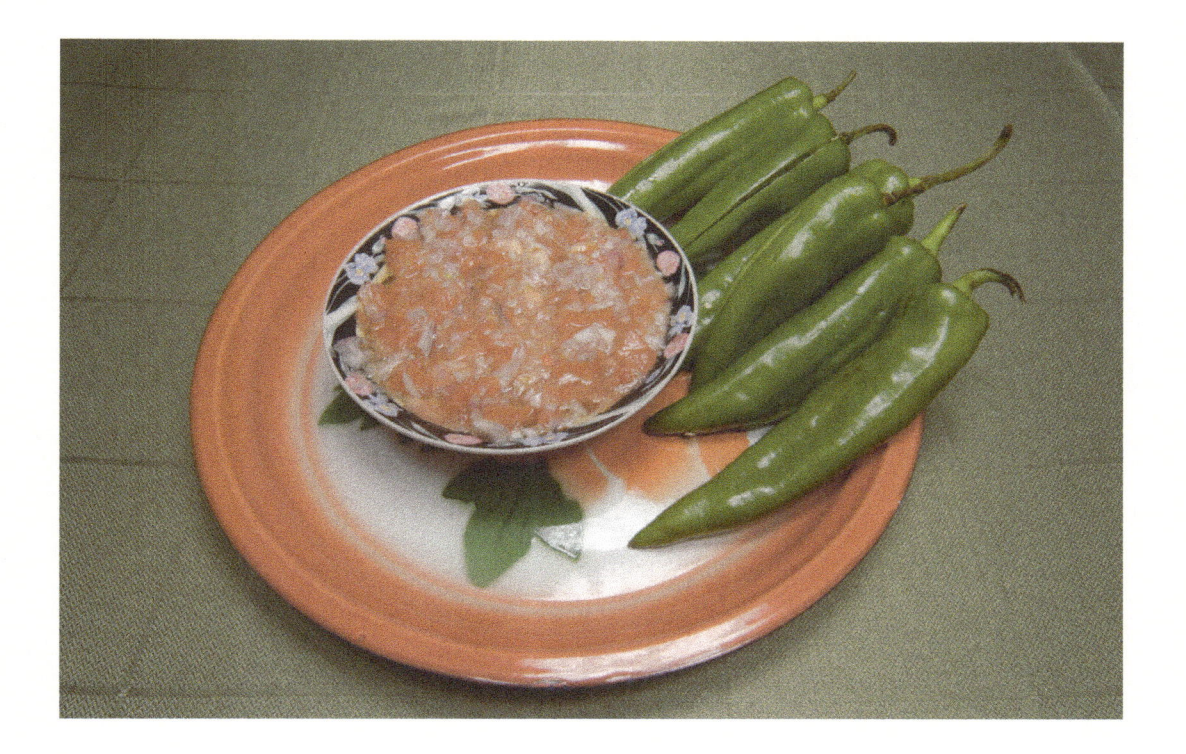

Straight From the Garden: Leaf and Root Vegetables

When I was growing up in Gindeberet, we had a garden where we would pick vegetables to cook. A fresh picked vegetable is so delicious. When I moved to Bellingham, I did not have a garden. But later, I started selling Ethiopian food by opening a stand at the Bellingham Farmers Market. Every Saturday, I brought my food to sell. I met so many kind people who enjoyed my food. And I met farmers! I would trade Yedoro Wat for beautiful vegetables to make into food for my family or to sell the next week at the market. I am spoiled by the good vegetables we have in the Pacific Northwest and I love them! I love the colors of carrots, beets, and kale. They look so beautiful on Injera and give a good feeling of health. For vegetarians and vegans, I have included lots of dishes in this chapter and the previous one, showing the many delicious ways we Ethiopians enjoy our vegetables.

Above: Filled peppers known as Qaria Sinig (p. 167).

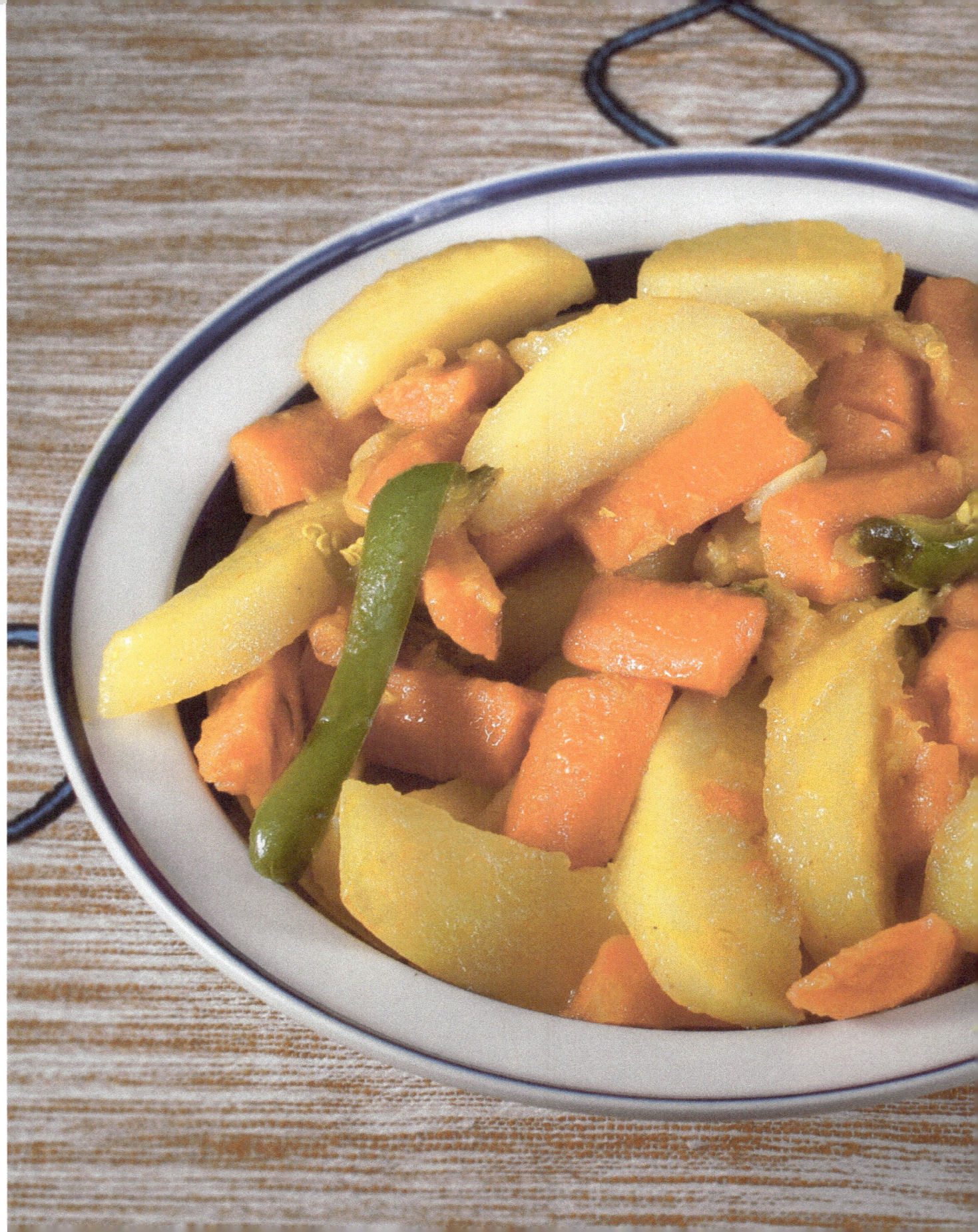

Leaf & Root Veggies

Potatoes and Carrots
የድንች ና ካሮት ወጥ
(Yedinich Na Carrot Wat) V VG GF DF

Time: 40 min
Serves: 6–8
Difficulty:

In Ethiopia, we eat potatoes with almost every meal. This recipe is for one of the most common ways in which they are served. We prize root vegetables because they do not need refrigeration.

Ingredients:
- Yellow onion, 1 large, cut in half and sliced into ¼ inch thick wedges
- Carrots, 4 large, peeled, quartered lengthwise, and cut into 2–3 inch lengths
- Red potatoes, 4 medium, peeled and cut into ¼ inch thick wedges
- Vegetable oil, ½ cup
- Turmeric, ½ tsp
- Salt, 1 tsp
- Ginger-Garlic Paste, 1 Tbsp (p. 23)
- Water, 1 cup
- Jalapeño pepper, 1, stemmed but not seeded, quartered lengthwise

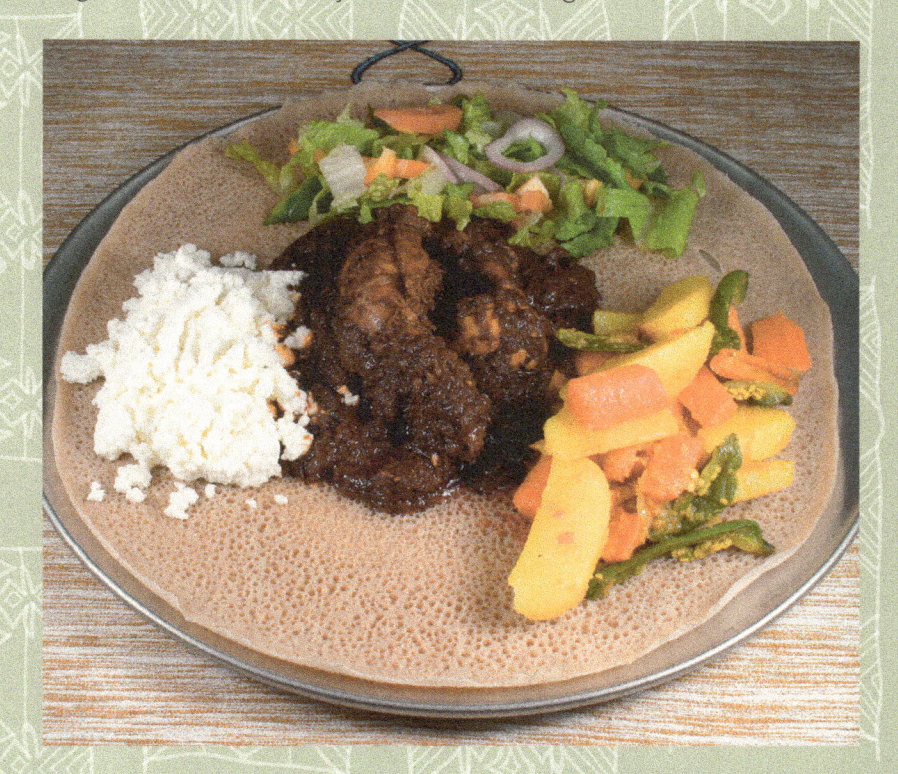

Directions:
1. Put onions in pot over high heat, add oil, turmeric, salt, and Ginger-Garlic Paste, and stir to mix. Cook 10 min, stirring frequently to prevent sticking.
2. Add carrots and cover, stirring every few min. Cook 10 min, during which time you can peel and cut the potatoes. (Keep the cut potatoes covered in cold water until ready to use).
3. Add ~⅛ cup water, stir, and cover. Repeat every min, until 1 cup water has been added.
4. When carrots are fork tender, drain potatoes and add to carrots.
5. Cook 10 min, then add jalapeño.
6. Cook several min longer until potatoes are tender, then serve.

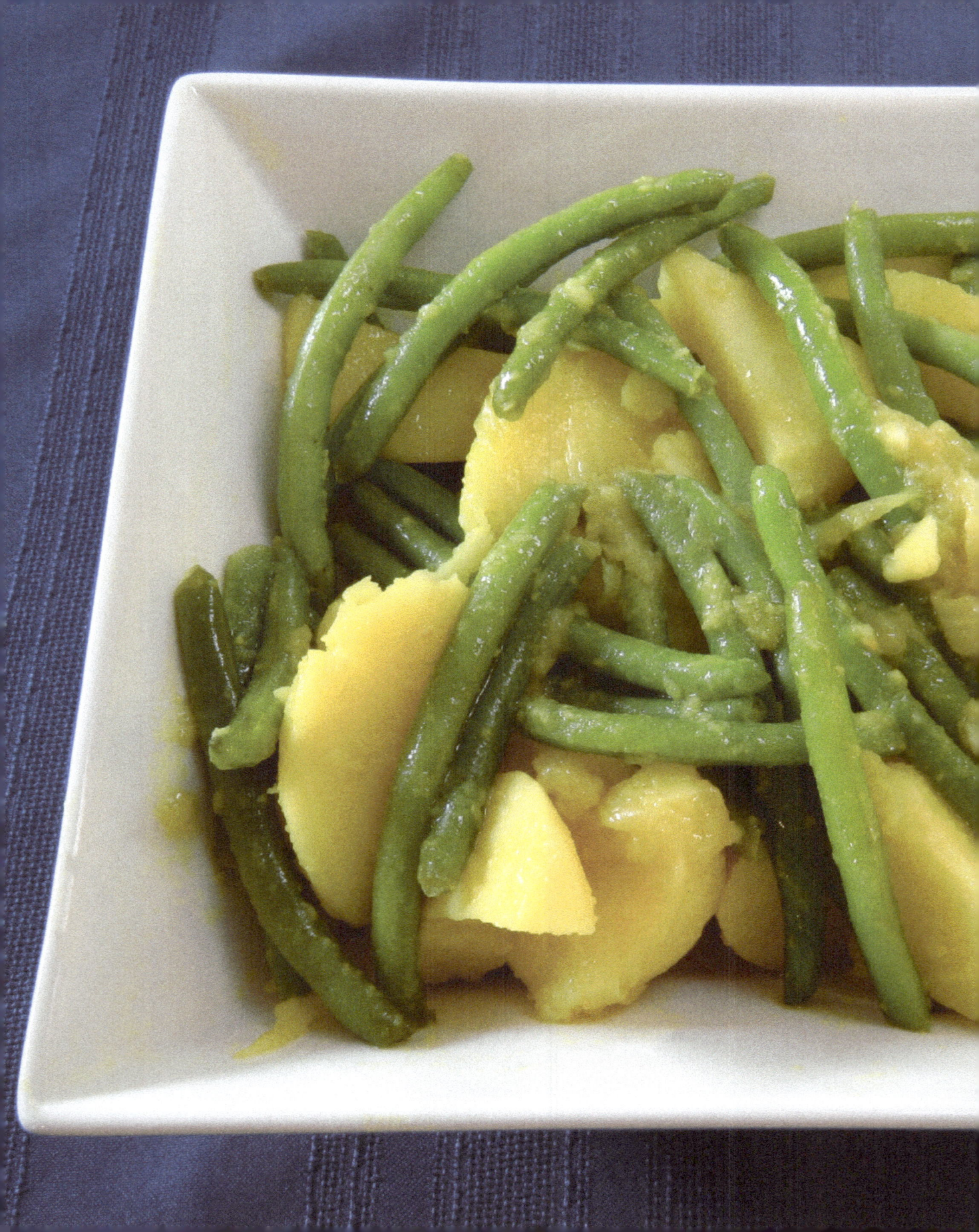

Leaf & Root Veggies

Potatoes and Green Beans
የድንች ና ምስር ወጥ
(Yedinich Na Miser Wat) (V) (VG) (GF) (DF)

Time: 30 min
Serves: 6–8
Difficulty:

This is a delicious way to eat your potatoes on Injera (p. 33).

Ingredients:

Yellow potatoes, 2 lb, peeled and cut into ¼ inch thick wedges
Yellow onion, 1 large, cut in half and sliced to ¼ inch thickness
Olive or vegetable oil, ½ cup
Ginger-Garlic Paste, 1 Tbsp (p. 23)
Turmeric, 1 tsp
Salt, 1 tsp
Water, 2½ cups
Green beans, 1 lb, washed trimmed
Jalapeño, 1, stemmed, cut into quarters lengthwise

Directions:

1. Peel and cut potatoes and place them in a bowl, covered with cold water.
2. Combine onions, oil, Ginger-Garlic Paste, turmeric and salt in a large pot. Cook 5 min over high heat, uncovered. Stir frequently.
3. Drain potatoes, add to onion mixture with ½ cup water. Cook 6 min, stirring occasionally.
4. Add 1½ cups water. Cover and cook 10 min.
5. Add beans and ½ cup water. Stir to combine and cook, covered, for 5 min.
6. Place in serving bowl and garnish with jalapeño.

The Crown Jewel of African Cuisine

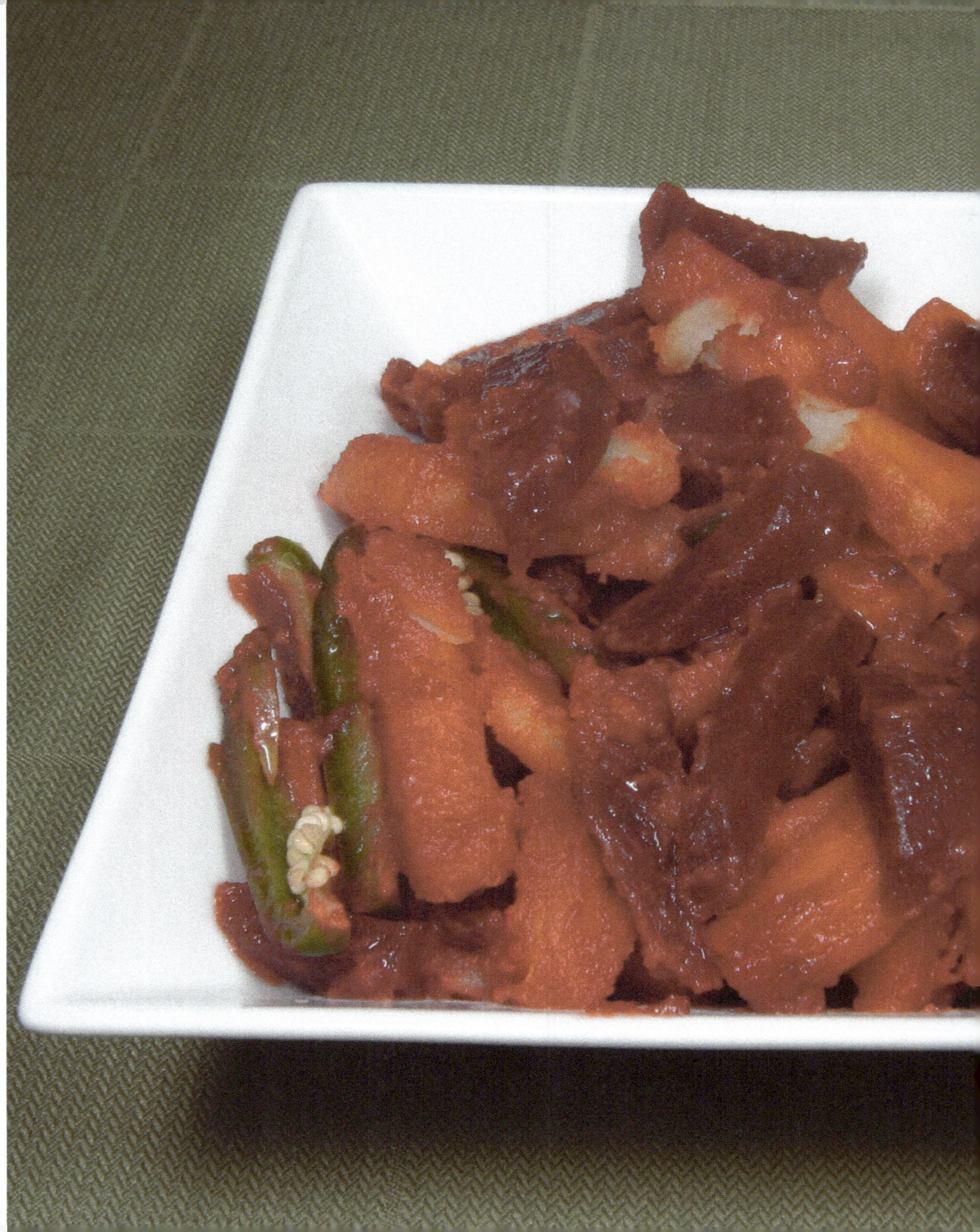

Beets, Potatoes and Carrots
የቀይስር, ድንች ና ካሮት ወጥ
(Yekeysir, Dinich Na Carrot Wat) (V) (VG) (GF) (DF)

Time: 1 hr 30 min
Serves: 6–8
Difficulty: ♦♦◊◊◊

In Ethiopia we like to eat beets, as they are considered to be especially good for your health, among vegetables.

Ingredients:
Red potatoes, 1 lb, peeled, cut in half, then cut into ½ inch slices
Beets, 2 lb, greens removed
Large yellow onion, cut in half, then cut into ¼ inch slices
Water, 5½ cups, divided
Ginger-Garlic Paste, 2-3 Tbsp (p. 23)
Salt, 2 tsp
Carrots, 1 lb, peeled, cut in half lengthwise, and then cut into 3 inch lengths

Directions:
1. Peel and cut potatoes and place them in a bowl, covered with cold water.
2. Place beets in a medium saucepan, cover them with water and cook 40 min over high heat for. Check occasionally to make sure the beets remain covered with water.
3. Remove beets from heat and run under cold water until cool enough to handle. Peel beets and cut into ½ inch dice.
4. Place onions in large pot with ½ cup water, Ginger-Garlic Paste and salt. Cook 3 min over medium-high heat, uncovered.
5. Add 1 cup water and cook 12 min.
6. Add beets and 2 cups water to onions. Stir and cook ~20 min, covered, until beets are tender. Stir occasionally to prevent sticking.
7. Add carrots, drained potatoes and 2 cups water. Stir and cook 20 min, covered, stirring occasionally to prevent sticking.

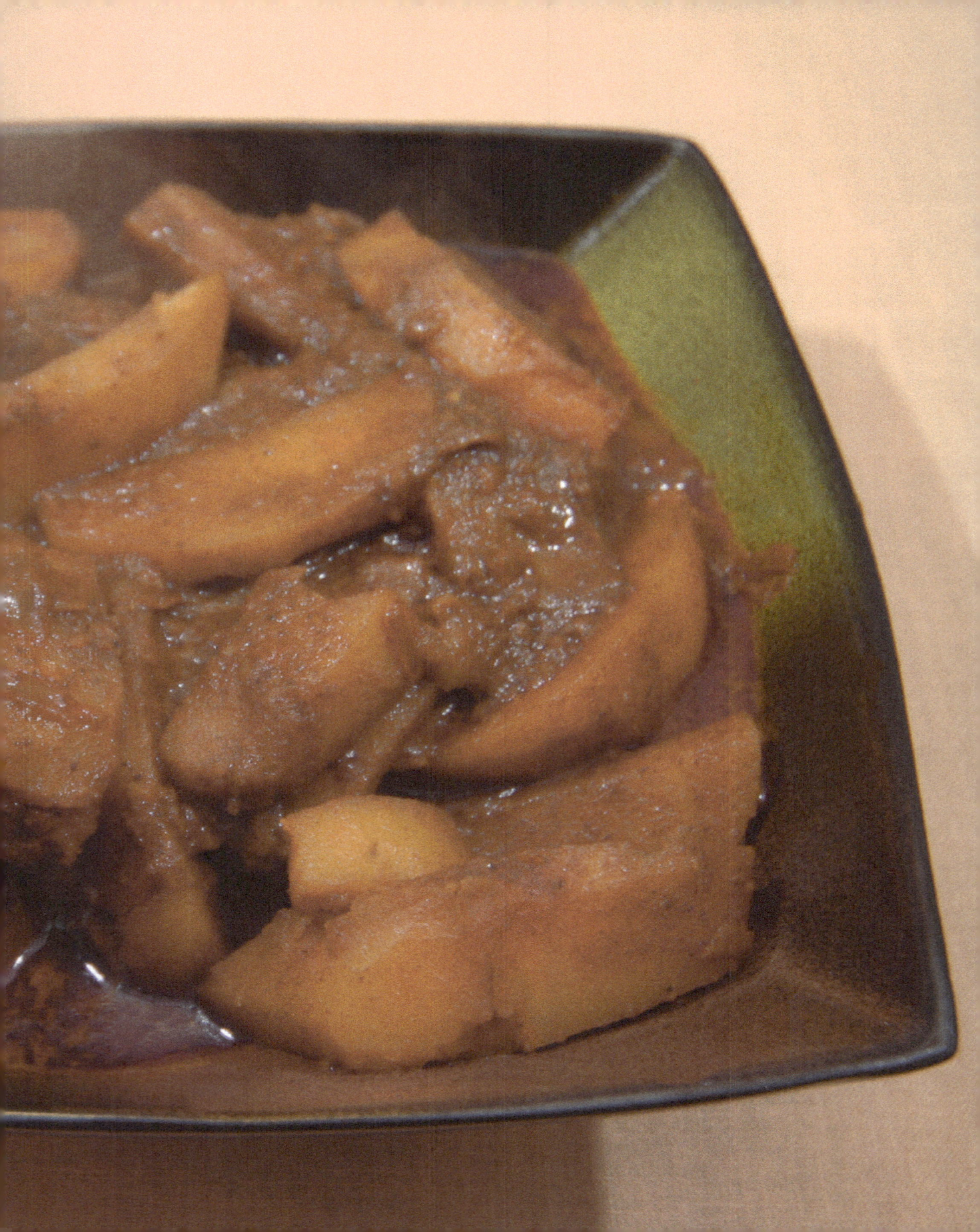

Spicy Potatoes and Onions
የድንች ቀይ ወጥ
(Yedinich Key Wat) (V) (VG) (GF) (DF)

Leaf & Root Veggies

Time: 50 min
Serves: 4–5
Difficulty: ♦♦♢♢♢

I love this dish because it is all vegetables, but still very hearty and comforting.

Ingredients:

Red potatoes, 6 large, peeled and each cut into 8 wedges
Yellow onion, 1 large, finely diced
Vegetable oil, ½ cup
Berberre paste, ½ cup (p. 29)
Water, 2 cups plus 2 Tbsp total
Ginger-Garlic Paste, 1 Tbsp (p. 23)
Salt, 1½ tsp

Directions:

1. Peel and cut potatoes and place them in a bowl, covered with cold water.
2. Place onions in a large pot and cook 4 min over high heat.
3. Add oil. Cook 5 min, uncovered, stirring to prevent sticking.
4. Add Berberre paste and 2 Tbsp water. Stir to combine and reduce heat to medium high. Cook 2 min.
5. Add Ginger-Garlic Paste, salt and ½ cup water. Stir to combine and cook 15 min. Stir occasionally to prevent sticking.
6. Drain potatoes and add them to the onion mixture, along with ½ cup water. Stir to combine and cook 7 min, uncovered. Cover the pot and cook 7 more min. Add ½ cup water and cook 7 more min or until potatoes are tender but not falling apart.

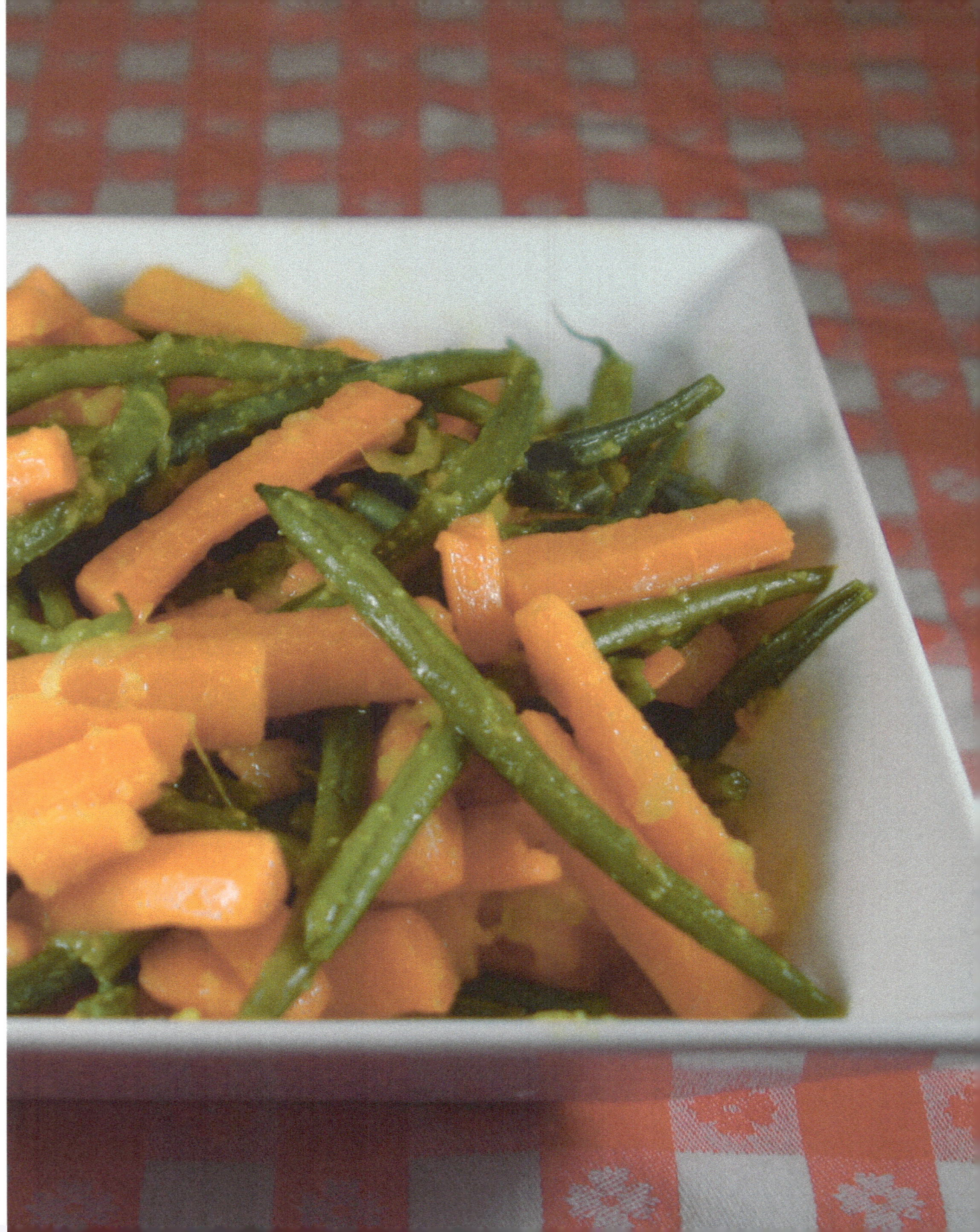

Leaf & Root Veggies

Carrots and Green Beans
የካሮት ና ምስር ወጥ
(Yecarrot Na Miser Wat) (V) (VG) (GF) (DF)

Time: 35 min
Serves: 6–8
Difficulty: 🥄

In Ethiopia, this is a favorite alongside Ethiopian Tripe Stew (p. 91).

Ingredients:
Yellow onion, 1 large, cut in half, then cut into ¼ inch thick wedges
Vegetable oil, ⅓ cup
Ginger-Garlic Paste, 1 Tbsp (p. 23)
Salt, 1 tsp
Turmeric, ½ tsp
Water, 1½ cup total
Carrots, 1½ lb, peeled, cut in half lengthwise, then cut into 3 inch lengths
Green beans, ¾ lb, washed and trimmed

Directions:
1. Place onions, oil, Ginger-Garlic Paste, salt and turmeric in small pot. Cook 5 min over medium-high heat.
2. Add carrots and ¼ cup water. Stir to combine. Cover and cook 15 min.
3. Add beans and 1¼ cup water. Cook 10 min, covered, stirring occasionally.

The Crown Jewel of African Cuisine

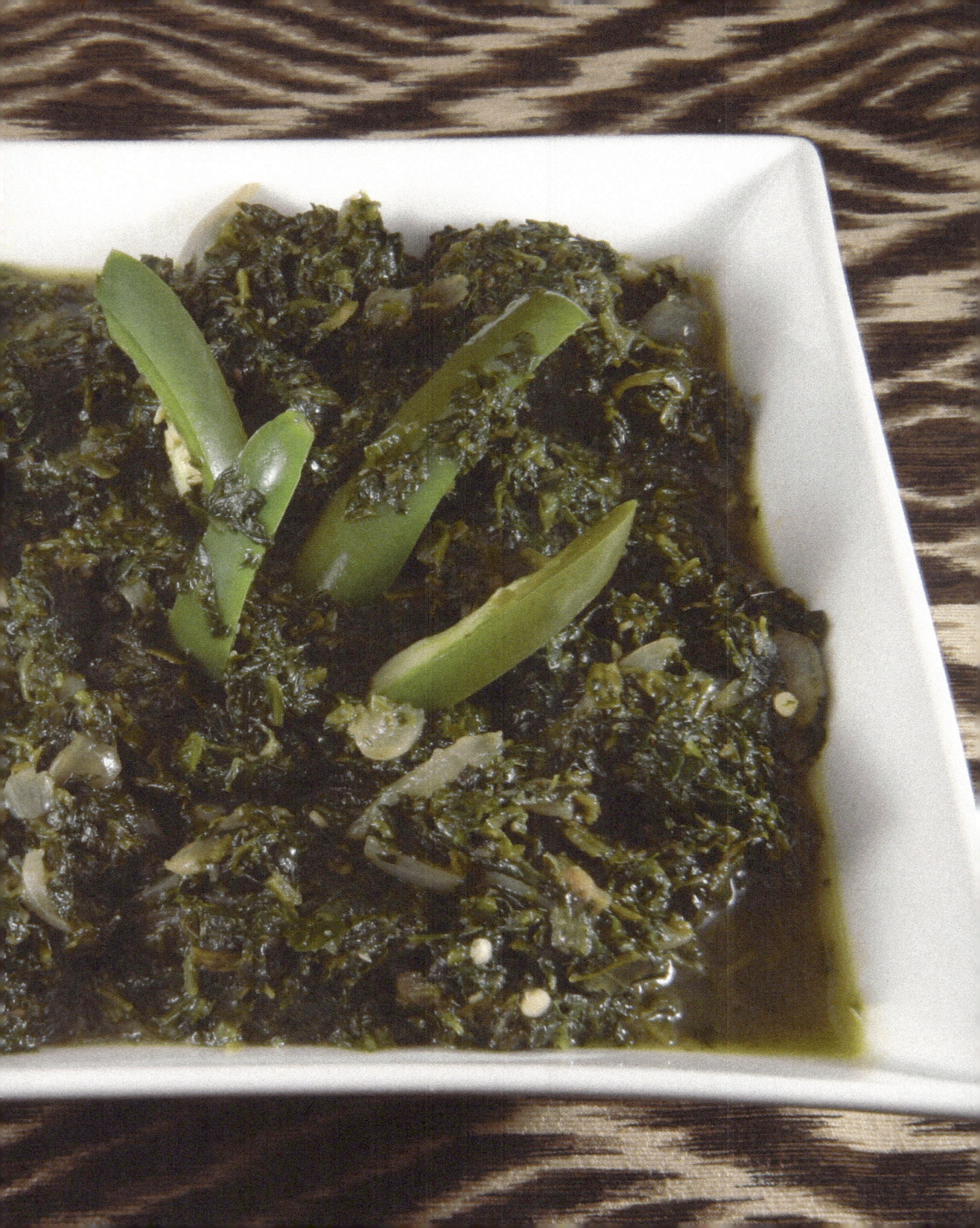

Ethiopian Spinach
ቆስጣ
(Qosta) Ⓥ ⓋⒼ ⒼⒻ ⒹⒻ

Leaf & Root Veggies

Time: 45 min
Serves: 8–10
Difficulty:

Spinach pairs well with all meats and lentils, so it is a very popular side dish in Ethiopia.

Ingredients:

- Yellow onion, 1 large, cut in half and then sliced into ¼ inch thick wedges
- Vegetable oil, 1 cup
- Salt, 2 tsp
- Ginger-Garlic Paste, 2–3 Tbsp (p. 23)
- Spinach, frozen chopped, 6 lb
- Jalapeño, 1, stemmed and quartered lengthwise

Directions:

1. Place onions, oil, salt and Ginger-Garlic Paste in large pot. Cook 7 min over high heat. Stir frequently to prevent sticking.
2. Spread onion mixture at bottom of pot. Place spinach on top of onion mixture without disturbing onion mixture. Do not stir. Cover and cook 13 min over medium high.
3. Increase heat to high. Stir to combine. Cook ~20 min, covered, stirring occasionally until onions are translucent.
4. Remove to serving bowl and garnish with jalapeño.

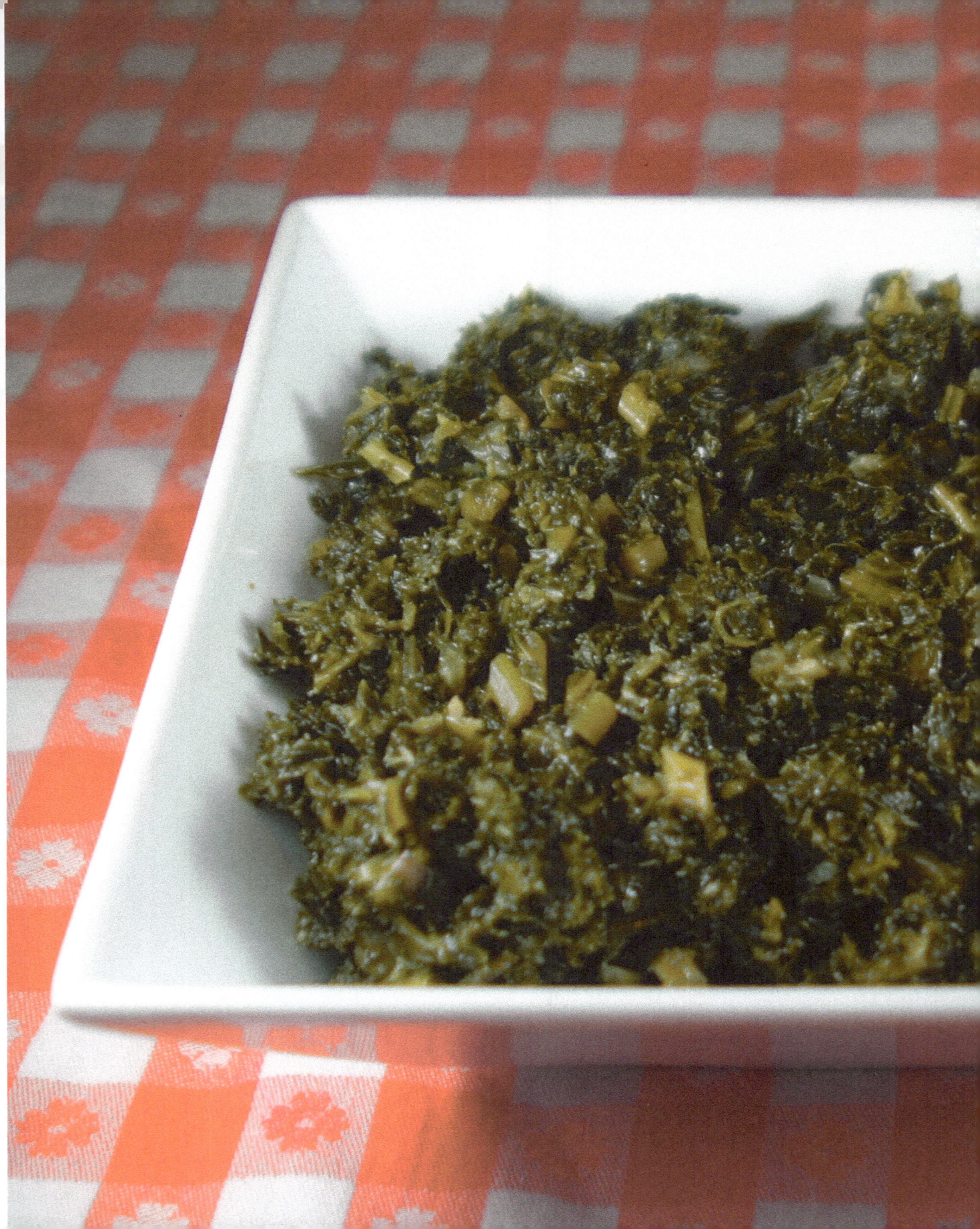

Leaf & Root Veggies

Ethiopian Kale
ጎመን
(Gomen) V VG GF DF

Time: **1 hr 15 min**
Serves: **8–10**
Difficulty:

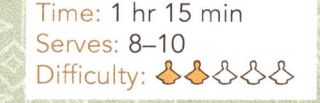

One of my favorite meals is this kale dish paired with shiro. My mouth waters just thinking about it!

Ingredients:

- Yellow onion, 1 large, cut in half, then sliced into ¼ inch thick wedges
- Water 2½ cups total
- Vegetable oil, ½ cup
- Salt, 1 ½ tsp
- Ginger-Garlic Paste, 1 Tbsp (p. 23)
- Kale, 3 bunches, washed, stemmed, and coarsely chopped
- Jalapeño, ½, stemmed and cut lengthwise into 2 pieces

Directions:

1. Place onion and ¼ cup water in large pot over medium-high heat. Cover and bring to boil. Reduce heat to medium and cook 15 min.
2. Add oil, salt, Ginger-Garlic Paste and ¼ cup water and stir. Spread this mixture on the bottom of pan. Increase heat to medium high. Place kale on top of onion mixture without disturbing. Do not stir. Cook 9 min, covered.
3. Stir to combine. Cook 6 min, covered.
4. Add ½ cup water. Cook 30 min, adding an additional ½ cup water every 10 min to keep mixture from drying out.
5. Add jalapeño and stir. Cook 10 min.
6. Reduce heat to low. Cook ~5 min, uncovered, until water has evaporated.

The Crown Jewel of African Cuisine

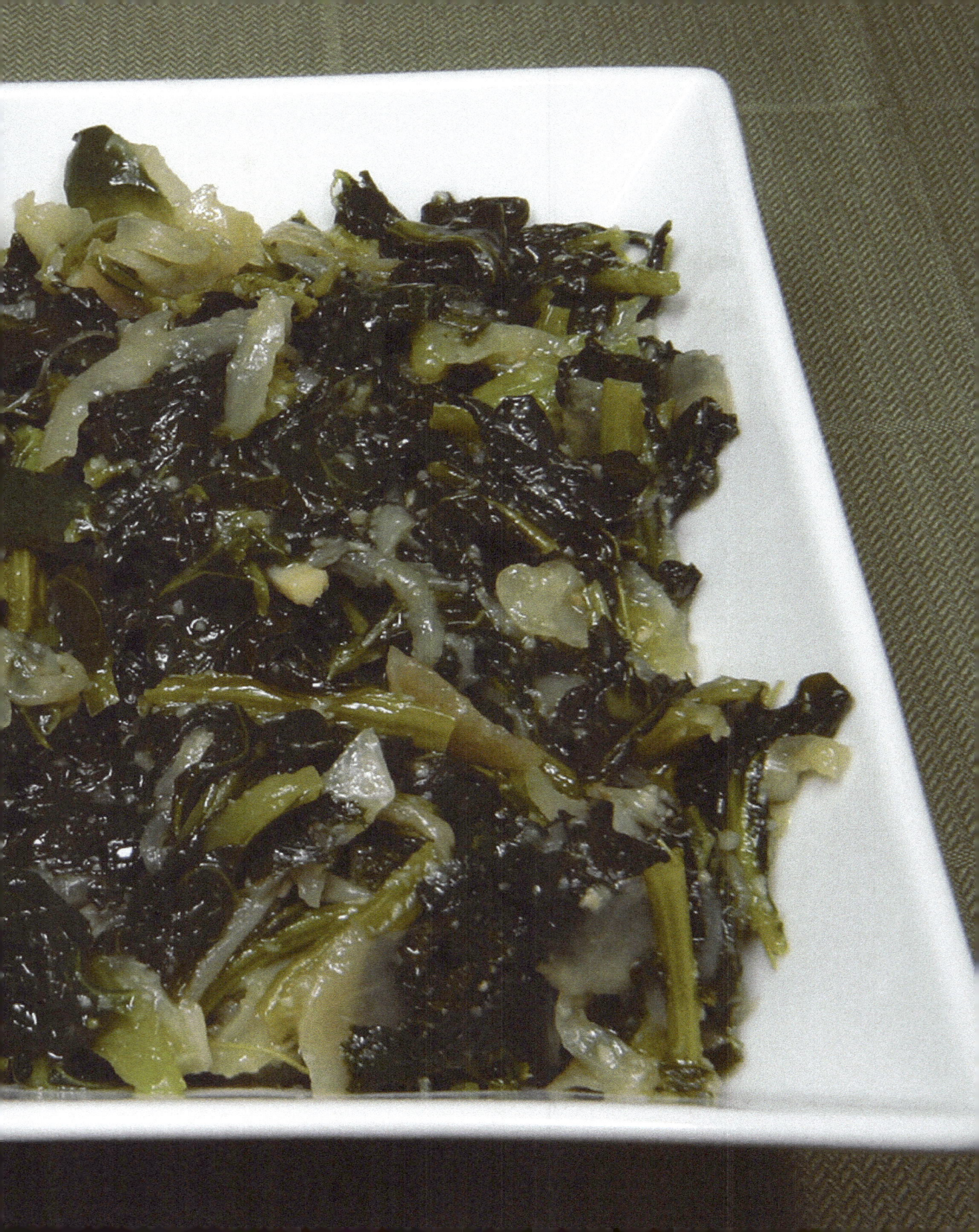

Ethiopian Collards
ጥቁር ጎመን
(Tiqur Gomen) V VG GF DF

Time: 1 hr 15 min
Serves: 6–8
Difficulty: ●●○○○

One of the vegetables we eat most in Ethiopia is collard greens. Most Ethiopians are Christians and during Lent, we eat plenty of Gomen.

Ingredients:

- Yellow onions, 1½ large, cut in half and sliced into ¼ inch thick wedges
- Vegetable oil, 1 cup
- Ginger-Garlic Paste, 3 Tbsp (p. 23)
- Salt, 2 t
- Water, ¼ cup
- Collards, 3 bunches, torn into bite-sized pieces, with string-like fibers peeled from small veins, and large midribs discarded
- Jalapeño, 1, stemmed and sliced lengthwise into eighths

Directions:

1. Combine onions, oil, Ginger-Garlic Paste, and salt in large pot over medium-high heat. Cook 7 min, uncovered, stirring often to prevent sticking.
2. Add water, scrape the bottom, and cook 1 min.
3. Add the collard pieces, mix with the onions, cover, and cook 8 min, stirring occasionally to ensure even cooking.
4. Add jalapeño slices.

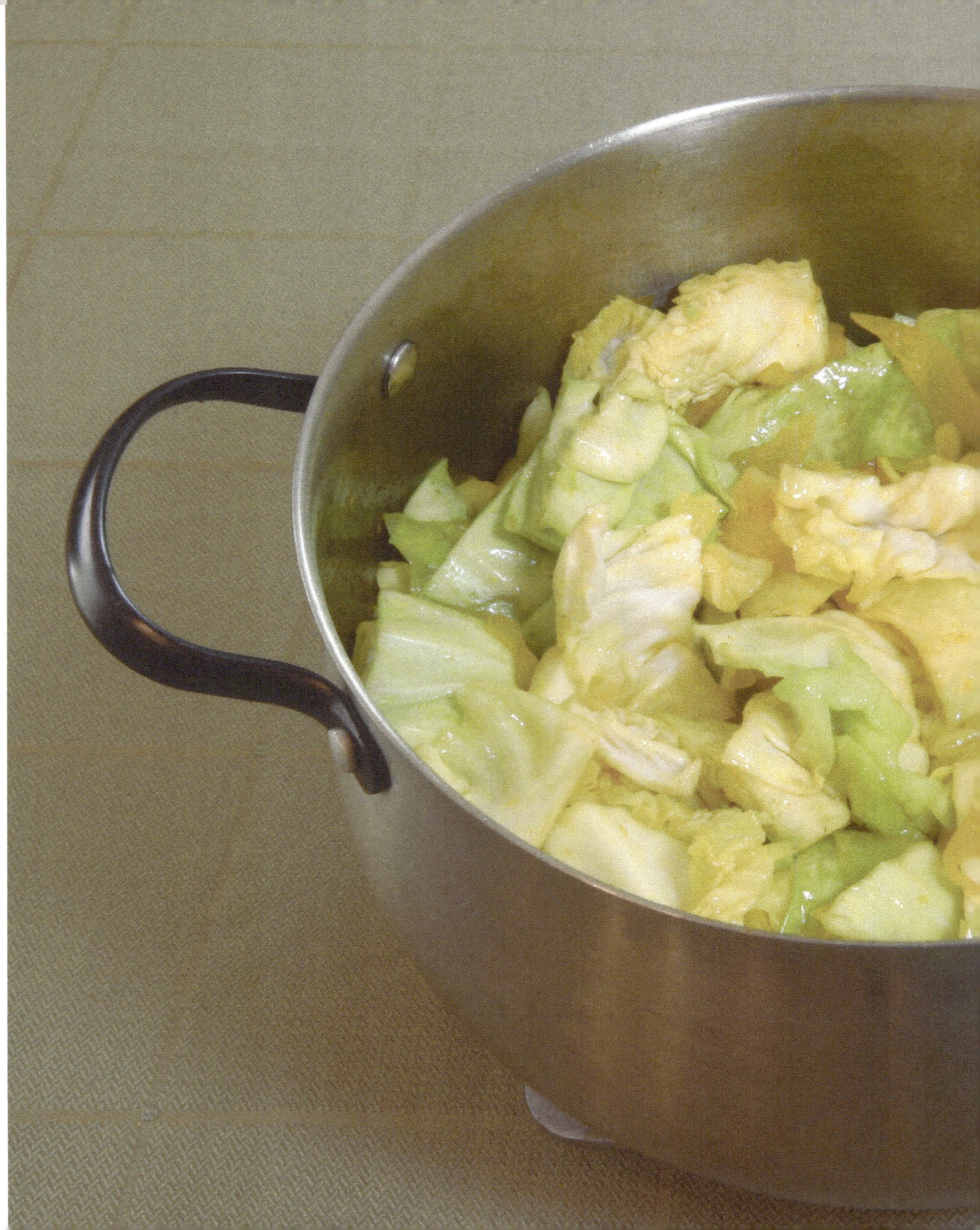

Leaf & Root Veggies

Ethiopian Cabbage
ጥቅል ጎመን
(Tiqil Gomen) (V) (VG) (GF) (DF)

Time: 25 min
Serves: 4–6
Difficulty: ♨♨♢♢♢

A nice, inexpensive side dish to have in the winter.

Ingredients:

- Yellow onion, 1 medium, coarsely chopped
- Olive or vegetable oil, ½ cup
- Turmeric, 1 tsp
- Ginger-Garlic Paste, 1 Tbsp (p. 23)
- Salt, 1 tsp
- Water, ½ cup
- Cabbage, 1 head, cored, coarsely chopped and separated

Directions:

1. Place onion, oil, turmeric, Ginger-Garlic Paste in a large pot. Cook 2 min over high heat.
2. Add ¼ cup water. Cook 3 min.
3. Add ¼ cup water and spread onion mixture over bottom of pot. Place cabbage on top of onion mixture without disturbing. Do not stir. Cook 3 min, covered.
4. Stir to combine. Cook 10 min, covered.

The Crown Jewel of African Cuisine

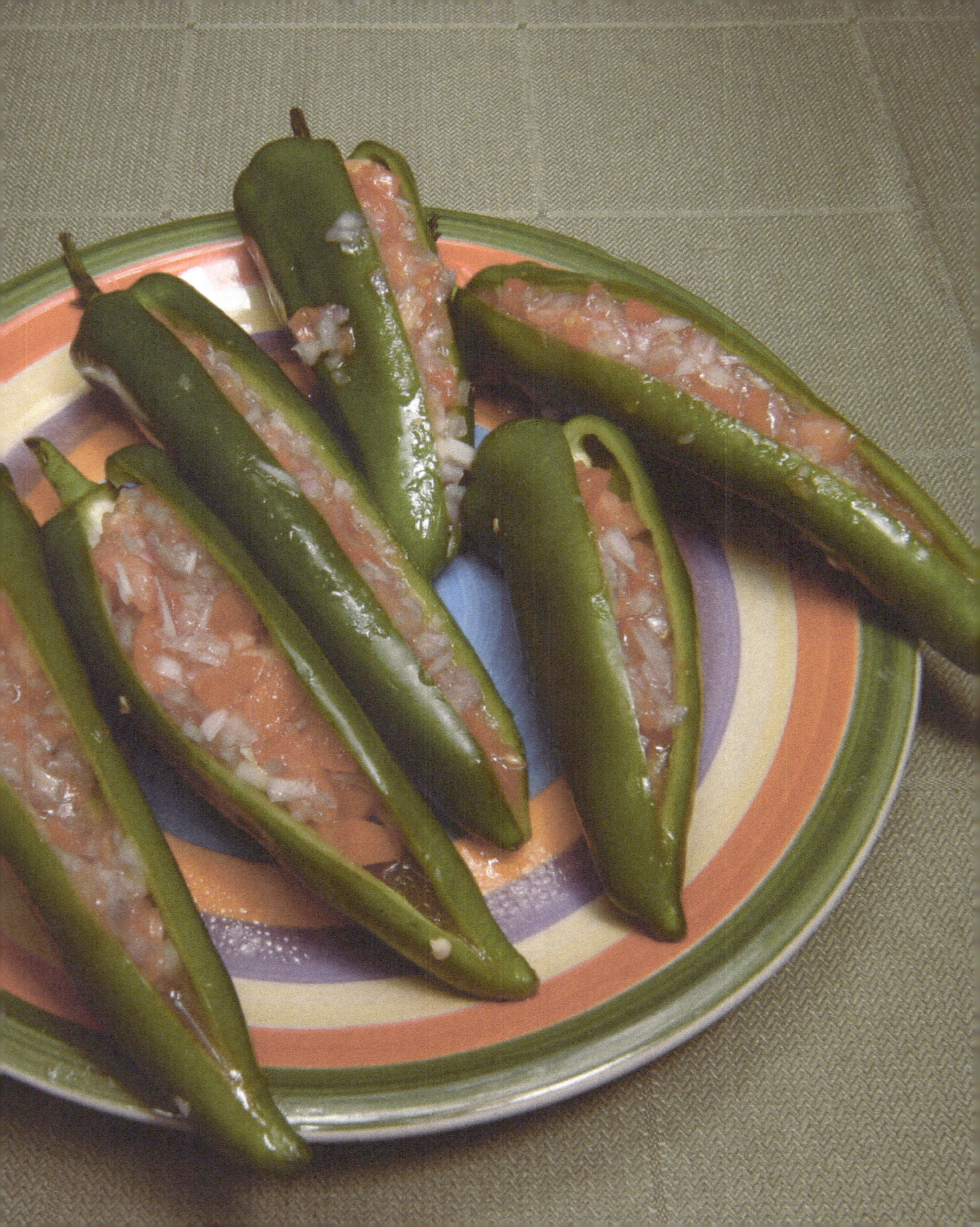

Leaf & Root Veggies

Filled Peppers
ቃርያ ሲፈግ
(Qaria Sinig) V VG GF DF

Time: 10 min
Serves: 6
Difficulty: ◆◇◇◇◇

This dish is one of the most colorful and festive-looking of Ethiopian dishes. I love it as a side dish for a party or celebration.

Ingredients:

Shallots, 2, finely diced
Tomato, 1 large, finely diced
Lime, 1, juiced
Salt, 1 tsp
Vegetable oil, ¼ cup
Anaheim peppers, 6

Directions:

1. Place shallots, tomatoes, lime juice, salt and oil in a small bowl. Mix and set aside
2. Make 1 lengthwise slice down the side of each pepper. Remove seeds and membrane from inside the peppers, being careful to keep the pepper intact.
3. With soup spoon, fill each pepper with the shallot tomato mix. Refrigerate until ready to serve.

The Crown Jewel of African Cuisine

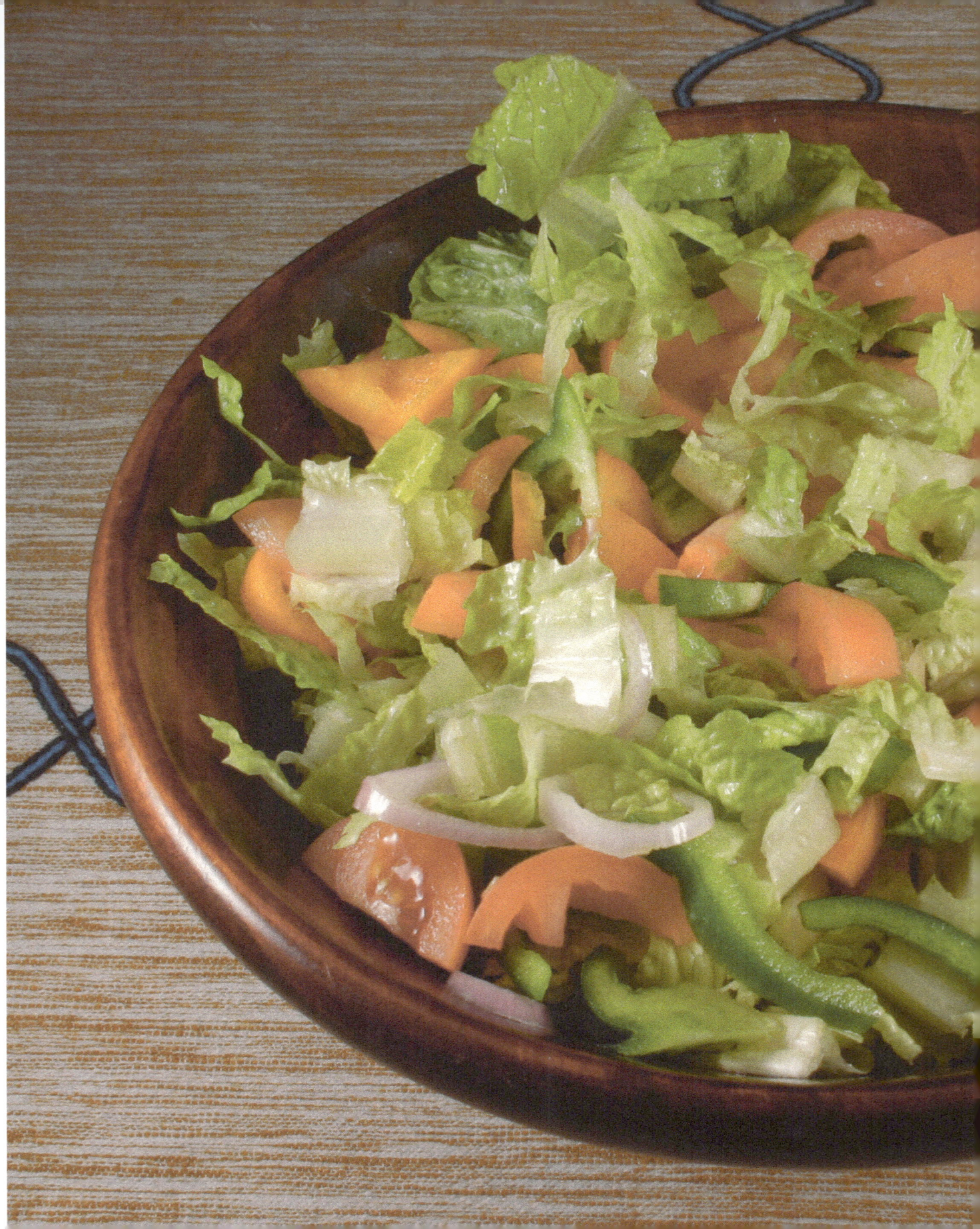

Lettuce, Pepper & Tomato Salad
የቲማቲም ሳላጣ
(Yetimatim Salata) Ⓥ VG GF DF

Time: 10 min
Serves: 4–5
Difficulty:

This salad is not traditionally Ethiopian, but I served it at the farmers market for years, as it goes perfectly alongside traditional dishes.

Ingredients:

For the salad:
Hearts of romaine, 2, coarsely chopped
Green bell pepper, ½, seeded, coarsely chopped
Orange bell pepper, ½, seeded, coarsely chopped
Plum tomatoes, 2, coarsely chopped
Shallot, 1 clove, sliced ¼ inch thick
Salt, 1 tsp

For the dressing:
White vinegar, 1 Tbsp
Olive oil, ¼ cup
Lime, ½, juiced
Salt, ½ tsp

Directions:

1. Whisk dressing ingredients in small bowl.
2. Place salad ingredients into large bowl. Add dressing and toss before serving.

Leaf & Root Veggies

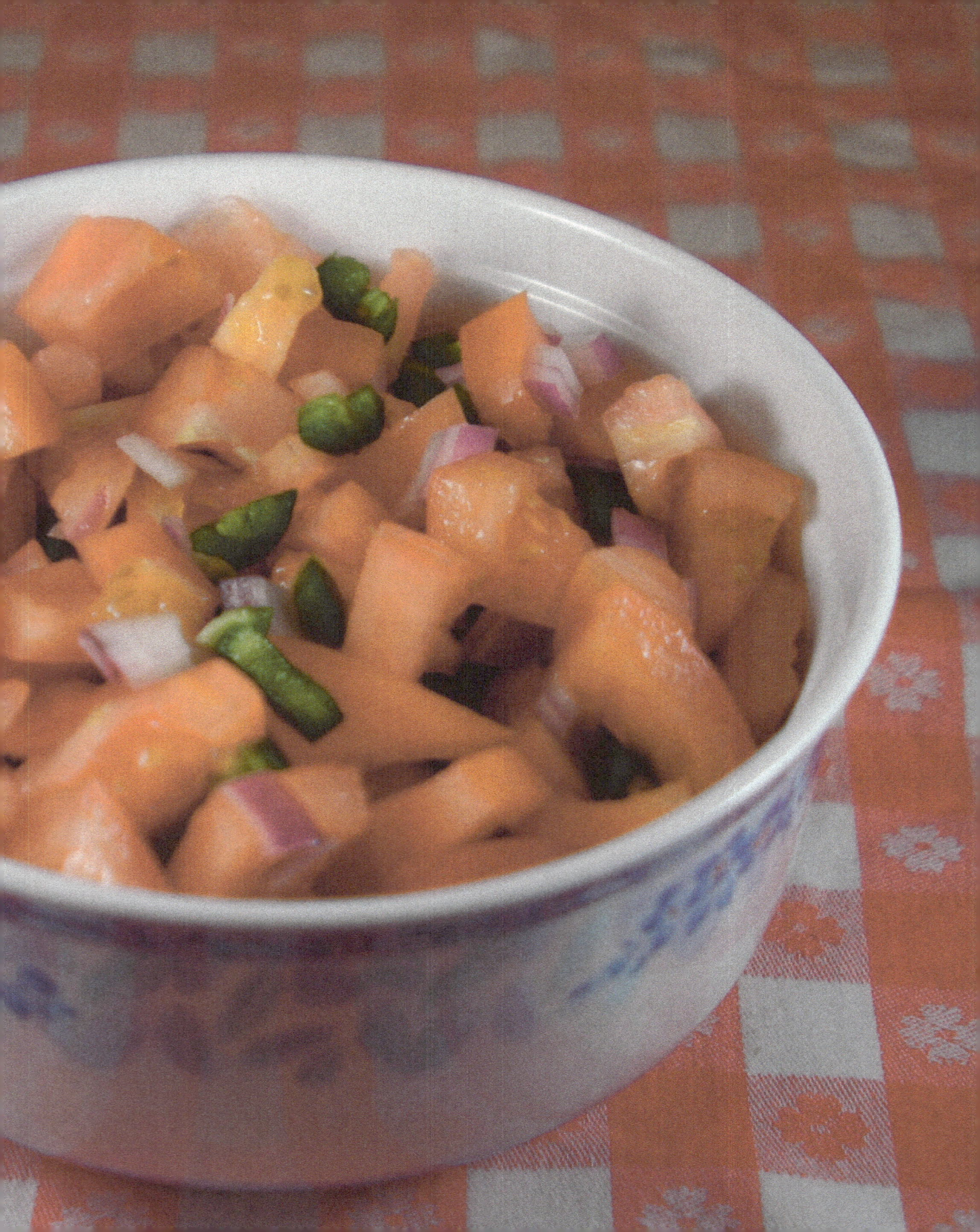

Leaf & Root Veggies

Fresh Tomato Salad
የቲማቲም ና ሽንኩርት ሳላጣ
(Yetimatim Na Shinkurt Salata) (V) (VG) (GF) (DF)

Time: 5 min
Serves: 4
Difficulty:

In Ethiopia, we serve fresh tomatoes, prepared this way, to complement vegetarian meals.

Ingredients:

For the salad:
- Large tomatoes, 2, cut into ½ inch dice
- Red onion, ½ medium, finely diced
- Jalapeño, 1, seeded, finely diced

For the dressing:
- Olive oil, 2 Tbsp
- White Vinegar, 1 Tbsp
- Lemon, 1, juiced
- Salt, ½ tsp

Directions:
1. Whisk dressing ingredients to combine.
2. Place salad ingredients into bowl. Add dressing and toss to combine before serving.

The Crown Jewel of African Cuisine

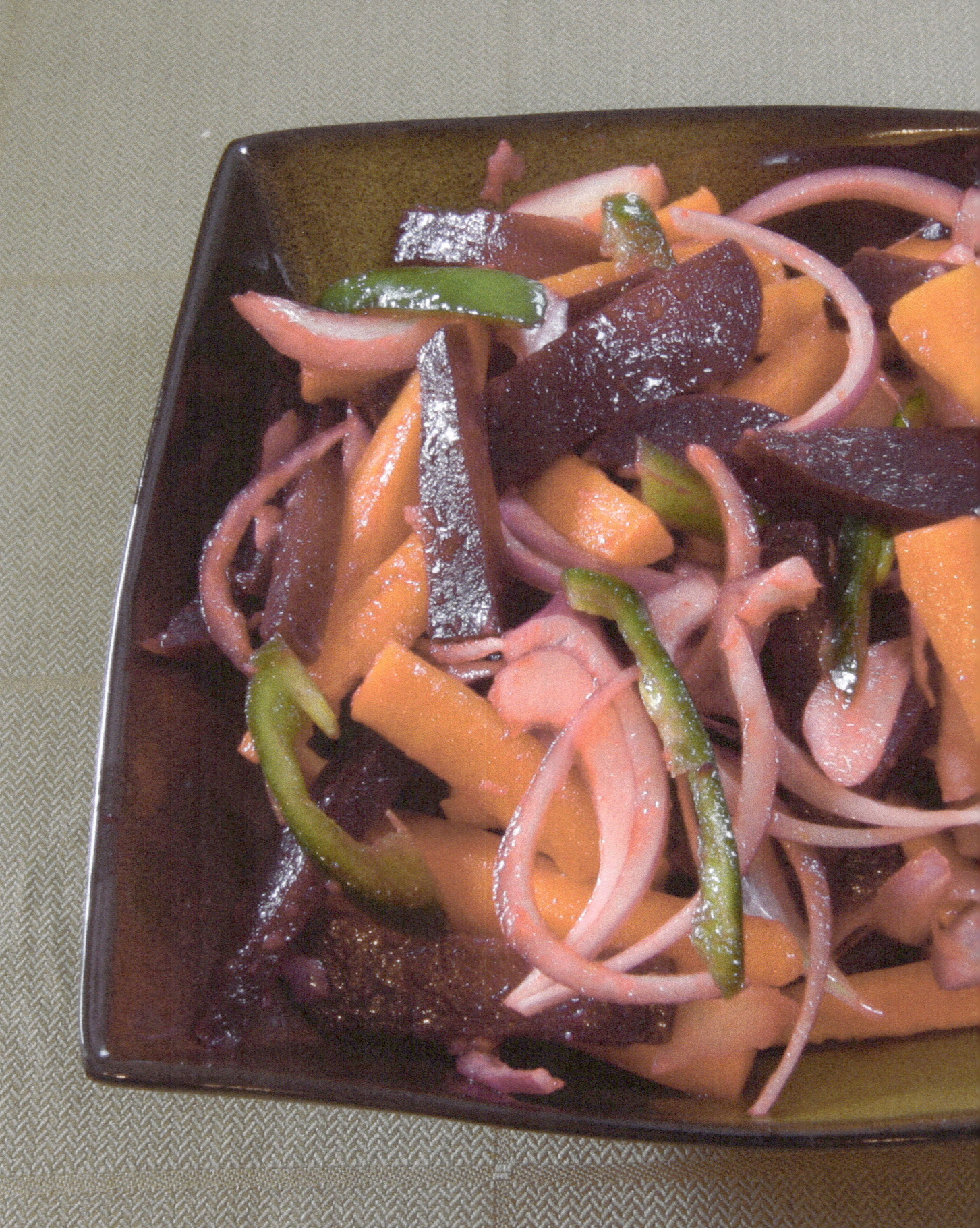

Cold Beet Salad
የድንች, ካሮት ና ቀይሥር ሳላጣ
(Yedinich, Carrot Na Keysir Salata) (V) (VG) (GF) (DF)

Leaf & Root Veggies

Time: 1 hr 15 min
Serves: 8–10
Difficulty: ♦♦◇◇◇

This Ethiopian dish is a summertime favorite at my restaurant.

Ingredients:

For the salad:
Beets, 3 medium, greens trimmed
Carrots, 6 medium
Red potatoes, 4 medium
Red onions, 1½ large, cut in half, then sliced into ¼ inch thick wedges, and the layers separated
Jalapeños, 2, seeded, cut into 2 inch by ¼ inch strips

Dressing:
Limes, 2, juiced
Olive oil, ¼ cup
White vinegar, ¼ cup
Salt, 1½ tsp

Directions:

1. Place beets, carrots and potatoes into separate small pots and cover with water. Cover and cook over high heat. Cook carrots 20–25 min or until tender. Cook potatoes around 40 min or until tender. Cook beets around 1 hour or until tender. When vegetables are done, remove each from heat and rinse with cold water until cool.
2. Place red onions in large serving bowl. Place jalapeños over onions.
3. Peel potatoes and carrots.
4. Cut carrots into 4 inch lengths, quartered lengthwise. Place on top of jalapeños.
5. Cut each potato into 8 wedges and layer on top of carrots.
6. Peel beets and cut into 8 wedges and later on top of potatoes.
7. Refrigerate bowl until ready to serve.
8. Immediately before serving, whisk dressing ingredients together in bowl. Pour over salad and gently toss.

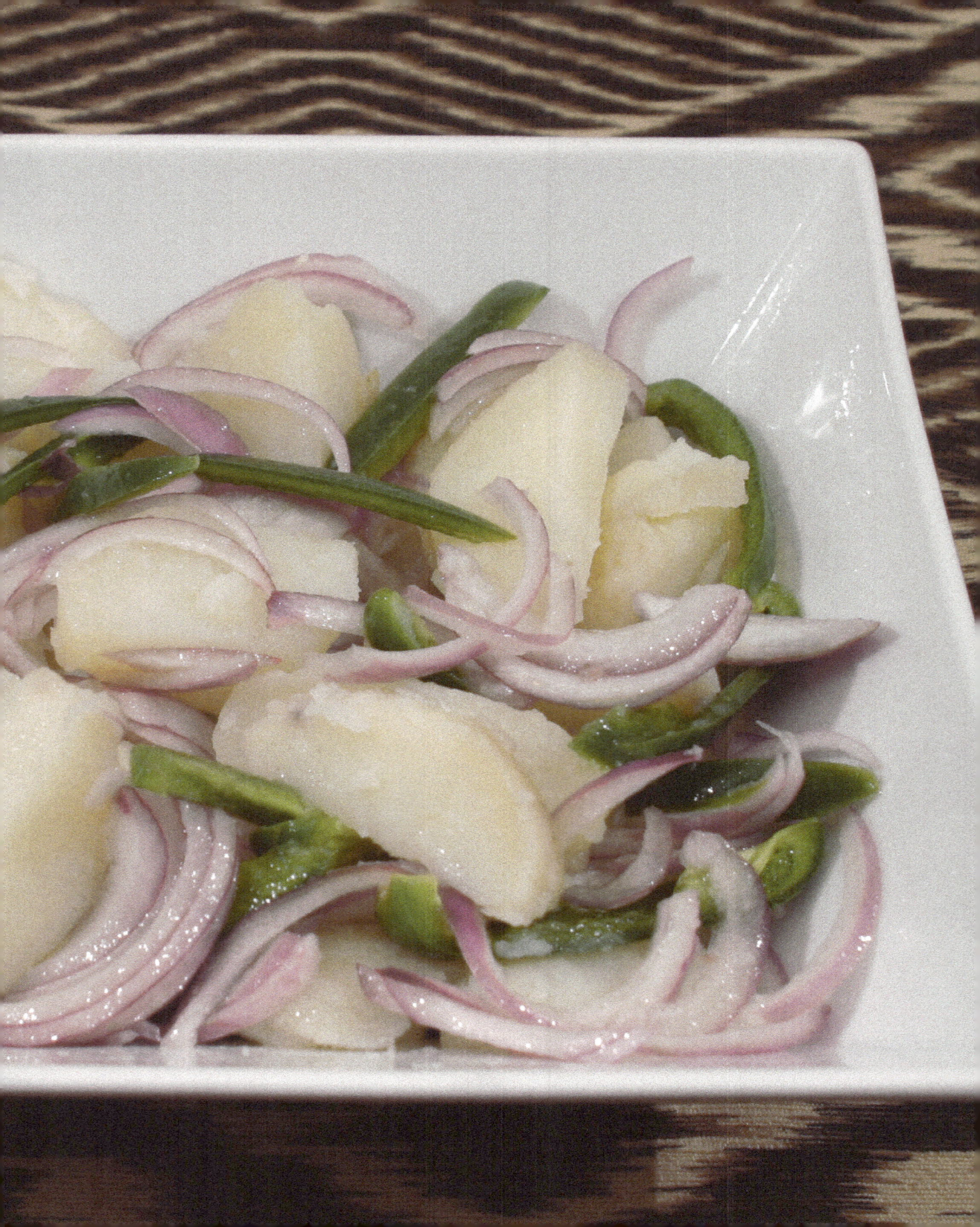

Ethiopian Potato Salad
የድንች ሳላጣ
(Yedinich Salata) (V) (VG) (GF) (DF)

Time: 1 hr
Serves: 4
Difficulty:

This Ethiopian Potato Salad is much lighter than traditional European potato salads.

Ingredients:

For the salad:
Red potatoes, 4 medium
Red onion, ½ medium, sliced into ¼ inch thick wedges
Jalapeños, 2, seeded, sliced lengthwise into ¼ inch thick slices

For the dressing:
Lime, 1, juiced
Olive oil, 1 Tbsp
Salt, 1 tsp

Directions:

1. Place potatoes into a medium saucepan and cover with water. Cook 45–50 min at a gentle boil over medium-high heat, uncovered, until tender.
2. Prepare other vegetables and dressing and combine in a serving bowl.
3. Drain the potatoes and rinse in cold water until they are cool enough to handle.
4. Peel potatoes, cut each into 8 wedges, and place them in the serving bowl.
5. Gently toss.

Leaf & Root Veggies

The Crown Jewel of African Cuisine

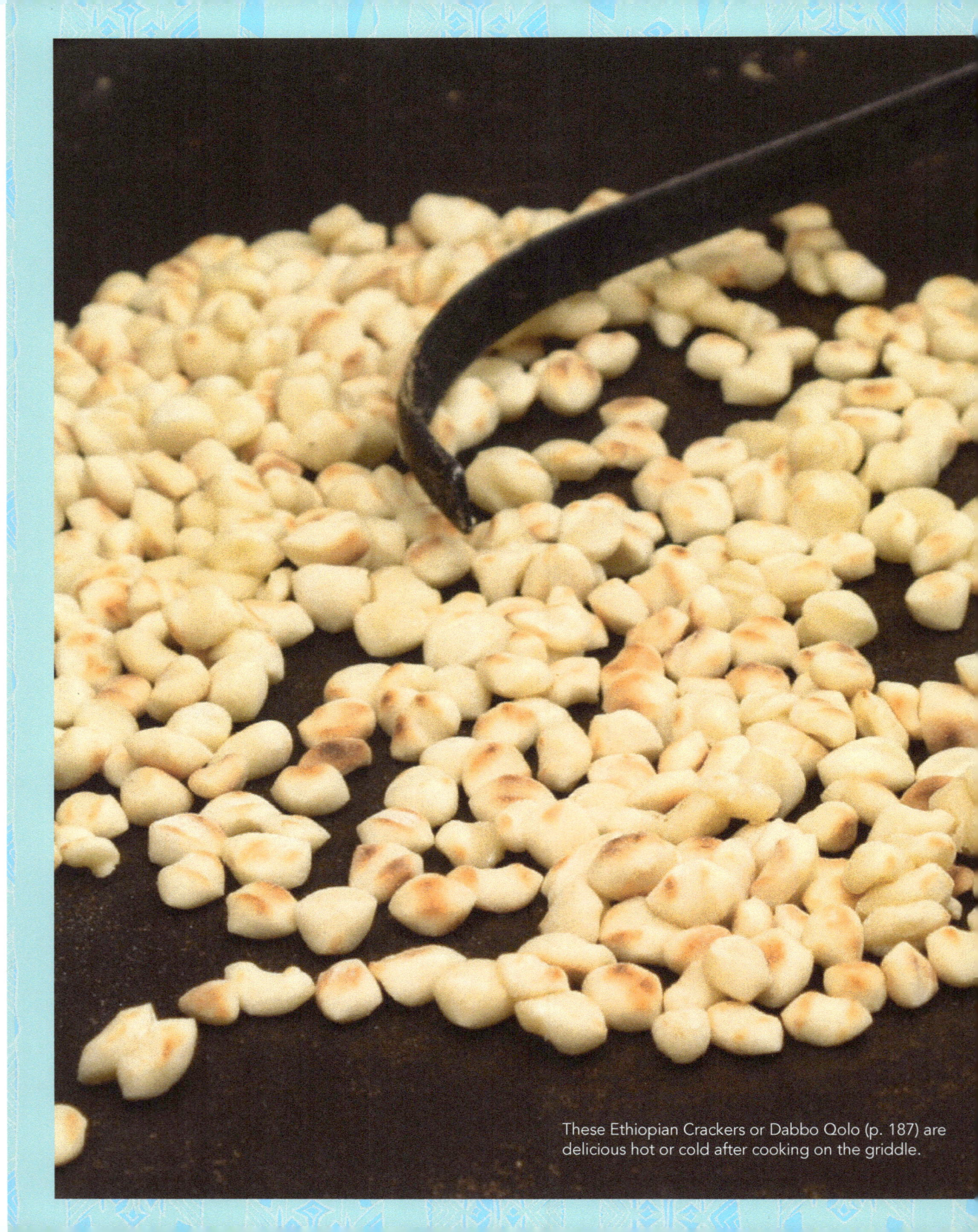

These Ethiopian Crackers or Dabbo Qolo (p. 187) are delicious hot or cold after cooking on the griddle.

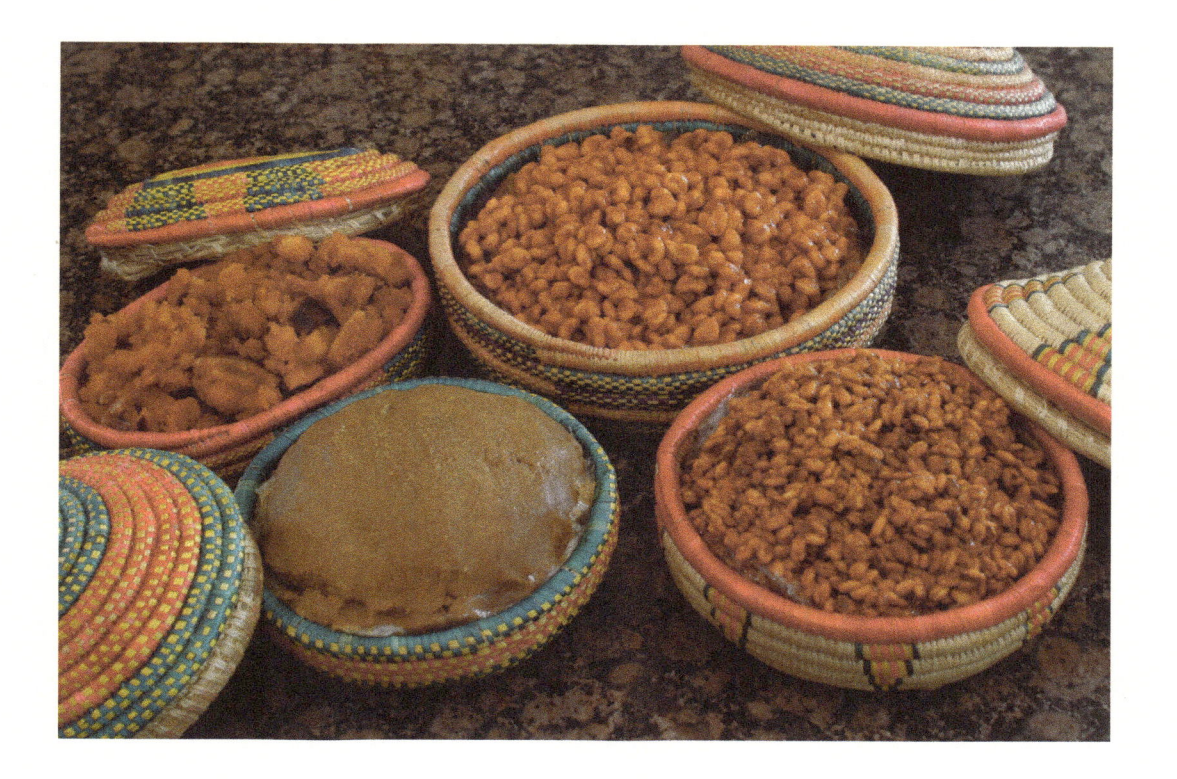

Just a Nibble: Snacks and Treats

These recipes are for all the foods we eat when it's not a regular meal. We serve these when a guest comes over and we want something small to eat while we have our coffee or tea. We eat some of these when we are on a trip. We cannot carry our Injera here and there, so we bring hearty foods that are easy to carry and can help us make our journey. My family loves many of these snacks, especially Ethiopian Chocolate!

Above (top left to bottom right): Spicy torn bread or chachabsa (p. 47); spicy crackers or dabbo qolo (p. 187); Ethiopian chocolate or chuko (p. 189); roasted barley or qolo (p. 185).

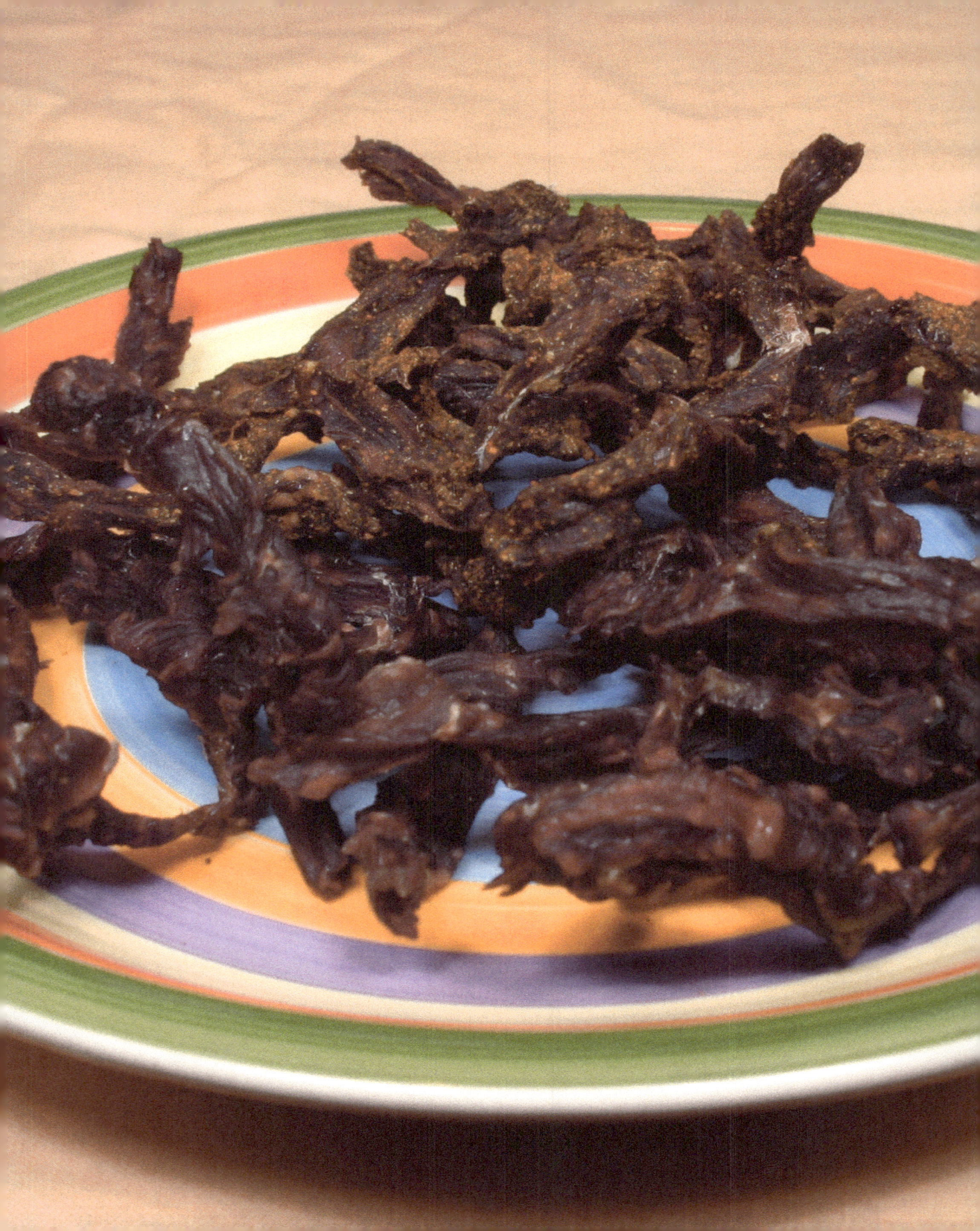

Spicy and Regular Beef Jerky
ቋንጣ ና ቋንጣ በምጥምጣ
(Quanta Na Quanta Be Mitmita) GF DF

Time: 15 min, plus 3 days to cure
Serves: 5
Difficulty:

In many cultures, people are not as familiar with drying meats as we are in Ethiopia. Please use caution, good hygiene and good sense if you use this recipe.

Ingredients:

Lean beef, 1¼ lb, (top round or eye of round are good choices)

Salt, ½ tsp

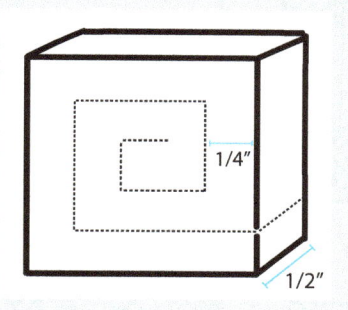

Directions:

1. Cut beef into long strips that are ¼ inch wide, as shown in illustration.
2. Toss meat well with salt.
3. Hang meat strips on clean dowel indoors for 3 days.
4. Cut into bite sized pieces.

For a spicy variation:

Instead of tossing with salt, toss with 1 tsp mitmita*.

*available at specialty stores and online, see p. 17

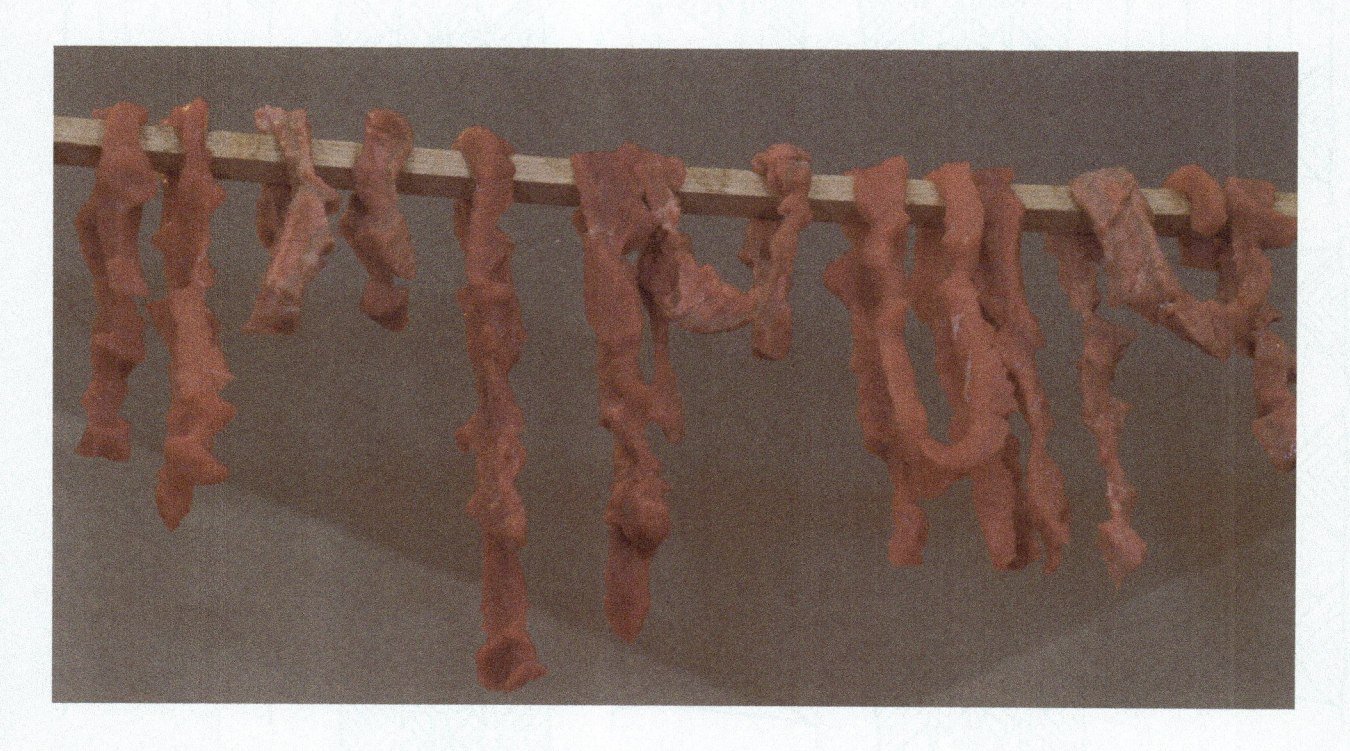

The Crown Jewel of African Cuisine

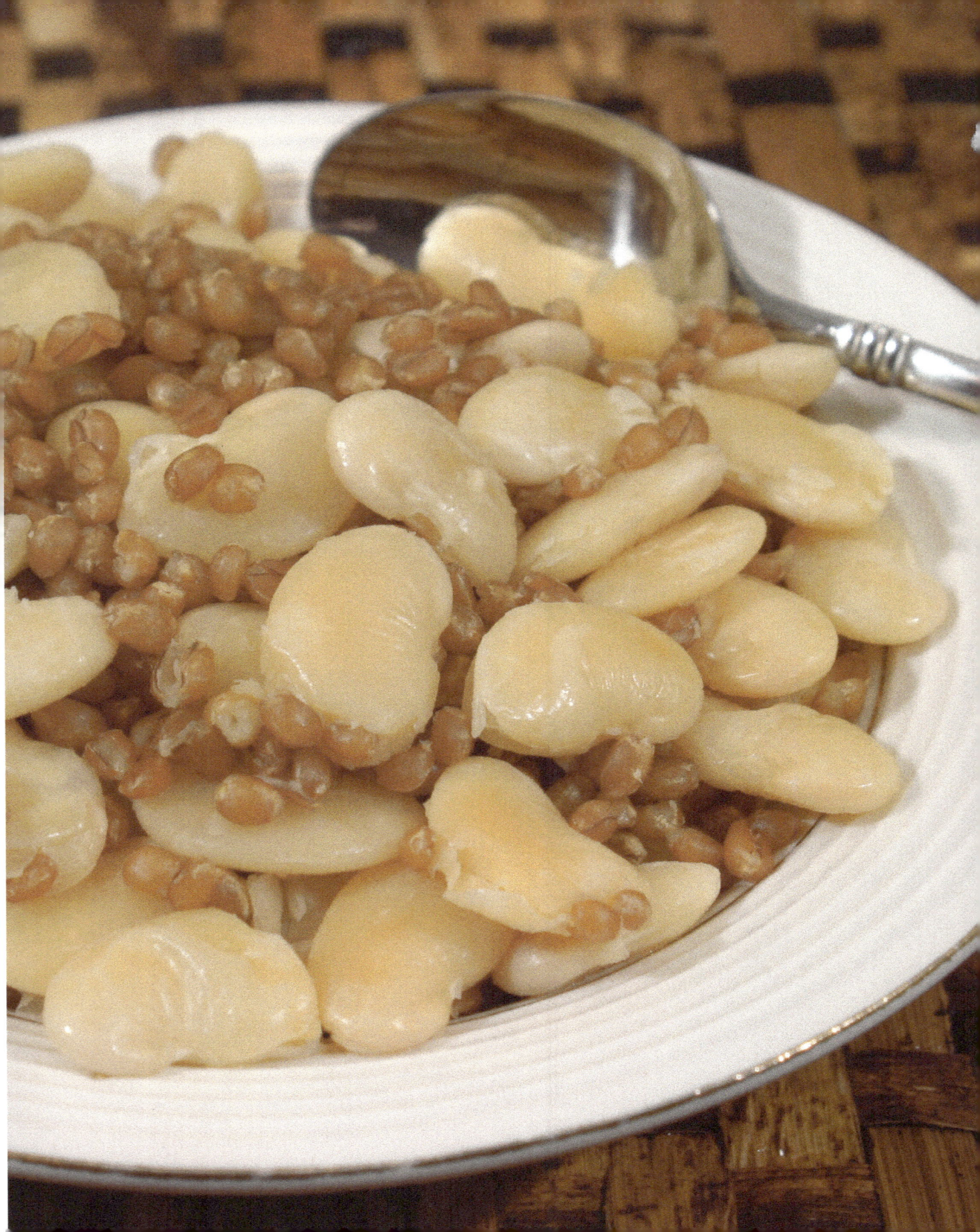

Snacks & Treats

Salted Beans & Grains, 4 Ways
ንፍሮ
(Nifro) (V) (VG) (GF) (DF)

Time: 3–5 hr
Serves: 6–8
Difficulty: 🌶

Nifro has two different and unusual roles in the lives of Ethiopians. People use it to supplement a diet if they can't afford to eat Injera (p. 33) daily. We also commonly eat it after funerals.

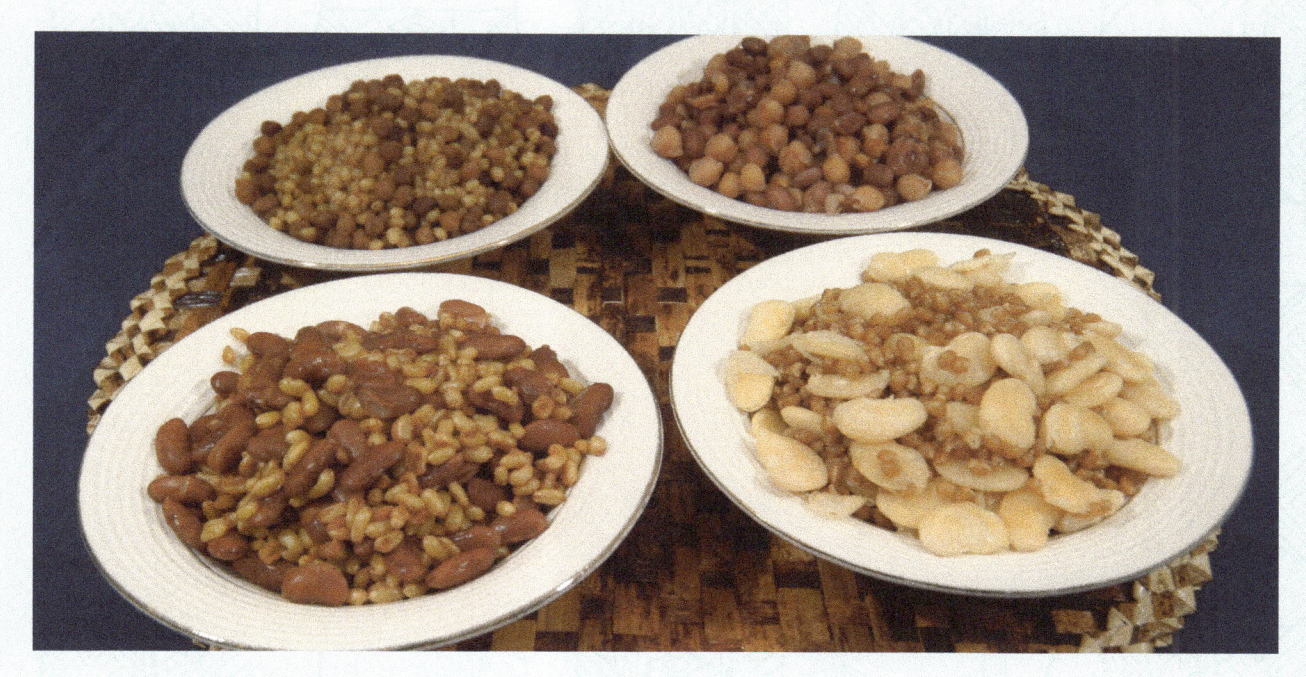

Version I. Wheat Berry and Fava Bean Nifro

Ingredients:

Dried wheat berries*, 1 cup, rinsed (remove any stones)

Dried fava beans, 1 cup, rinsed (remove any stones)

Water to cook

Salt, 1 tsp

*available at specialty stores and online, see p. 17

Directions:

1. Two hours ahead of cooking, soak wheat berries in a medium bowl.
2. One hour prior to cooking, soak fava beans in a separate medium bowl.
3. Drain wheat berries and place in a large pot with 6 cups water over high heat. Cook 30 min, covered.
4. Reduce heat to medium high. Cook 30 min, partially covered.
5. Drain fava beans beans and add to pot. Add 4 more cups water. Cook 1 hour.
6. Add salt, reduce heat to low, and cook 25 min or until water is gone.

The Crown Jewel of African Cuisine

Snacks & Treats

Version II.
Chickpea and Kidney Bean Nifro

Directions:

1. Two hours ahead of cooking, soak dried chickpeas in a medium bowl.
2. One hour prior to cooking, soak kidney beans in a separate medium bowl.
3. Drain chickpeas and place in large pot with 6 cups water over high heat. Cook, covered, for 30 min.
4. Reduce heat to medium high. Cover and cook 30 min with lid ajar.

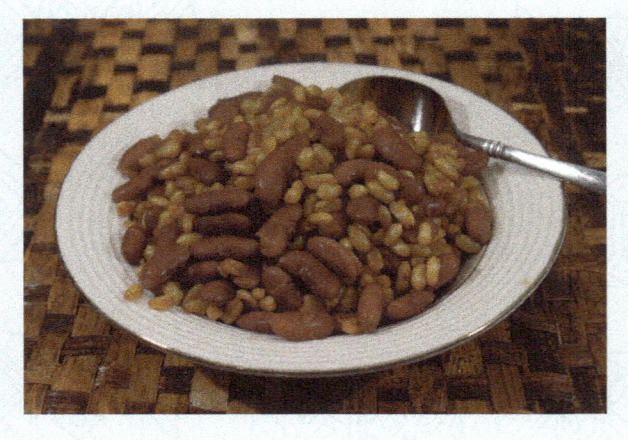

Ingredients:

Dried chickpeas, 1 cup, rinsed (stones removed)
Dried kidney deans, 1 cup, rinsed (stones removed)
Water to cook
Salt, 1 tsp

Version III:
Kamut Berry and Kidney Bean Nifro

Directions:

1. Two hours ahead of cooking, soak dried kamut berries in a medium bowl.
2. One hour prior to cooking, soak kidney beans in a separate medium bowl.
3. Drain kamut berries and place in a large pot with 6 cups water over high heat. Cook, covered, for 30 min.
4. Reduce heat to medium high. Cook 30 min, partially covered.
5. Drain kidney beans and add to pot. Add 4 more cups water. Cook 1 hour.
6. Add salt. Reduce heat to low and cook 25 min or until water is gone.

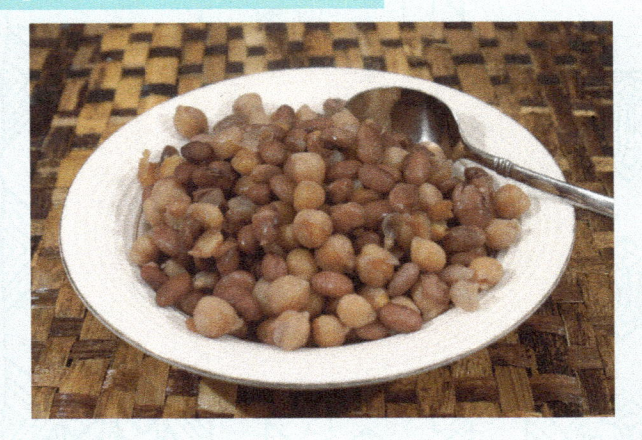

Ingredients:

Dried kamut berries*, 1 cup, rinsed (stones removed)
Dried kidney beans, 1 cup, rinsed (stones removed)
Water to cook
Salt, 1 tsp

*available at specialty stores and online, see p. 16

Snacks & Treats

Version IV:
Chickpea and Wheat Berry Nifro

Directions:
1. Two hours ahead of cooking, soak dried chickpeas in a medium bowl, and soak wheat berries in separate bowl.
2. Drain chickpeas and wheat berries and combine in a large pot with 8 cups water and salt over high heat. Cook 30 min, covered.
3. Reduce heat to medium high. Cook 1 hour 40 min, covered.
4. Reduce heat to low and cook 25 min or until water is gone.

Ingredients:
Dried chickpeas, 1 cup, rinsed (stones removed)
Dried wheat berries*, 1 cup, rinsed (stones removed)
Water to cook
Salt, 1 tsp

*available at specialty stores and online, see p. 17

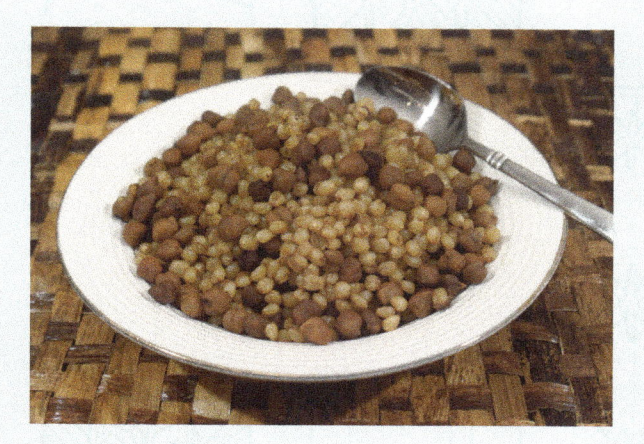

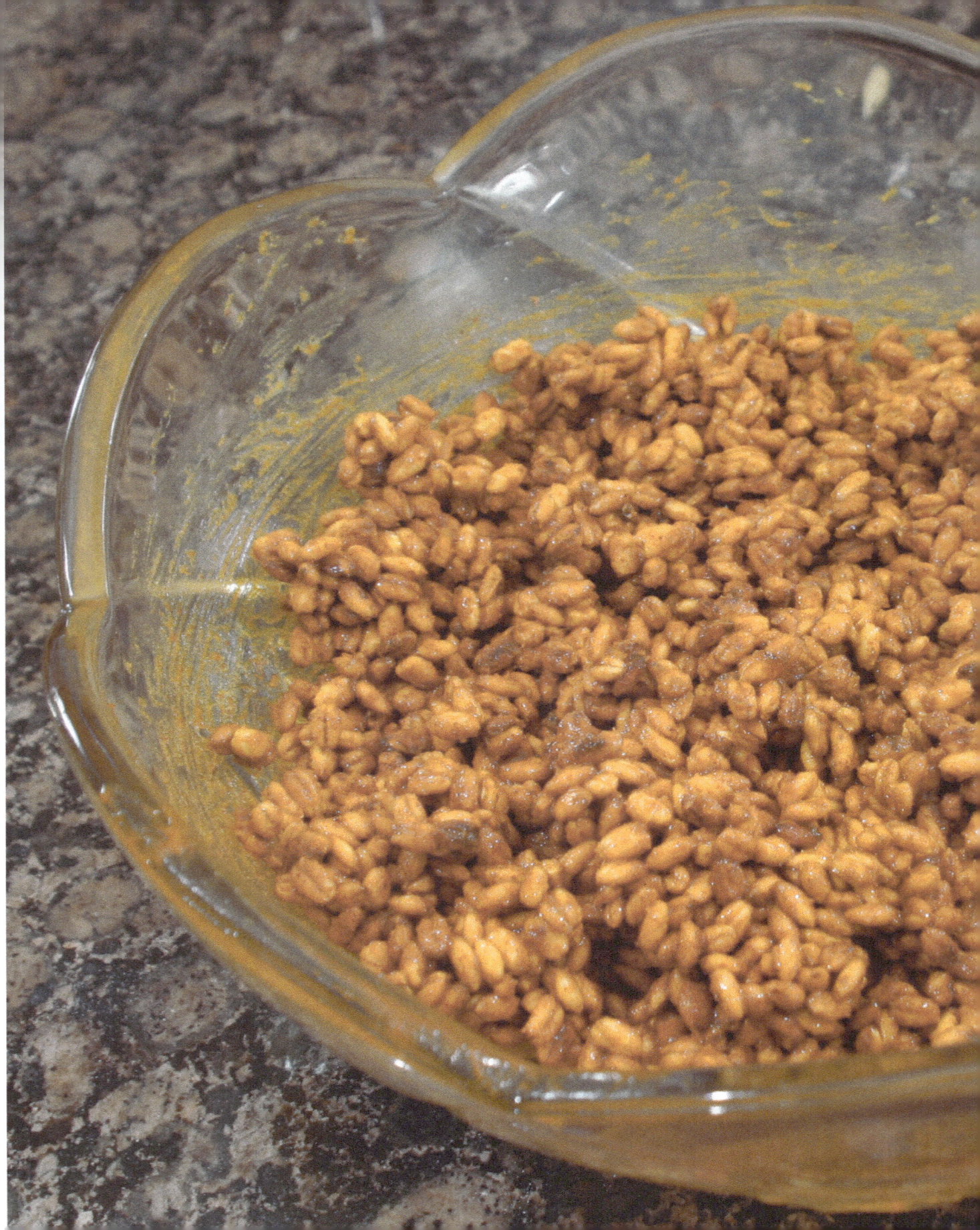

Snacks & Treats

Roasted Barley
ቆሎ
(Qolo) Ⓥ ⓋⒼ ⒼⒻ ⒹⒻ

Prep Time: 15 min
Serves: 6
Difficulty: ♦◊◊◊◊

We eat Qolo as a snack, serve it to guests, and often buy it as street food. It can be served spicy or unspiced by leaving out the Berberre paste.

Ingredients:

Pearl barley, 3 cups
Niter Kibe, ½ cup (p. 21)
Salt, pinch
Berberre paste, 1 tsp (p. 29)

Directions:

1. Heat a frying pan over medium-high heat.
2. Place barley into pan and dry roast for 6–8 min, stirring constantly. Some of the barley will pop during this time.
3. Remove to a bowl and set aside to cool.
4. Melt Niter Kibe in the pan, then add salt and Berberre paste. Pour over the roasted barley. Mix to coat evenly.

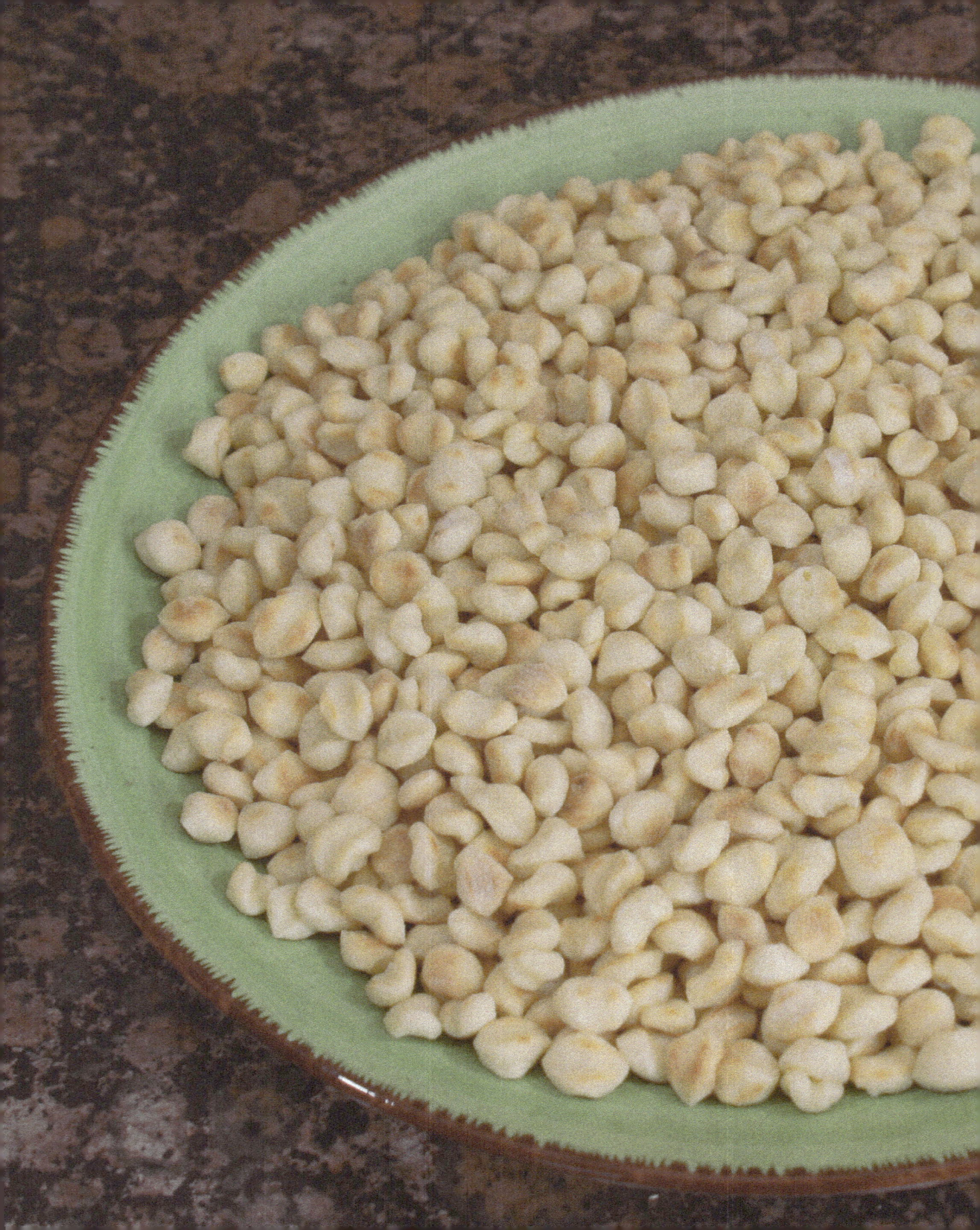

Snacks & Treats

Ethiopian Crackers, 3 Ways
ዳቦቆሎ
(Dabbo Qolo) (V) (VG) (DF)

Time: 25 min
Makes: 3 cups
Difficulty: ♦♦♢♢♢

Ethiopian people eat these crunchy crackers between meals or bring them as a gift of food when traveling long distances to visit someone. They are perfect for long trip, as they do not spoil quickly.

Ingredients:
- Bleached flour, 2 cups
- Sugar, 1 Tbsp
- Vegetable oil, 1 Tbsp
- Salt (a pinch)
- Water, ⅔ cup

Directions:
1. In a bowl, combine the flour, sugar, oil, salt, and water, working it together to form a ball.
2. Turn the dough out onto a floured surface, and knead 4 min with the heel of your hand.
3. Break off a small piece of the dough, and roll it into a long cord that is about ¼ inch thick. Repeat until all dough has been turned into cords.
4. With scissors, cut the cords into ¼ inch lengths over a lightly floured dish. Shake the dish every once in a while to coat the pieces with flour, so that they do not stick together.
5. Heat a large non-stick frying pan over medium-high heat.
6. Once the pan is hot, add half of the dough pieces to the pan, and reduce the heat to medium.
7. Using a spatula, turn the dough pieces frequently, until they are golden-brown on all sides (12–14 min total). During this time, break up any clusters of pieces that may clump together.
8. Remove the crackers to a plate to cool, and repeat with the remaining dough pieces.

These crackers are often eaten plain. To give them extra flavor, try:

Spicy Ethiopian Crackers (above right):

After the crackers have cooled, place them in a bowl. In a separate small bowl, combine 1 Tbsp Berberre powder* (or if you want it even spicier, use mitmita*), a pinch of salt, and ½ cup Niter Kibe (melted) (p. 21), pour it over the crackers, and mix thoroughly by hand.

Turmeric-seasoned Ethiopian Crackers (below right):

Before forming the dough, add a pinch of turmeric to the water used to form the dough. Crackers seasoned in this manner are not typically used for the spicy variation.

*available at specialty stores and online, see p. 16-17

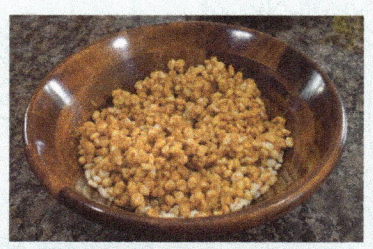

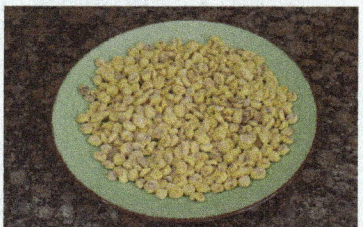

The Crown Jewel of African Cuisine

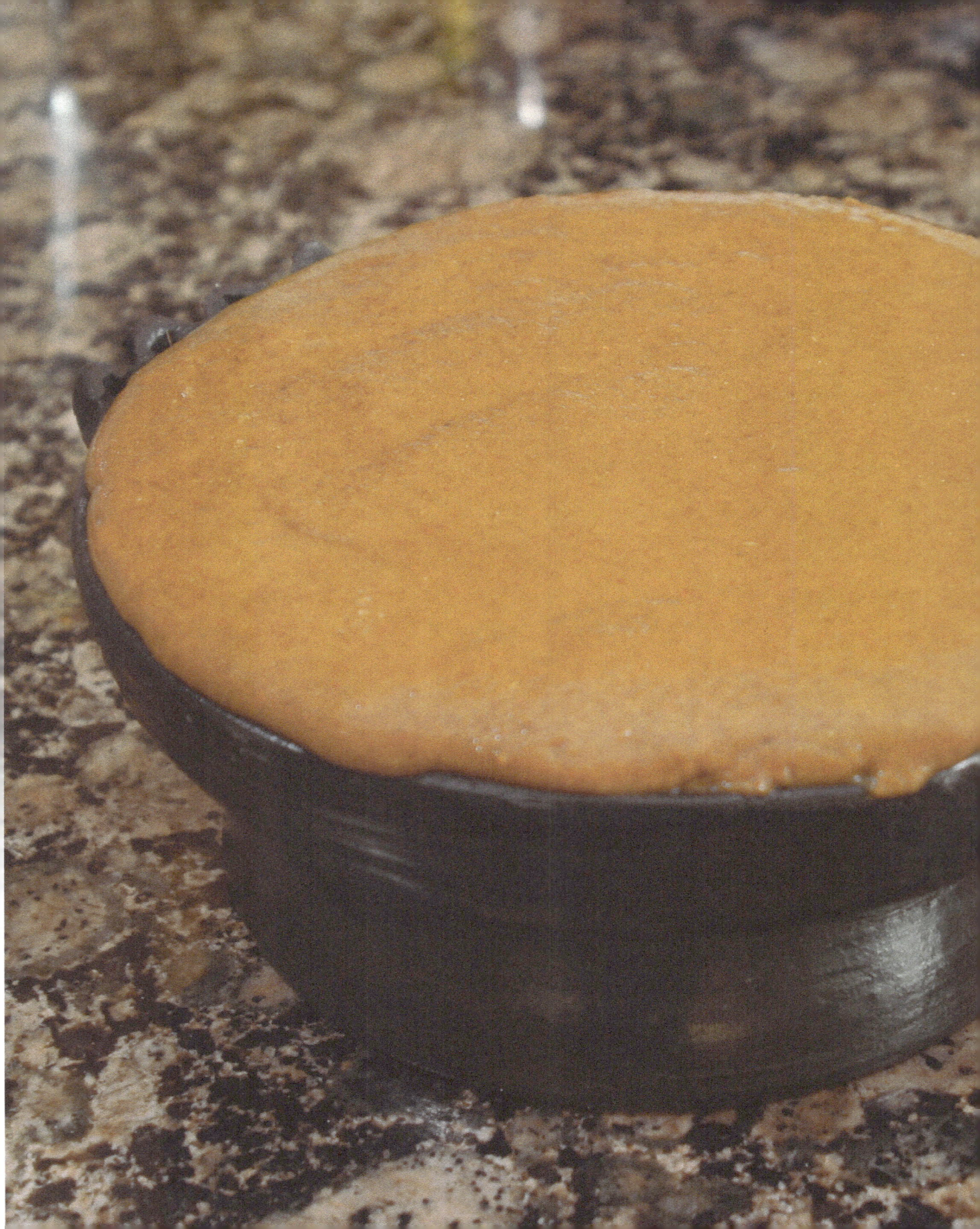

Snacks & Treats

Ethiopian Chocolate
ጭኮ
(Chuko) V VG GF DF

Time: 5 min
Serves: 6–8
Difficulty:

Chuko is really not chocolate at all, but it has a consistency similar to fudge. We love it more than any chocolate though, especially as travel food.

Ingredients:

Besso*, 2 cups

Niter Kibe, 1 cup, melted (p. 21)

Berberre powder* (or if you want it even spicier, use mitmita*) 1 Tbsp

Salt, ⅛ tsp

K'olo, a few Tbsp (optional, if you want a crunchier snack) (p. 185)

*available at specialty stores and online, see p. 16

Directions:

1. Combine all ingredients in a medium-sized bowl. Pat down until forms a solid mass.
2. Cut into bite-sized pieces to serve.

The Crown Jewel of African Cuisine

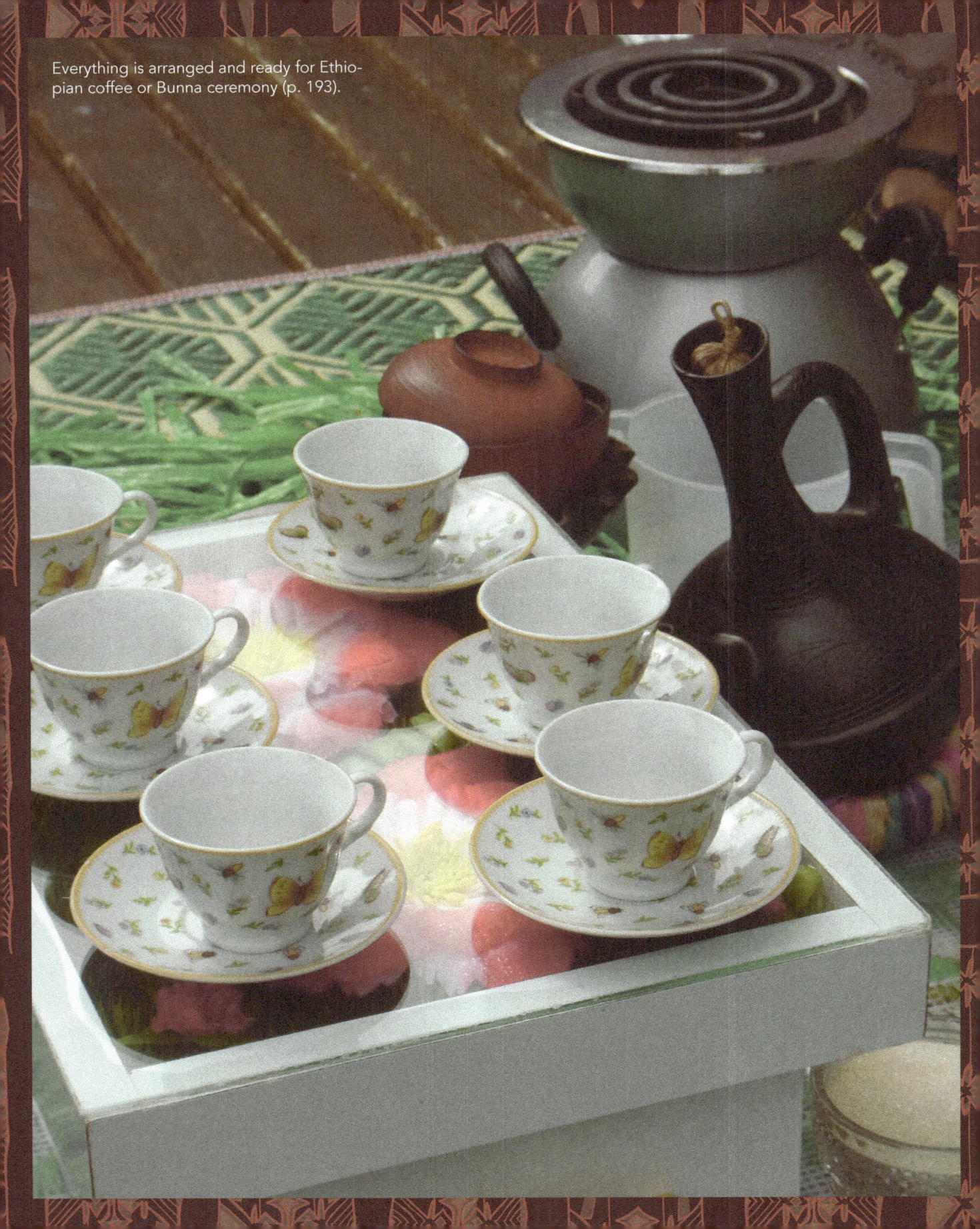

Everything is arranged and ready for Ethiopian coffee or Bunna ceremony (p. 193).

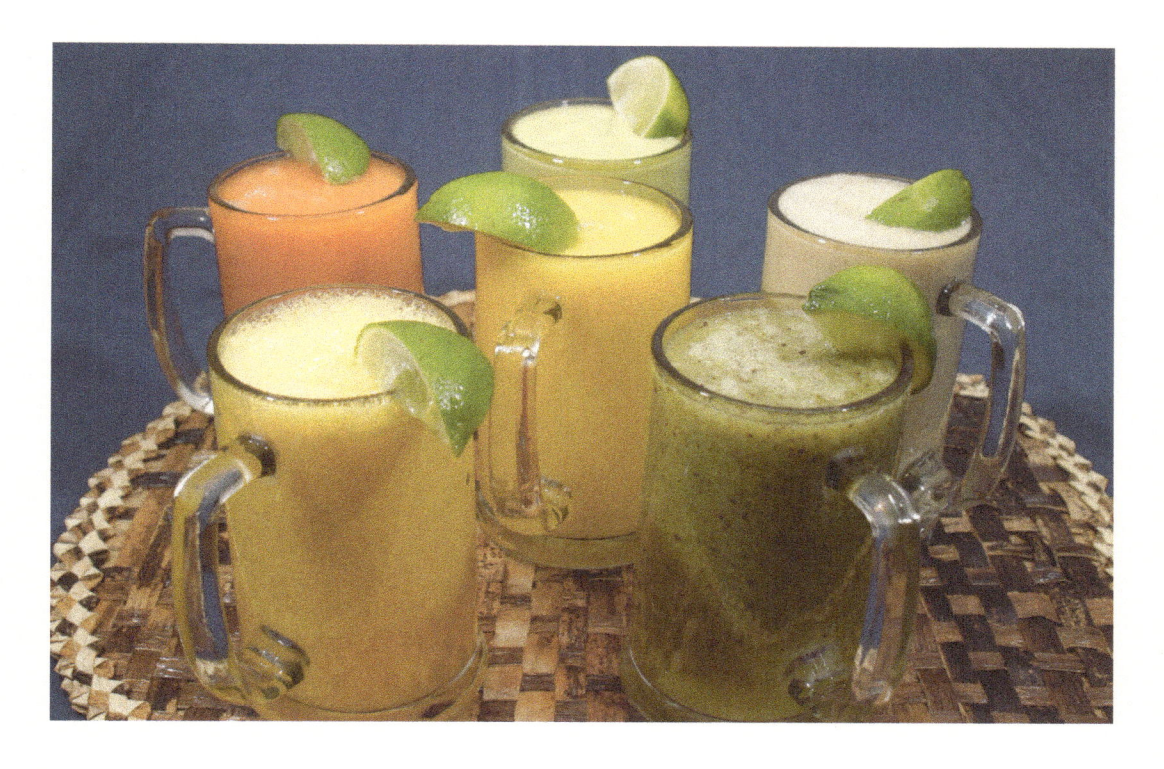

Thirst Quenchers: Ethiopian Drinks

Did you know that coffee originally comes from Ethiopia? So of course, we have a very strong love for coffee. In America, people like to get a quick cup of coffee and go, go, go! In Ethiopia, when we have coffee, it is a time to sit and be with friends. We slowly roast the green coffee beans while we talk, sharing stories and spending time while the beans get smoky and dark. We boil the coffee water in a beautiful clay pitcher and talk. And then of course, we drink. But we do not only drink coffee. Sometimes we drink tea! And remember, Ethiopia is a hot place to live. We enjoy fresh fruit drinks very much. So I have also included some of my favorite smoothie drinks.

Above: An array of Ethiopian fruit smoothies (p. 199).

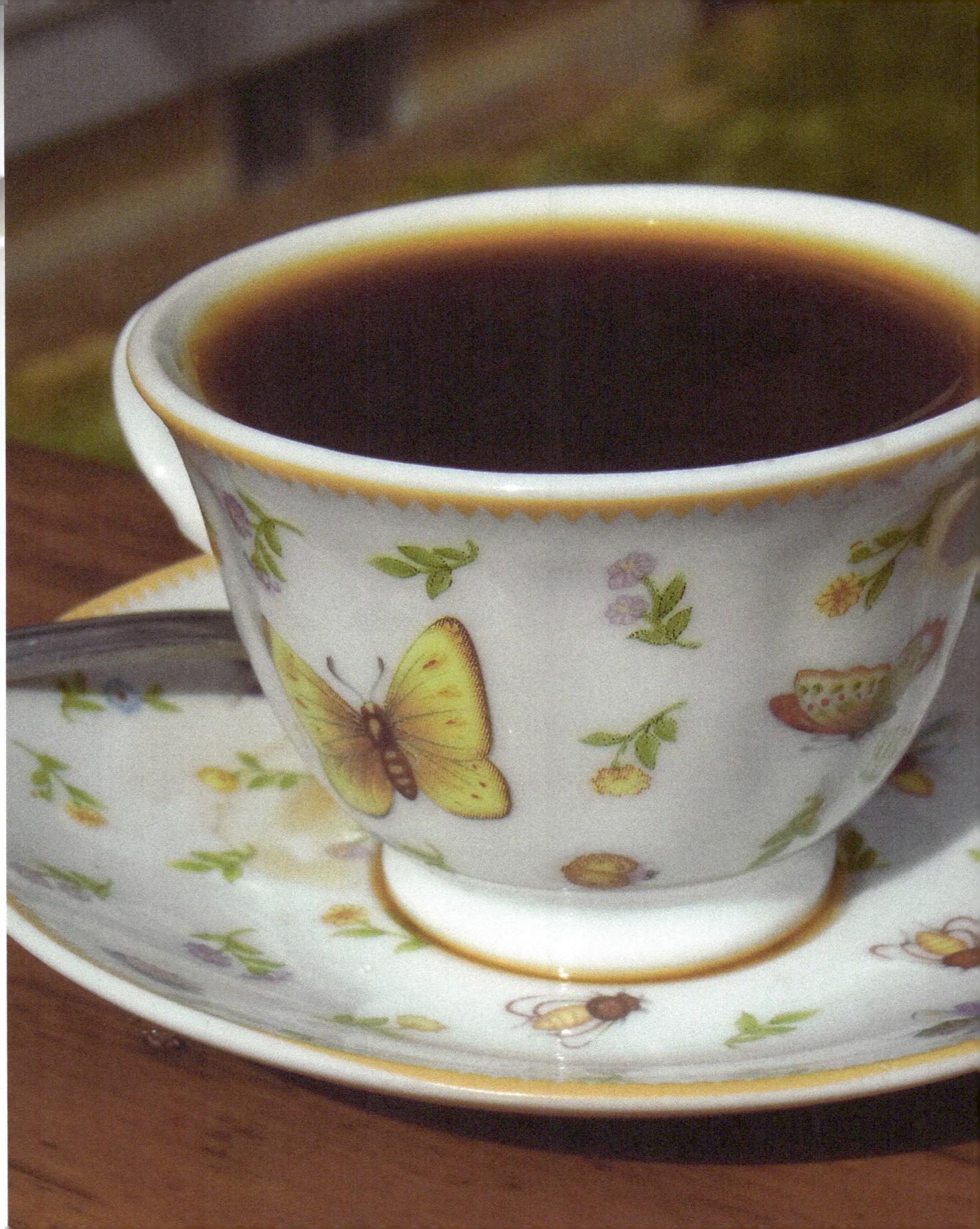

Ethiopian Drinks

Ethiopian Coffee
ቡና

(Bunna) V VG GF DF

Time: 20 min
Serves: 4
Difficulty:

The Ethiopian coffee ceremony is a very important part of our culture. We begin by roasting green coffee beans and end by serving the coffee in a demitasse.

Ingredients:

Yirgacheffe or green Ethiopian coffee beans*, 1 cup
Water, 4 cups

*available at specialty stores and online, see p. 17

Directions:

1. Place coffee beans in small skillet. Roast dry over medium-high heat until dark brown and fragrant.
2. Grind coffee beans in a spice or coffee grinder and pour the grounds into a pot.
3. Heat water to boiling and pour it over the coffee grounds.
4. Let the coffee brew to desired strength. Pour slowly into demitasses, without disturbing the grounds at the bottom of the pot. Serve with or without sugar, to taste.

The Crown Jewel of African Cuisine

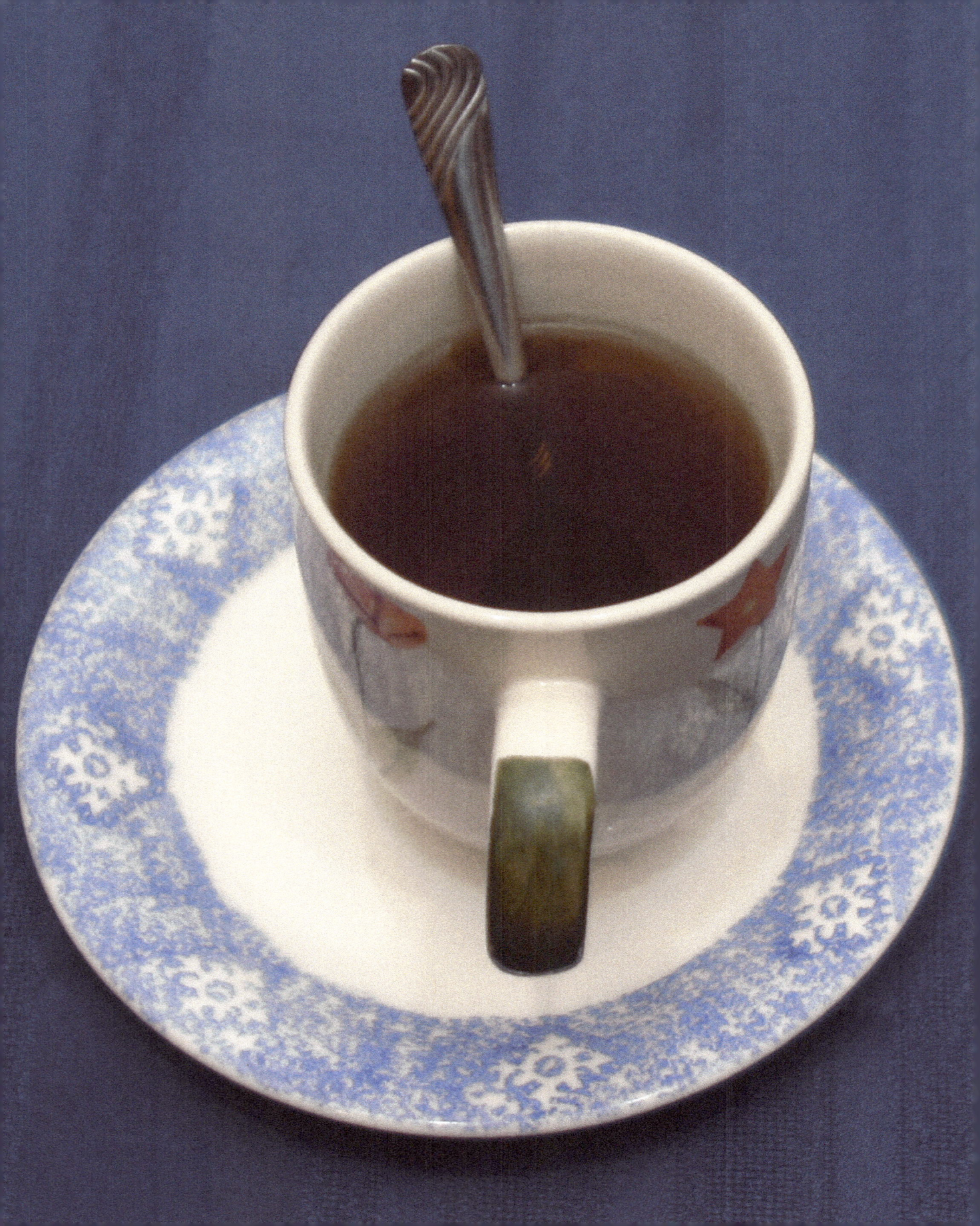

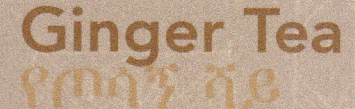

Ethiopian Drinks

Ginger Tea
የጠሳኝ ሻይ
(Yetosayn Shai) (V) (VG) (GF) (DF)

This is a comforting tea. We like to drink it for an upset stomach.

Time: **1 hr 15 min**
Serves: **4**
Difficulty:

Ingredients:
Ginger root, 1 oz, finely diced
Whole cloves, 4–5
Cinnamon, 1 inch piece
Water, 4 cups
Decaffeinated or caffeinated black tea, 2 bags

Directions:
1. Place ginger root, cloves, cinnamon and water into a small saucepan and simmer for 1 hour.
2. Pour through a strainer into a second saucepan. Add bagged tea and steep to desired strength.

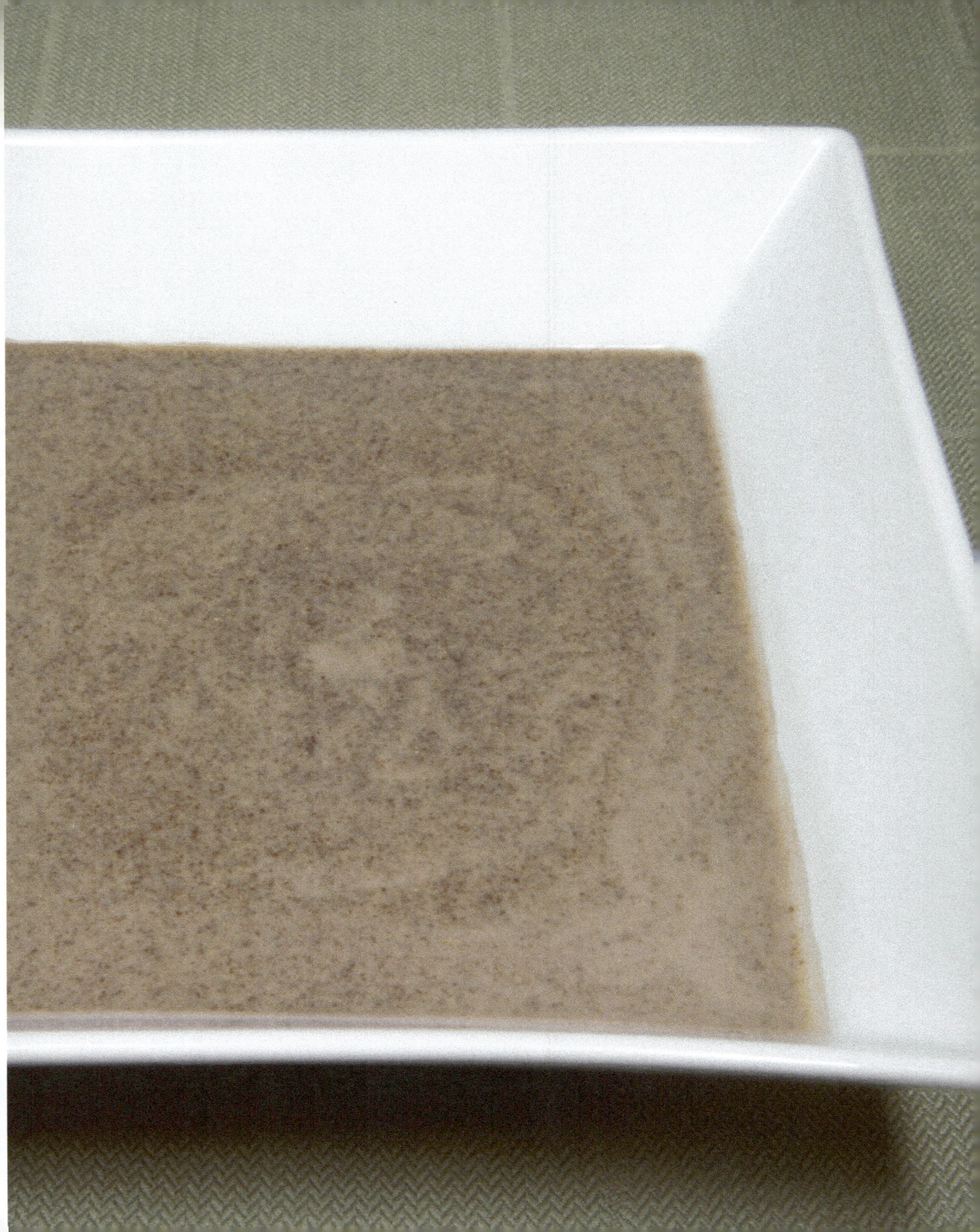

Ethiopian Drinks

Flax Seed Porridge
ተልባ
(Telba) (V) (VG) (GF) (DF)

Time: 15 min
Serves: 5
Difficulty: ♦♦♢♢♢

Telba and Ethiopian Collards (p. 163) are my father's favorites during Lent. Be aware, telba has a laxative effect.

Ingredients:

Flax seeds*, ⅔ cup
Water, 2 cups
Salt, 1 tsp

*available at specialty stores and online, see p. 16

Directions:

1. Warm an electric skillet to 350° F.
2. Pour the flax seeds onto the skillet, stirring constantly for 3 min. When the seeds begin to crackle, hold a lid above the skillet to prevent the seeds from flying around the kitchen!
3. After 3 min, the seeds should be fragrant, and some should have opened. At this time, turn off the heat, and continue stirring the seeds on the skillet for 2 min more.
4. Remove the dry-roasted seeds to a bowl and set aside to cool.
5. Grind the seeds to a powder in a spice grinder (or coffee grinder) in batches (15 seconds per batch). The resulting powder should be fine enough to pass through a flour sifter.
6. Combine the flax powder (you should have about 1 cup of powder after grinding all of the seeds) with 1½ cups water and the salt, and whisk.
7. After the mixture has thickened somewhat, add ½ cup more water, whisk again, and refrigerate until serving.

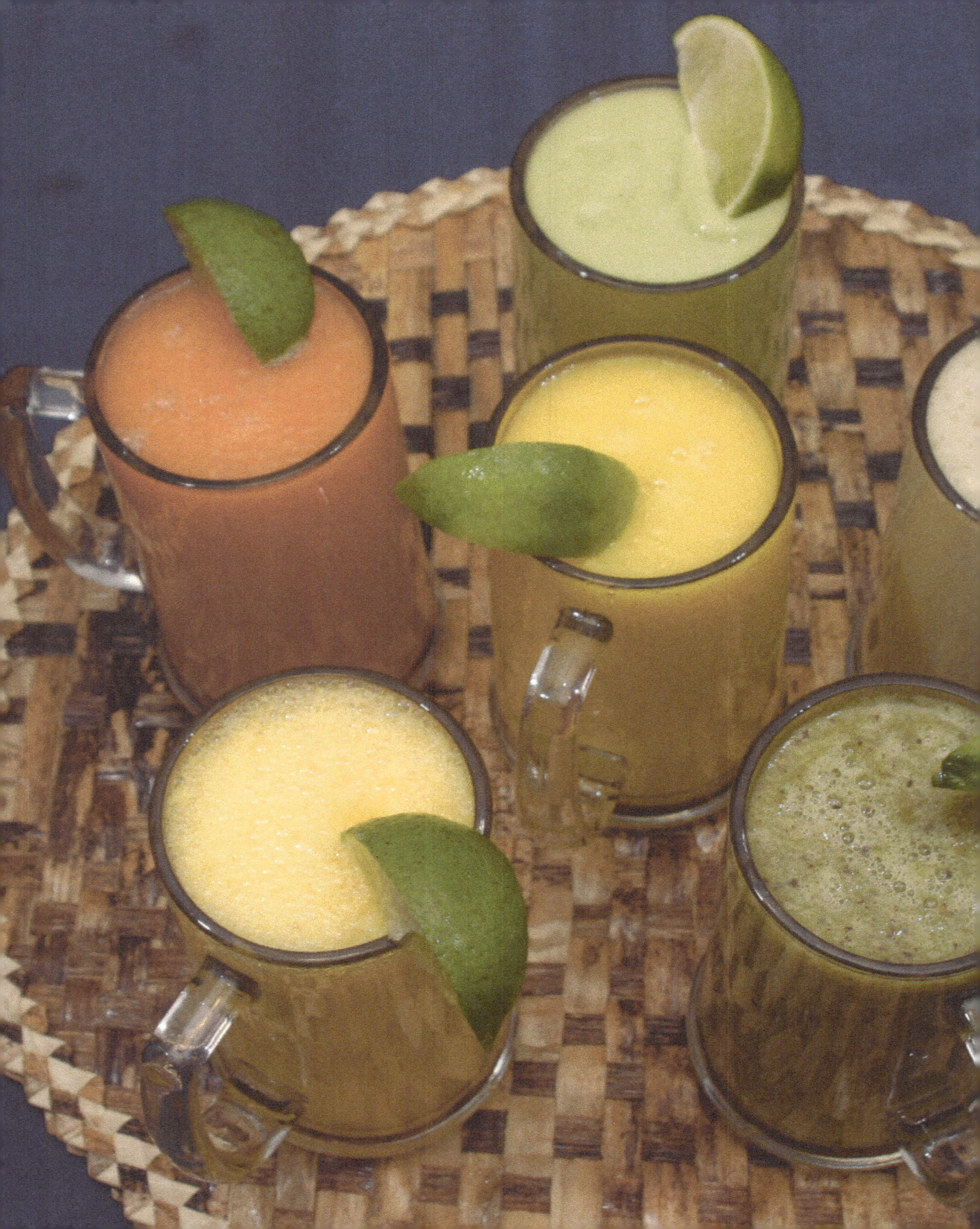

Ethiopian Drinks

Fruit Smoothies, 6 Ways
የፍራፍሬ ጭማቂ
(Yefrafre Chimaqi) V VG GF DF

Time: 25 min
Makes: 2 large drinks
Difficulty:

These refreshing drinks are made with fruits that are commonly found in Ethiopia - except kiwi, I added that for fun. Smoothies in Ethiopia have very little sweetener, so add sugar or agave if you like it sweet!

Ingredients:
Ripe papaya, large (~2 lb)*
Lemon, ¼, juiced
Lime, ¼, juiced
Sugar, 1 Tbsp
Water, ½ cup

*or substitute other fruit, as described in the recipes below

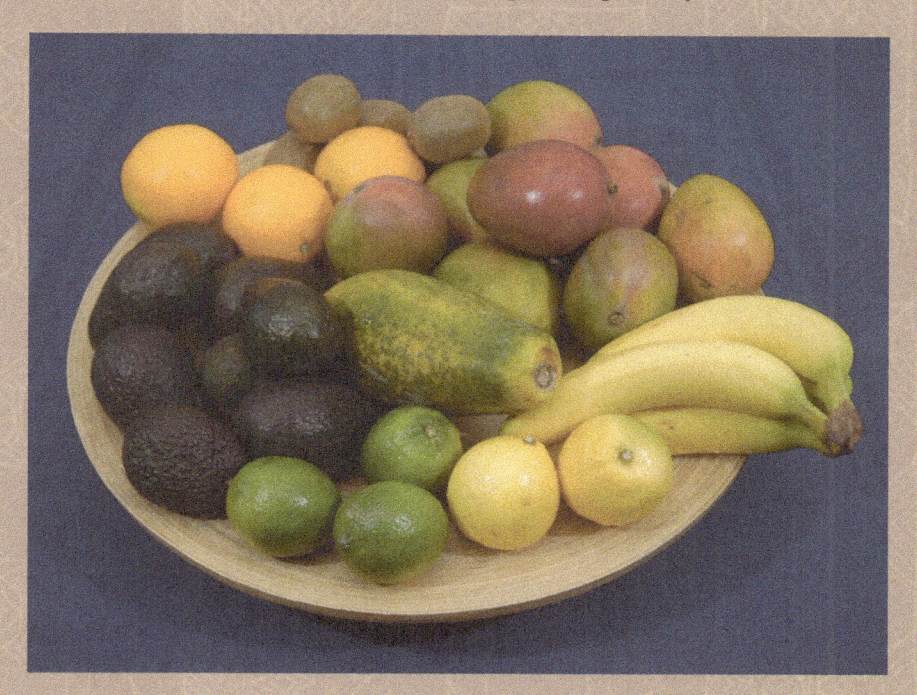

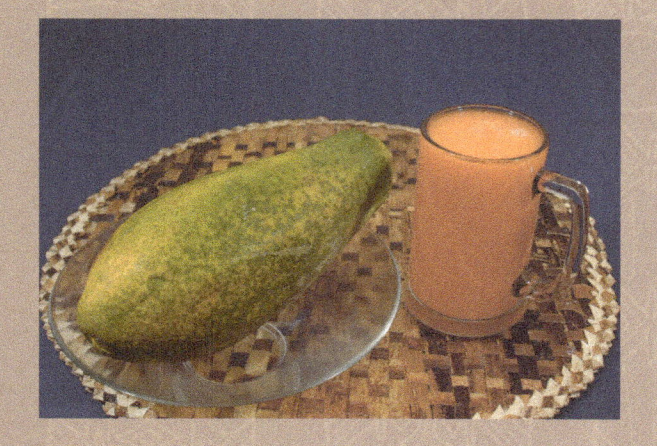

Directions:

Papaya Smoothies

1. Cut the papaya in half lengthwise, and again crosswise. Remove the seeds and the peel.
2. Add the fruit and the other ingredients to a blender, and blend 30 seconds until smooth.

The Crown Jewel of African Cuisine

Ethiopian Drinks

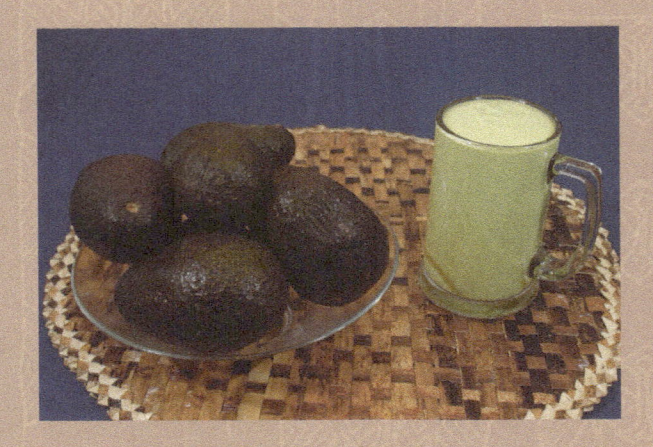

Avocado Smoothies
Substitute 3 large ripe avocadoes for the papaya, pitting and peeling them before adding them to the blender with the remaining ingredients. Also, increase the amount of water to 4 cups total. (Makes 3 large smoothies.)

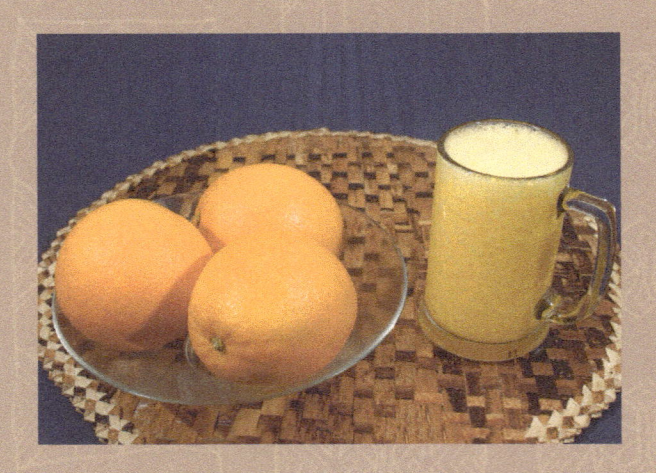

Orange Smoothies
Substitute 3 large navel oranges for the papaya. Cut the rind off of the orange to expose the flesh, trim off any excess bits of white pithy flesh, cut the orange in half lengthwise, and remove the white core before adding the orange pieces to the blender with the remaining ingredients. (Makes 2 large smoothies.)

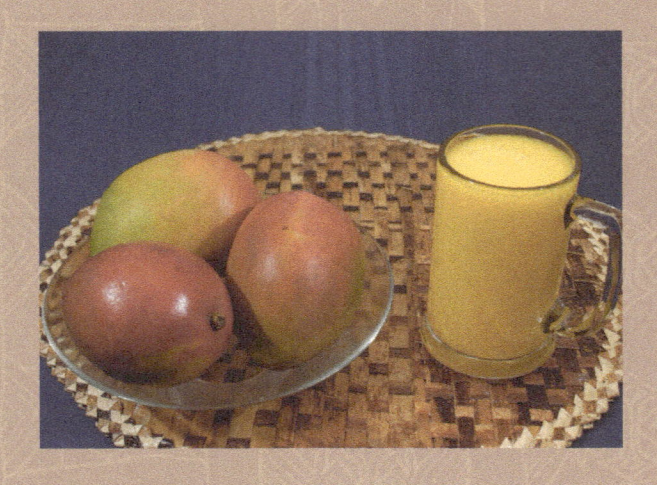

Mango Smoothies
Substitute 2 ripe mangoes (~1 lb, total) for the papaya. Peel the mangoes, remove their seeds, then cut the flesh into chunks and add it to the blender with the remaining ingredients, increasing the water to 1 cup total. (Makes 2 large smoothies.)